Illness and Immortality

Illness and Immortality

Mantra, Maṇḍala, and Meditation in the Netra Tantra

PATRICIA SAUTHOFF

OXFORD
UNIVERSITY PRESS

OXFORD
UNIVERSITY PRESS

Oxford University Press is a department of the University of Oxford. It furthers the University's objective of excellence in research, scholarship, and education by publishing worldwide. Oxford is a registered trade mark of Oxford University Press in the UK and certain other countries.

Published in the United States of America by Oxford University Press
198 Madison Avenue, New York, NY 10016, United States of America.

Library of Congress Control Number: 2021949460
ISBN 978-0-19-755326-8

DOI: 10.1093/oso/9780197553268.001.0001

1 3 5 7 9 8 6 4 2

Printed by Integrated Books International, United States of America

To Corey

Contents

Acknowledgments

At the risk of appearing grim, I would like to begin by acknowledging all the friends I lost suddenly during the process of writing this book. Sudden death has occurred around me my entire life. Clearly this has had a profound impact on my areas of interest. When I began this work, people found my interest in illness and immortality odd. Now that I finish it in the midst of a global pandemic that has claimed more than four million lives and counting across the world, it seems more relevant than ever.

Lyra, of everyone, your death was the most traumatic. You were taken too soon and too violently. I treasure the years I spent working by your side and I will cherish those memories for the rest of my life. Max, Jeff, and Brian, I am so sorry that you felt it necessary to take your own lives. I miss you and I wish there had been something I could have done to keep you with us a little longer. David, your art hangs on my wall and I am so glad to have a piece of your last series. Thank you for always being a shoulder on which to cry and for being so good at packing up a house! Michael, I still haven't accepted that you are gone and will continue to listen for your voice and your laugh in my headphones. Dana and Pete, you are missed.

As for the living, thank you for using your valuable time to read this book. I hope you enjoy it.

Like all written works, this one would not exist were it not for intellectual, social, and emotional support. Thanks to Dagmar and Dominik Wujastyk, Chloe Peacock, Daniel Simpson, Sundari Johnson, Anya Golovkova, Olivia Katbi Smith, Jason Wilson, Alexander Reid Ross, Alex Smith, and Farren Stanley for giving me all three over the years. Thank you to Richard Morgan and Peter Breslin for the friendship and the memes. Jane Allred, you have no idea what having another woman around to talk to during this covid lockdown has meant to me.

Thank you to Dagmar Wujastyk and the AyurYog team for bringing me aboard and supporting me with your patience and genius during the final stages of this work. This work would have been impossible without the generous support of so many colleagues. I want to thank my thesis supervisors Dr. Ulrich Pagel, Dr. Renate Söhnen-Thieme, and Dr. James Mallinson, all of whom guided me in the production and completion of this work. I would like to extend my special thanks to each of them for the many hours they took painstakingly editing, reiterating fine points of Sanskrit, and urging me to read the texts in different ways.

I also want to extend a special thank you to Alexis Sanderson and the Movement Center in Portland, Oregon. Professor Sanderson read several difficult passages of the *Netra Tantra* with me and was generous enough to allow me to attend his weekly lectures at the Movement Center.

Drs. Judit Törzsök and Péter-Dániel Szántó read and commented thoroughly on a very different version of my thesis. This helped me exorcise the text of many errors and assumptions. Your guidance helped in more ways that I can count.

I was able to present the preliminary findings in this work and various conferences and want to especially thank Dr. Harunaga Isaacson, Dr. Dominic Goodall, and Dr. Jung Lan Bang for their especially astute and helpful feedback. Thank you to the International Indology Graduate Research Symposium, World Sanskrit Conference, American Academy of Religion, and Society for Tantric Studies for inviting me to present research related to this project. Thanks also to the Brough Sanskrit Award for funding conference travel. Dr. Kengo Harimoto allowed me to access the Nepal German Manuscript Cataloguing Project's manuscript copies of both the *Svacchanda* and *Netra* Tantras, which I hope to examine with more depth in the future. I would also like to thank all my Sanskrit teachers, Drs. James Carey, Renate Söhnen-Thieme, Alastair Gornall, Paolo Visigalli, Sadananda Das, James Mallinson, and Professor Alexis Sanderson for their patience and persistence. Drs. David Gray and Jun Lan Bang offered clarifications to several of my questions in the course of casual conversation and I appreciate their willingness to discuss their work with me. I am particularly indebted to Lorilliai Biernacki, who unwittingly set me on this path many years ago.

This project would not have been possible without the support of my colleagues. Thank you to Ryan Dunch and everyone in the University of Alberta's department of History, Classics, and Religious Studies. You adopted me immediately and encouraged me throughout my time in Canada. Thank you to the European Research Council for allowing the AyurYog project to move to Canada, which allowed me to join. Thank you also to the Singhmars, whose generosity meant that I could continue the work of the AyurYog project for more than a year after the project officially ended.

I would also like to thank my friends at Mediagazer. Especially Lyra McKee, Andria Krewson, and Gabe Rivera, who allowed me the time I needed to travel in support of Sanskrit language acquisition and conference presentation, and who took me back when I needed cash. A special shoutout goes to my colleagues at Nalanda University: Andrea Acri, Aleksandra Wenta, Sean Kerr, Garima Kaushik, Noemie Verdon, Ranu Roychoudhuri, Sraman Mukherjee, Max Deeg, Aditya Malik, Kashshaf Ghani, Smita Polite, and our fearless leader, Gopa Sabhrawal. Many thanks also to the students of Nalanda, who helped make the best of a crazy situation and whose continued friendship fills me with joy. I am also so proud of everything so many of you have accomplished in the last few years. To Amartya Sen, your vision for Nalanda was a wonderful one and I hope we achieved it, even if only for a fleeting moment.

Thank you to my friends around the globe on whose sofas I crashed and whose music and art inspired me throughout the writing process. And finally, thank you to Corey Pein: husband, copyeditor, cook, cat dad, computer repair man, travel companion, and the love of my life.

Abbreviations

ĀgnG	*Āgniveśya Gṛhya Sūtra*
ĀpŚS	*Āpastamba Śrautasūtra*
AŚ	*Arthaśāstra*
AVŚ	*Atharva Veda Saṃhitā, Śaunakīya recension*
BGP	*Baudhāyana Gṛhya Paribhāṣa Sūtra*
BGŚ	*Baudhāyana Gṛhya Śeṣa Sūtra*
BraYā	*Brahmayāmala Tantra*
BS	*Bṛhat Saṃhitā*
BU	*Bṛhadāraṇyaka Upaniṣad*
ChU	*Chāndogya Upaniṣad*
CS	*Cakrasamvara Tantra*
DSĀ	*Dharmasūtra of Āpastamba*
DSB	*Dharmasūtra of Baudhāyana*
GS	*Guhyasiddhi*
HT	*Hevajra Tantra*
ĪPPV	*Īśvara Pratyabhijñā Vivṛti Vimarśinī*
ĪU	*Īṣa Upaniṣad*
JG	*Jaiminīya Gṛhya Sūtra*
KĀ	*Kamikāgama*
Kauś	*Kauśika Sūtra*
KauśS	*Kauśikapaddhati on Kauśika Sūtra*
KC	*Śrīkaṇthacarita*
KhV	*Khecarīvidyā*
KJ	*Kaulajñānirṇaya*
KP	*Kālikā Purāṇa*
KSTS	Kashmir Series of Texts and Studies
KubjT	*Kubjikā Tantra*
KV	*Kalāvilāsa*
LK	*Lakṣmīkaulārṇava*
LT	*Lakṣmī Tantra*
MāU	*Māṇḍūkya Upaniṣad*
MBh	*Mahābhārata*
MP	*Mṛgendrapaddatīkā*
MS	*Manusmṛti*
MT	*Mṛgendra Tantra*
MU	*Maitrī Upaniṣad*

MVT	*Mālinīvijayottara*
NAK	National Archives Kathmandu
NGMCP	Nepal German Manuscript Cataloguing Project
NS	*Nayasūtra*
NT	*Netra Tantra*
NTU	*Netratantroddyota*
ParT	*Parākhya Tantra*
PBY	*Picumata Brahmayāmala*
PG	*Pāraskara Gṛhya Sūtra*
PH	*Pratyabhijñāhṛdaya*
PhT	*Phetkāriṇī Tantra*
PS	*Paramārthasāra*
PSC	*Paramārthasāra* [commentary]
PTV	*Parātrīśikā Vivaraṇa*
Rām	*Rāmāyaṇa*
ṚV	*Ṛgveda*
ṚVi	*Ṛgvidhāna*
SP	*Skanda Purāṇa*
SpK	*Spanda Kārikās*
SpN	*Spanda Nirṇaya*
SpV	*Spandavivṛti*
SS	*Suśruta Saṃhitā*
SU	*Saṃvarodaya Tantra*
SVB	*Sāmavidhāna Brāhmaṇa*
SvT	*Svacchanda Tantra*
SvTU	*Svacchanda Tantra Uddyota*
SYM	*Siddhayogeśvarīmata*
ŚB	*Śatapatha Brāhmaṇa*
ŚS	*Śiva Sūtras*
ŚvetU	*Śvetāśvatara Upaniṣad*
TĀ	*Tantrāloka*
TĀV	*Tantrāloka Vivarana*
TB	*Taittirīya Brāhmaṇa*
TS	*Taittirīya Upaniṣad*
TSB	*Tantrasadbhāva*
TU	*Taittirīya Upaniṣad*
VaiG	*Vaikhānasa Gṛhya Sūtra*
VBh	*Vijñānabhairava*
VDhP	*Viṣṇudharmottara Purāṇa*
VŚT	*Vīṇāśikha Tantra*
YH	*Yoginīhṛdaya*

Introduction

In ninth-century Kashmir, spirit possession caused illness, sudden death, and the obstruction of worldly gains. Only through a series of optional rites (*kāmya*) meant to bring about worldly enjoyments (*bhoga*) could a practitioner assuage these evils. The *Netra Tantra*, a text with at least two clear layers of redaction,[1] describes rites that sought to alleviate these ills.

Like other texts categorized as Tantras, the early ninth-century[2] *Netra Tantra* presents itself as a work of divine origin in the form of a dialogue between the god Śiva and goddess Pārvatī. The *Netra Tantra* is a fairly conservative Tantra that does not explicitly call for heterodox practices and belongs to the path of mantras (*mantramārga*). Its rites are accessible to ascetics and married householders alike.[3] The *Netra Tantra* clearly derives from the *Svacchanda Tantra*, which White dates to the seventh century at the latest.[4] This places the *Netra Tantra* well after the earliest *mantramārga* Śaiva Tantras, the fifth-century *Niśvāsatattvasaṃhitā*,[5] and several hundred years prior to its eleventh-century commentator, Kṣemarāja. The *Netra Tantra* often alludes to the *Svacchanda Tantra* and assumes familiarity with the ritual technicalities that appear throughout the *Svacchanda Tantra*. As such, this work is a study of the *Netra Tantra* but also includes translations and analysis of the *Svacchanda Tantra* where necessary. Though the rites are accessible to many, the *Netra Tantra*'s audience is the Śaiva officiant who performs the ritual duties on behalf of another. Its main audience is a royal officiant who protects the king and his family through rites of appeasement (*śānti*) and carries out a lustration (*nīrājana*) to empower the monarch and his armies.[6]

Both the *Svacchanda* and *Netra Tantra*s belong to the category of Bhairava Tantras. Their main deities are manifestations of Śiva in his fierce Bhairava form. In the *Netra Tantra*, Bhairava's ultimate manifestation is Amṛteśa, a formless deity who bestows relief from ailments to a ritual benefactor and conquers death. Amṛteśa carries many names, including Mṛtyujit and Mṛtyuñjaya.

This monograph explores the iconographies, initiations, and rites described in previously unexamined sections of the *Netra Tantra*. The text

Illness and Immortality. Patricia Sauthoff, Oxford University Press. © Oxford University Press 2022.
DOI: 10.1093/oso/9780197553268.003.0001

describes a world in which invisible supernatural beings cause illness, and where the appeasement of a deity leads to the aversion of death. It examines the relationship between the professional *mantrin* and the benefactor on whose behalf he performs these rites. It also explains how Tantra functioned in the Himalayan courts and reveals the role of the *mantrin* in the operation of the kingdom.

Large parts of *Netra Tantra* remain uncharted. A two-volume edition appeared in 1926 and 1939. It relies on two privately held manuscripts from Kashmir. According to the editor, neither manuscript is very old, dating perhaps to the early nineteenth century.[7] The Nepalese-German Manuscript Cataloging Project holds microfilms of twenty manuscripts that bear the title *Netrajñānārṇavatantra*,[8] and three manuscripts that carry the names *Amṛteśatantra*,[9] *Mṛtyujitāmṛtīśamahābhairavatantra*,[10] and *Mṛtyujidamṛt eśatantra*.[11] At present, Flood, Wernicke-Olesen, and Khatiwoda are nearing a complete critical edition and translation of the Nepalese manuscripts.[12] Brunner's (1974) summary of the *Netra Tantra* is the first substantial study of the text since its editions in the 1920s and 1930s. While Brunner considers it hugely helpful as a navigational tool, she is dismissive of the text as being less polished than the *Svacchanda Tantra*. This may explain why it has yet to receive the same level of attention as the *Svacchanda Tantra*.

Padoux's (1990) study of mantras relies on the *Netra Tantra* as well as a wide range of other Tantric literature to understand the power and energy of language in Tantra. Much of Padoux's focus is on the *Netra Tantra*'s twenty-first chapter. Sanderson's (2004) article on religion and the state provided the first in-depth translation of part of the text and provides a likely date of final redaction. More recent work by White (2012) focuses on the demonological aspects of the *Netra Tantra*; it helps to reveal the sorts of spirits that might cause various illnesses and presents the *Netra Tantra*'s own mythology about Śiva. Bäumer's (2018, 2019) translation of Chapters 1, 7, and 8 presents the highest two levels of yoga. Bäumer approaches the work from the perspective of a modern-day practitioner rather than a historian.

In contrast to Bäumer's focus on yoga, I explore the theory and ritual practice discussed in the text. I expand on Padoux's study of Tantric mantras[13] through a translation and analysis of the *Netra Tantra*'s discussion of the nature of mantra. This enables me to argue in favor of the view that Kṣemarāja sees mantras themselves as speech acts, at least as described in the *Netra Tantra*. Where Padoux employs the *Netra Tantra* as one of many texts that offers him the opportunity to weave together a comprehensive study on Tantric mantras, I focus on the *Netra Tantra* and its own discussion of mantra. This approach allows me to apply Padoux's findings on the mantric system to an individual mantra and demonstrate its unique properties. I also follow Sanderson's work on the *Netra Tantra*, which centers on the relationship between the monarch and the *mantrin*. I argue that the lowest, physical (*sthūla*) form of practice is the most important to the attainment of worldly ends, such as good health, prosperity, and the continued rule over a kingdom. The responsibility for the efficacy of the rite lies solely with the *mantrin*. It also demonstrates that the *maṇḍala* acts as a microcosm for the physical body. This offers the *mantrin* an outlet for constant practice while the monarch continues the affairs of the kingdom.

Iconographies are vital to the Tantric rites of the *mantramārga*. The large body of Sanskrit texts associated with the *mantramārga* presents an archetypal Śiva who lives in the cremation ground and bears human skulls. In the Bhairava Tantras, Śiva takes on a terrifying and ecstatic form. He surrounds himself with goddesses, *yoginīs*, demons, and other supernatural creatures.[14] Within the Bhairava Tantras, deities appear in multiple forms, sometimes manifesting as mantras and at others resembling their Purāṇic forms. The practitioner uses these scriptural depictions of deities to call forth a visualized form that appears on the ritual diagram, the *maṇḍala*. He then performs sacrificial rites in which he presents ritual offerings to the deity and asks for salvation (*mokṣa*) or worldly enjoyments (*bhoga*).

Overview

Oṃ juṃ saḥ. When used properly, this simple mantra cures all illnesses and offers immortality. Of course, this is no simple task.

The central questions of this work focus on illness and immortality. What does the *Netra Tantra* mean by immortality? How does one attain it? How do the rites described within the text alleviate illness? What role does the deity play in the reduction of illness and attainment of immortality? Who has access to these rites?

To answer these questions, I interrogate five key concepts: mantra, iconography, identity, ritual, and yoga. The majority of the translations used to examine these concepts come from the *Netra Tantra*. On a few occasions I turn to the *Svacchanda Tantra*, an earlier and related work that the *Netra Tantra* itself builds on.

The efficacy of all Tantric rites relies on mantras. Without mantra, rituals become empty actions that have no impact on the world. So great is their power that mantras are encoded within texts so that they do not fall into use by one who does not fully understand their nature and strength.

Chapter 1 introduces the reader to Tantric mantras. It situates them within ritual and meditation and offers a brief overview of their form. I then contextualize the mantra *oṃ juṃ saḥ* within the Tantric canon and compare it to a Vedic mantra that shares both its name and its intended outcome. Finally, I translate the section of the text in which the mantra is encoded. This provides the reader with an example of mantric encoding. It also demonstrates that each component of the mantra can be defined by sound, shape, and movement. These elements are far from arbitrary. Instead, we see that mantras are essential parts of the cosmos. They exist for us to discover, not to create. Even our in- and out-breaths can be understood and utilized as mantra.

Chapter 2 examines the nature of mantra. I first explore ideas of mantras as magic utterances and examine ritual language. This leads to a theoretical discussion in which I argue against Staal's assertion that mantras are not speech acts.[15] While Staal's work is incredibly useful to understanding mantras, I argue that the *Netra* and *Svacchanda Tantra*s anticipate his argument and offer a counter explanation. The perspective they offer is unique to these two texts and the *Netra Tantra*'s twenty-first chapter provides a philosophically rigorous examination into the composition, characteristics, power, and productiveness of mantras. The text offers a tripartite explanation of mantras as formless, disembodied, and embodied or unmanifest potential, potential, and limited potential. Through this discussion, we learn the most important feature of mantras: that no matter their form (or lack thereof), the mantra and the deity are inseparable. This too helps explain the importance of encoding the mantra within the text. The chapter ends with a brief section on the practicalities of mantric recitation, namely, in the eleven types of sequences that protect the mantra from impurities such as mispronunciation or incorrect usage. Further, we find a type of semantic analysis called *nirvacana* that uses the roots of words to demonstrate the eternal nature of the text itself.

In Chapter 3 I turn away from the theoretical to introduce the focus of devotion: the god Śiva or Bhairava as manifested in the forms of Amṛteśa and Mṛtyujit. Bühnemann[16] and Sanderson[17] note several sculptures of Mṛtyujit that had earlier been misidentified. After briefly discussing representations of the deity and his female companion found in bronze and temple statuary,

I return to the textual tradition to locate the deity in the wider corpus of Sanskrit literature. I first situate Śiva as outside of Vedic orthodoxy, instead living and worshipping in the charnel ground. This associates the deity with death and the ability to overcome it. I then examine references to Mṛtyujit and the conquering or cheating of death within the Purāṇas. We find references to Mṛtyujit in several Purāṇas, which demonstrates that he is known outside of the Tantric canon. The stories told within these texts help build the mythology and visual characteristics of the deity. Again returning to the *Netra Tantra*, I then translate sections of text that describe the physical forms of Amṛteśa and Mṛtyujit. Key characteristics identify the forms of these deities. They appear in subsequent chapters that allow one to worship Amṛteśa and Mṛtyujit using the mantra *oṃ juṃ saḥ* in the form of Sadāśiva, Bhairava, Tumburu, Nārāyaṇa, Viṣṇu, Sūrya, Viśvakarman, Rudra, Brahmā, and Buddha. Additionally, I have translated some sections that describe the female companions of these deities. I have not translated these sections in full because the companions generally share the physical attributes of the god and the repetition does little to further iconographical analysis. That said, during visualization practices, it is vital that the worshipper include the consort alongside the deity. The practice of worshipping Amṛteśa in the guise of other Brahminical deities allows the practitioner to use the protective *mṛtyuñjaya* mantra while simultaneously adhering to calendrical rites and festivals that center on those other deities. I translate the texts' descriptions of deities, from Amṛteśa to Mṛtyujit, to different forms of Viṣṇu, Sūrya, and even the Buddha. I then compare these accounts with the physical records of the Himalayan region. Many of these depictions are unique to the region. This demonstrates the limited geographic influence of the *Netra Tantra*. It also corroborates evidence that the *Netra Tantra* had a place of prominence in Himalayan court life.

Chapter 4 examines the interrelationship between religion and society for followers of the non-dual Tantric Śaiva tradition. First, I examine the creation of the Tantric identity as separate from social and religiously orthodox identities. I explore the new Tantric identities created through initiation and ask how these new identities impact the larger social experience of practitioners. I do this by analyzing the function of transgression within the Tantric milieu. This leads to a discussion of the ways in which its members negotiate or retain caste status. I then reflect on the origin of Tantric practice and map how Tantra seeks to subvert the social caste paradigm. I examine the theories about the historical spread of Tantric practice—whether it was a practice that began with kings and priests, reaching the lower castes in discourse, or a practice that commenced among the lower castes and worked its way up through society. For this, I consult textual descriptions of practices that are prescribed for members of different castes. This leads to an examination of the removal of caste by means of initiation. I also reflect on the internal hierarchy of initiatory statuses that replace caste. This offers a humanizing look at the individual needs and actions of practitioners. I contrast this with the non-Tantric sphere. Social and religious ties existed between Tantric writers and the upper echelons of Kashmiri society. I argue that caste erasure was limited to the ritual sphere and was therefore symbolic. I compare the philosophical ideal of the vanquishment of caste distinction with the social necessity for hierarchy. This illuminates the ways in which Tantric practice bestows power to the individual religious initiate. I also explore the nature of auspicious and inauspicious symbols related to initiation. These symbols appear in the *Svacchanda Tantra* when it charts the preliminary rites that precede initiation and help explain how the *mantrin* judges the initiand's preparedness for entry into the Tantric sphere.

Again, Chapter 5 turns toward the theoretical. I examine the use of mantra within initiation (*dīkṣā*) rites and how Sanskrit phonemes connect to the hierarchy of realities (*tattva*) through which one passes during initiation. This again offers an example of how the text describes the divine nature of sound. Initiation also offers a practitioner the ability to adopt a new identity. The process of initiation symbolically destroys the initiand's body, unbinding his soul, and offering him the gift of liberation. I analyze sections of the *Netra Tantra* that speak to both the theoretical and practical elements of initiatory rites.

Chapter 6 examines the socio-historical practicalities of a monarch participating in the Tantric sphere. The twelfth-century chronicle *Rājataraṅgiṇī* offers a useful guide. Its narratives demonstrate how practitioners who have shed caste identity through initiation still retain it in the social world. Its author, Kalhaṇa, focuses largely on monarchs, disapproving of their participation in Tantric rites. I discuss literary evidence that demonstrates the widespread agreement on what qualifies as prohibited and the penalties for transgressions. Next, I briefly discuss literary evidence of royal patronage before turning to specific rites related to the king. First, I translate and analyze passages related to the protection of the king. These rites include marking the body and food of the king with preventative ritual objects and mantras and large-scale rituals that protect everything under the king's purview. I contrast these public or semi-public rituals with the private rituals to maintain the monarch's health. In this section we again return to semantic analysis to understand how objects, such as variously colored mustard seeds, are by the nature of their names beneficial to ritual.

In Chapter 7, I trace the historical development of possession to argue in favor of a literary tradition that undermines the argument that such beliefs were held only by the disempowered. Instead, I show that exorcism and demonic possession have a long history in literary Tantra and therefore must not have been an idea that existed only among the non-elite. I then briefly explore ideas of immortality and the conquering of death in the Sanskrit literary tradition. I supplement this with similar rites in the Tibetan Buddhist tradition and explore the places in which the rites overlap. This sheds light on the corporeal yoga tradition of the *Netra Tantra*. The first of three chapters on yoga, the *Netra Tantra*'s sixth chapter offers a detailed description of ritual oblation to escape death. The translated passage offers a look at the natural products—honey, milk, ghee, trees, and seeds—offered to the ritual fire. These objects must be protected with enveloping mantras and accompanied by recitation.

Chapter 8 continues the translation of Chapter 6 of the *Netra Tantra* as the topic shifts from oblation to *maṇḍala*. The theoretical basis for my analysis relies on understanding the nature of mantras from Chapters 1 and 2 and the initiation rites of Chapter 5. Because the *Netra Tantra* itself offers only practical information about *maṇḍala* use in ritual, I turn to two other texts, the *Mālinīvijayottaratantra* and *Cakrasamvara Tantra*, to examine the written form of the mantra and colors of the *maṇḍala*. Here we see how the embodied mantra is placed onto the *maṇḍala*, thus activating it. Again, proper performance is necessary for the correct outcome. The colors of the ritual objects and *maṇḍala*s point to their efficacy.

Finally, in Chapter 9, I turn my focus to the *Svacchanda Tantra* to translate a section of the text focused on visualized meditation meant to conquer both time and death.[18] This meditation uses the breath and instructs the practitioner to visualize Brahmā, Viṣṇu, and Rudra in order to attain longevity. It then offers further visualization of the self washed over with nectar. I compare the imagery of the *Svacchanda* and *Netra Tantra*s to offer a more complete understanding of immortality within the Śaiva canon.

Death rites dominate Chapter 6 of the *Netra Tantra* and Chapter 7 of the *Svacchanda Tantra*. Their performance reveals the spiritual and social power of the *mantrin*. The *Netra Tantra* describes mantras and *maṇḍala*s that the priest conducts on behalf of the dying. This contrasts with a visualization practice found in the *Svacchanda Tantra*. It contains instructions for meditation that offers its user a direct means to conquer death and overcome time.[19] The *Netra Tantra* sets out to grant success in the world of men, to confer benefits, to bring an end to sickness, to destroy untimely death, and to bring about peace and nourishment.[20]

Throughout this work, I trace Śaiva Tantric rituals to their *kāpālika* roots. In doing so, I connect the exorcistic and apotropaic rites found in the *Netra Tantra* to orthodox texts, including the *Atharva Veda* and *Chāndogya Upaniṣad*. I compare the *mṛtyu vañcana* rites of the *Netra Tantra* to complementary rituals found in the Buddhist *Cakrasamvara*. This allows me to compare ritual specifics, such as colors and sacrificial ingredients.

In addition, I examine the conception of the body in medieval India. This body was vulnerable to demons and reliant on deities for its continued existence. For the Tantric practitioner, the divinized body is part of a psychophysical organism. Through practice, the *mantrin* moves from the gross or corporeal (*sthūla*) body to the subtle (*sūkṣma*) through breath practices and consciousness until he reaches its highest manifestation (*para*). The body (*deha*) is less important than form (*rūpa* or *svarūpa*). Form includes the physical body as only a small part of the individual. A person's form includes their *sthūla*, *sūkṣma*, and *para* manifestations as well as their social bodies, including caste and name. The protective rites of the *Netra Tantra* reveal that the name of an individual overcome with illness works as a ritual substitute for that person. This is not to say that the physical body of the person is not important. The body is central to ritual practice. When the *mantrin* places the mantra upon the body (*nyāsa*), he creates a Tantric body that itself becomes a ritual tool. The body and the mantra become fused. This allows the mantra to heal the body.

I should note that the study utilizes the Kashmir Series of Texts and Studies edition of the *Netra Tantra*. Published in 1927 and 1939, this text is based on manuscripts much later than those preserved in Nepal. Therefore, my focus is on the text as it has been transmitted recently, rather than an examination of the earliest edition and may have been changed at a later date to reflect subsequent innovation. This study was never intended as a work of philology. Instead, it is meant to be an interdisciplinary look at how one group of practitioners approached illness and immortality.

1

The Mantra

Oṃ Juṃ Saḥ

At its most simple, Tantra defines itself as the path of mantras (*mantramārga*).[1] The efficacy of Tantric rites lies in mantras, which call forth the gods and ultimately lead practitioners to salvation. Padoux says, "There is no possible understanding of the tantric phenomenon without an examination and understanding of a particular use of forms of speech that are mantras."[2] Like many Tantric mantras, the seed (*bīja*) mantra of the *Netra Tantra* appears deceptively simple. With just three syllables, the mantra *oṃ juṃ saḥ* can do what no medicine can do: it can alleviate pain, exterminate illness, and even bring about immortality.

Tantric Mantras

Before I examine the use of the *oṃ juṃ saḥ* mantra, I want to first put it into the context of mantras in general—both Tantric and non-Tantric. Mantra has long been an integral part of Indian religious traditions, beginning with Vedic mantric compositions and moving into nearly all other Indian religions. Staal demonstrates that comparison between the similarities of Vedic and Tantric mantras is more fruitful than a focus on the differences.[3] Both types of mantras appear in ritual and meditation—two practices that are sometimes impossible to distinguish—and can be recited aloud, inaudibly, mentally, or left unenunciated.[4] Vedic mantras are typically verses of the Vedas themselves and come directly from Sanskrit verses. Tantric mantras are instead made of phonemes that have no obvious syntactic value. In the Tantric system, practitioners consider mantric phonemes to be identical with deities. In addition to aural expression, the initiated teacher (*mantrin*)[5] places (*nyāsa*) mantras on physical objects. He (and the *mantrin* is almost certainly a he) manifests the mantric phonemes on the bodies of other practitioners as well as on *maṇḍalas*, *cakras*, *yantras*,[6] and other ritual objects.

Illness and Immortality. Patricia Sauthoff, Oxford University Press. © Oxford University Press 2022.
DOI: 10.1093/oso/9780197553268.003.0002

A Mantra to Conquer Death

The ninth-century *Netra Tantra* instructs its *mantrin* to both recite and write its primary mantra while performing various rites meant to alleviate the pain of illness, cure illness altogether, or attain immortality. In Chapter 2, the *Netra Tantra, oṃ juṃ saḥ* reveals its mantra in an encoded form. The text further describes the mantra's phonemic technical associations in Chapter 22. This mantra, *oṃ juṃ saḥ*, is not unique to the *Netra Tantra*. It appears in a variety of Tantric texts where it is closely associated with conquering death (*mṛtyuñjaya*), both as a rite and a deity.[7] The *Netra Tantra* itself also appears under the names *Mṛtyuñjaya* and *Mṛtyujit* Tantra.[8] This mantra shares a name with the Vedic *mahāmṛtyuñjaya* mantra (also called the *trayambaka* mantra), but nothing more.[9]

In the *Netra Tantra*, the act of placing mantras on *maṇḍalas* and bodies empowers the physical sphere by demarcating ritual space.[10] The religious marking of bodies occurs in various forms across world religions.[11] In Hinduism, we often find such markings on the forehead (*tilaka*). These marks indicate one's alliance to Śaiva, Vaiṣṇava, or other religious orders.[12] Other religious identity markers include clothing and religious ornaments. Often, such identifications are temporary and can be supplanted in the case of conversion, excommunication, or a change in institutional position—such as the attainment of a higher initiatory status. They also indicate the acceptance of the practitioner by other members of the religious group. LaFleur offers two categories of possible modification: that which does not violate the surface of the body and that which does: such as cutting, piercing, or fasting.[13] The placement of mantra (*nyāsa*) in the Tantric context clearly conforms to this first category as it leaves no visible markings. The *mantrin* uses his hands, formed into specialized gestures (*mudrās*), to place mantras onto the body or ritual objects.[14] It is only when one writes or visualizes mantras that they are able to be seen.[15] Both types of mantras—visible and non-visible—have the power to transform the physical world because they call forth deities that are inherent within them. These deities protect the bodies of practitioners from the epidemics and illnesses inflicted upon them by demons. These demons too are invisible but physical. I discuss the iconography of the deities in Chapter 3. For now, I only note that there has been an eagerness on behalf of Western art historians to sanitize such images in order to make them more presentable to the modern viewer.[16] For the Śaiva practitioner, deities and their imagery do not represent something else (i.e., they are not symbolic).

Instead, they are both imbued with significance and agency[17] and very real forces that can be combated through ritual. For the medieval Śaiva practitioner, deities, mantras, icons, and *maṇḍalas* are aesthetic manifestations or corporalizations of that which already exists. They are not a creation of something new.[18] The complexity of such a world reinforces the Tantric tendency toward a professional class of practitioners who work in secrecy. Combating demons and calling forth deities is specialist and time-consuming work. *Mantrins* are trained first through initiation and then[19] learn how to call upon and interact with deities and demons.[20]

Encoding the Mantra

Like much of the medieval Tantric canon, the *Netra Tantra* utilizes the narrative form of a dialogue between the goddess Pārvatī and the god Bhairava (Śiva).[21] The *Netra Tantra*'s introductory chapter praises Śiva as the Eye (*netra*) of the Lord and recounts the widespread mythological story of Śiva consuming the god Kāma with a fire from his third eye.[22] It then offers synonyms for *amṛta*: highest abode (*paramaṃ dhāman*), highest or nectar of immortality (*parāmṛta*), highest bliss (*paramānnda*), highest place (*paramaṃ pada*), absolute knowledge (*niṣkalaṃ jñana*), or conquering death (*mṛtyjit*).[23]

The second chapter begins with a request from the goddess that Śiva reveal to her the remedy for ailments that afflict both divine and worldly beings. Among these maladies she lists anxiety (*ādhi*), fear of disease (*vyadhibhaya*), terror (*udvigna*), poison (*viṣa*), demons (*bhūta*), fear (*bhaya*), tetanus (*ardita*), sudden death (*apamṛtyu*), a hundred injuries (*śatākīrṇa*), fever (*jvara*), cough (*kāsa*), and wasting away (*kṣaya*).[24] Śiva responds that no one has ever before asked such a question and therefore he has never before revealed the answer.[25] He emphasizes the importance of the *mṛtyuñjaya* mantra and the *Netra Tantra*'s tripartite approaches of mantra, yoga, and knowledge.[26] Śiva adds to Pārvatī's list of maladies a group of supernatural beings that cause illness: Bhūtas, Yakṣas, Grahas,[27] Unmādas, Śākinīs, Yoginīs, Gaṇas, Bhaginīs, Rudramātṛs, Ḍāvīs, Ḍāmarikās, Rūpikās, Apasmāras, Piśācas, Brahmarṣas, and Grahas, as well as the afflictions of sudden (*apamṛtyu*) and natural death (*kālapāśa*).[28] Finally, Śiva reveals that protective practices should be carried out first for the king, then the king's sons, then all living creatures beginning with Brahmins, and finally all those tormented with the fear of illness (*doṣa*).[29] This discussion of the supernatural beings who cause disease demonstrates that invisible forces affect the world in observable ways. In order to counter these forces, Śiva reveals another invisible but observable element, mantra. This also shows how mantras cross boundaries to affect the corporeal (*sthūla*) and subtle (*sūkṣma*) bodies of practitioners. Śiva himself acts as a representative of the highest (*para*) body to encapsulate the tripartite nature of the world. This threefold paradigm appears throughout the *Netra Tantra* and connects to its practices of mantra, yoga, and knowledge (*jñāna*).[30]

In addition to revealing the *mṛtyuñjaya* mantra—*oṃ juṃ saḥ*—Śiva speaks about two other important elements of mantric practice. First, he describes the *mātṛkā*, the source for all mantras, and explains how to write the *mātṛkā* mantra on a lotus flower. In his eleventh-century commentary on the *Netra Tantra*, Kṣemarāja uses the *mātṛkā* to explain the technicalities of the *mṛtyuñjaya* mantra. This explanation relies on several aspects of the corporeal world: the earth, organic matter, and the phonemes of the *mātṛkā*[31] (*a*, *ka*, *ca*, *ṭa*, *ta*, *pa*, *ya*, and *śa*). The *mantrin* uses organic matter to create a ritual space on a pure plot of earth by drawing a lotus. He then places the *mātṛkā* onto the petals at the eight cardinal and inter-cardinal directions. Padoux notes that the five gross physical elements[32] spring from the corporeal (*sthūla*), the senses from the subtle (*sūkṣma*), and vital breath (*prāṇa*) from the highest (*para*).[33]

> The pure-souled *ācārya*[34] should draw an eight petaled lotus on smooth, pure earth smeared with sandal and aloe wood, and scented [with] fragrant camphor and strong saffron. After he has drawn [the lotus] with a great undertaking, [the *mantrin*,] decorated and adorned with a crown, smeared with sandalwood, [writes] the *mātṛkā*. Having placed *oṃ*[35] in the middle [on the pericarp of the lotus], he should draw [the phonemes of the *mātṛkā* on the petals] starting in the East. (NT 2.17–19)[36]

The *mātṛkā* mantra appears across Tantric literature.[37] Most explain it as the source of all other mantras.[38] Each phoneme of the *mātṛkā* mantra represents the first phoneme of its traditional phonological category. Therefore, it contains the complete alphabet.[39] By associating each phoneme with a cardinal or inter-cardinal direction, the categories of vowel, velar, palatal, etc., correspond to the compass points, here in the shape of a lotus flower. The lotus commonly forms the core of *maṇḍala*s and *yantra*s, with the petals oriented to the cardinal and inter-cardinal directions. This allows for the placement of the deities in their appropriate positions.[40] A *mantrin* first writes *oṃ* in the center of the lotus before placing the *mātṛkā* phonemes in their respective positions. During protective rites, rather than writing *oṃ*, the *mantrin* writes the name of the person afflicted with illness in the center of the lotus. The name—and therefore the person—afflicted with illness is then surrounded and protected by the mantra.

The physical creation of the mantra allows the practitioner to extract and worship the *mātṛkā* as a goddess. Both the *Siddhayogeśvarīmata* and *Svacchanda Tantra* describe the worship of the goddess named Mātṛkā as the power of Rudra (Śiva). Because Rudra possesses all the letters of the alphabet, he is the source of the categories of phonemes (*vargas*).[41]

> [The *mantrin*] should worship the mother of mantras with the highest devotion (*bhakti*), with multitudes of flowers, perfume, etc., O Devī. He should extract the deity invoked by the mantra (*mantradevatā*) [using the mantra]. Beginning with the all-pervading (*viśva*) and ending with manifold (*viśvarūpa*) [*oṃ*], [he should] always [worship with] the nectar of a white flower. The bright sound is highest Śakti, [who] resembles one-in-the-same Śiva. By this [worship] the pearls [of the mantra] are all bound in a cord. (NT 2.20-22ab)[42]

Once *oṃ*, from which all mantras emanate, is in place, the *mantrin* then constructs the rest of the *mṛtyuñjaya* mantra. The *Netra Tantra* does not give the mantra outright. It reveals it through the attributes of its phonemes and by common associations, such as that of *saḥ* with *amṛta*.[43] The exposition of the mantra concludes with two references to the cessation of death. The first is the association of non-death/immortality/the nectar of immortality (*amṛta*)[44] with the phoneme *sa*, which is a common Tantric connection.[45] The second is the description of *visarga* as the sixteenth vowel. The *Netra Tantra* equates *visarga* with the *kalā* nectar, or the nectar of the sixteenth phase of the moon. This moon nectar is *amṛta*, the nectar of immortality.[46]

> From this [*oṃ*], the seventy-million (*saptakoṭi*) mantras[47] arise, which possess [their own] authority. The terminal letter shining with various light,[48] [which is the] split belly of the moon [*j*], is placed upon a hook [*u*], and yoked with the last rising horizon [i.e., the wind or last labial nasalization][49] [*ṃ*]. That which is described is celebrated in the world as the supreme

> *amṛta* [*sa*]. This is the highest dwelling place. It is the highest *amṛta*. Joined with the *kalā* nectar [*visarga*], filled with the splendor of the moon, it is the highest abode [of Śiva]. That is the supreme word. That is supreme strength, that is supreme *amṛta*. The highest of splendors is the highest light of light. The divine Lord is the supreme cause of all the world. [He] is creator (*sraṣṭṛ*), supporter (*dhartṛ*), and destroyer (*saṃhartṛ*), none are more powerful than him. He is the receptacle of all mantras, the abode of all perfections (*siddhi*) and characteristics (*guṇa*). (NT 2.22cd-28ab)[50]

The *Netra Tantra* describes *j* as hanging on the hook of the letter *u*. In the *śāradā* script, which was used in Kashmir from approximately the eighth to twelfth centuries, *j* consists of two semicircles. The text reads this as the moon, split into two, its tail set upon the hook of the *u*. However, it may also refer to the shape the tongue takes when it produces the sound *j*. To form this sound, the tongue curves toward the top of the palate into a half circle. The hook of *u* is then either the stroke that signifies *u* or the forward momentum of the lips and breath as they move from *j* to *u* in a hook-like shape. Finally, this component of the mantra ends on the *anusvāra*, which is written as a dot (*bindu*) rising above the horizon of the characters or with the closing of the resting lips, pursed and causing both the ceasing of breath and sound. The mantra reveals its depth and importance by referencing both the written and mouthed shapes of the sounds. In both forms, the mantra's physical shape and characteristics are important and meaningful. Through the connection of the components of the mantra's kinetic and written forms, the text gives the mantra a body in the physical world. Simultaneously, it places the mantra into the body of the speaker through the movement of the tongue and lips as well as the cycles of breath. Through usage, a mantra becomes inseparable from its user. Once the connection between mantra and breath is made clear, the *Netra Tantra* then teaches that the mantra is Śiva.

In addition to the connection of *sa* and *saḥ* with *amṛta*, the *Netra Tantra* associates *sa* with the location of the divine. Both *sa* and *visarga* indicate highest abode/resting place (*paramaṃ dhāman*) of Śiva. In other words, when one reaches the resting place of Śiva, he also attains *amṛta*. Abhinavagupta explains the connection between the abode of Śiva and the physical body in the *Paramārthasāra*, where he explains that the thirty-six principles (*tattvas*) and the sense organs make up the divine body and all of the worldly constructions that come with having a body:

> The divine abode for him is his own body—endowed with the thirty-six principles, and replete with œils de bœuf [viz., the sense-organs], constructions inset in the body—or [if not his own, then] the body of another, or even an object, such as a jar. (PS 74)[51]

Of course, Abhinavagupta's reading is from a Trika non-dualist perspective. This means that for him there is no difference between the deity and the practitioner. While the *Netra Tantra* is itself a dualist text, Kṣemarāja's reinterpretation of it through a non-dual lens demonstrates that this ontological difference is minor. The shift in metaphysical outlook from dualist to non-dualist makes little difference on the performance of rites to cure disease and attain longevity (i.e., immortality).

As Abhinavagupta notes, the divine abode/physical body are endowed with thirty-six principles (*tattvas*). In the next chapter I explain how these *tattvas* are inherent within mantras and help to bring meaning to them. These meanings demonstrate the essential power of the mantras. Use of the mantra inspires spontaneous grace within the deity, which then drives out the demons that cause illness out of the body.

The last phoneme of the *mṛtyuñjaya* mantra, *visarga*, appears in written form as two dots, stacked one on top of another. This signifies the inhalation and exhalation of breath.[52] The word *visarga* also indicates a final emission breath and refers to liberation. *Visarga* completes the mantra, which begins with highest sound of Śiva and Śakti and ends with the *amṛtra.*

The *Netra Tantra* then praises the deity as the supreme cause of the world. This renders him more powerful than the creator (*sraṣṭṛ*), traditionally associated with Brahmā, the supporter (*dhartṛ*) Viṣṇu, and the destroyer (*saṃhartṛ*) Śiva. When the practitioner meditates on the *haṃsa* mantra during his quest to vanquish death (as described in the *Svacchanda Tantra*) he first gains the power of Brahmā, then Viṣṇu, and Rudra/Śiva. When he attains Śiva's power, he conquers death.[53] The *Netra Tantra* places the deity Mṛtyujit (Conquerer of Death) higher than Śiva, though he is also a manifestation of, and therefore the same as, Śiva.

Aṅgamantra

Finally, the text discusses the six limbs of the *aṅgamantra*, which *mantrins* use to place (*nyāsa*) mantras on the body and ritual objects to bring forth the deity.[54] This is a subordinate step, performed before the main rites.[55] If not done at all or performed incorrectly, the subsequent rites are rendered ineffective. The six *aṅgamantra*s are eye (*netra*), heart (*hṛd*/*hṛdaya*), head (*śiras*), topknot (*śikhā*), cuirass or breastplate (*kavaca*), and weapon (*astra*).[56] They emanate from, and are identical with, Śiva's own body. Through their use, the worshipper aligns the body with that of the deity. The *mantrin* places the phoneme of each *aṅgamantra* on the corresponding part of his or another's body, often onto the hands.[57] The *Kāmikāgama*[58] describes the placement of the *aṅgamantra*s beginning with the palm and moves either from the little finger to the thumb or in the reverse depending on whether one is a forest-dweller/renouncer (*mumukṣu*) or a householder (*bubhukṣu*).[59] The *Svacchanda Tantra* says a practitioner is to begin by consecrating a clay bath with the *aṅgamantra*s and should envelop the body with the mantra, beginning at the head and ending with the feet.[60] The *mantrin* offers foods such as sesame and mustard seeds while he recites the mantras associated with each *aṅga*.[61] This placement of the *aṅgamantra*s transforms the body. They prepare it for further ritual by surrounding the body in protective mantras. This creates a body that Davis describes as "parallel to that of Śiva,"[62] which coexists with Śiva and therefore can then act as Śiva during ritual performance. Once one has bathed in clay and been consecrated seven times with the *astramantra*, the clay will blaze like the sun. Kṣemarāja clarifies that the *mantrin* should allow the clay to be touched by the rays of the sun or that he is to touch it with his breath.[63] The worshipper then recites *oṃ* and performs the daily rites, which consist of mantra repetition and drinking water in order to remove impurities (*mala*).[64] Several more steps include placing consecrated clay on different parts of the body and reciting the mantra in various directions.[65] Once he has performed the *nyāsa*, the *mantrin* is able to personify the embodied mantra.

The *Netra Tantra* encodes the *aṅgamantra*s using the *mātṛkā* mantra and its position on an eight-petaled lotus. In his commentary, Kṣemarāja decodes the mantra and gives the phonemes outright.

> Now, I shall explain the limbs (*aṅga*). Armed with these, he achieves perfection.
>
> The *hṛdaya* mantra, [which] confers all perfections, [begins its encoding] in the south [i.e., with the sound *ca*],[66] with the sound in the middle [*j*], followed by the fifth vowel [*u*], and summits with the conclusion of wind [i.e., the nasal sound] [*ṃ*].

The *śiras* is the last sound of *soma* [i.e., the semi-vowels] [*v*] joined with that from fire [*y*] and yoked with *oṃ*.

Śikhā is taught as *māyā* [*ī*] joined with the cessation of wind [*ṃ*].

The *kavaca* is] the final syllable [*h*], rising *īśvara* [*ṃ*]and joined with an elevated half of twelve [i.e., the sixth vowel] [*ū*]. Now, with sound joined with Śiva and Śakti, he is enveloped and supreme.

The *netra* [*aṅgamantra*], [which is] most powerful and destroys all faults, begins with Bhairava [*j*], and an *oṃ*, situated with a head always in motion [i.e., the first semi-vowel] [*y*].

That *astra* mantra is proclaimed *ajīvaka* [*pha*] joined with *ṭa*.

The six *aṅgas* of the *mantrarāṭ* [i.e., the *mṛtyuñjaya mantra*], which confers *siddhi*s, is declared. (NT 2.28cd-33)[67]

The *aṅgamantras* are *hṛdaya* (*juṃ*), *śiras* (*vyom*), *śikhā* (*īṃ*), *kavaca* (*hūṃ*), *netra* (*jyom*), and *astra* (*phaṭ*).

The chapter ends with a reinforcement that the *mṛtyuñjaya mantra*, also called the *mantrarāṭ*, confers supernatural powers (*siddhi*s) on those who use it. In this case, the user is both the *mantrin* who performs the rites and the client on whose behalf he carries out the worship.

2
Language, Physicality, and Mantra

The Nature of Mantra

By definition, mantras are thought instruments.[1] According to traditional sources, mantras should be spoken and not written.[2] Tantric works often encode mantras in ways that emphasize the importance of vocal articulation.[3] Through repetition, mantras act as the most effective means of reaching salvation because they are by nature the divine Word and therefore synonymous with the deity they call forth.[4] In most cases, mantras can also be considered the equivalent of ritual acts.[5] However, Tantric and Vedic traditions understand mantric repetition (*japa*) differently. The Vaidika's foremost concern is accurate vocalization of the mantra during rites that involve ritual fires (*homa*).[6] Tantric innovation adds mantric repetition as inner visualization of the technicalities of semiotic insight taught in authoritative texts and by traditional teachers.[7]

The word "mantra" contains the root √*man*, meaning "to think," and the suffix "*-tra*," which signals instrumentality.[8] Padoux notes that in Tantric texts, *-tra* relates to the root √*trai*, meaning "to save." This makes mantras salvific thoughts, which can then be uttered, written, or otherwise utilized.[9] For Tantric practitioners, the mantra is identical with the deity. Liberation comes about from the will of that deity. Thus, mantras must be treated with care. It is not enough to know that the mantra is identical to the deity. Instead, one must recognize how the divine manifests in its mantric form.

To understand mantric forms, one must understand not only what mantras are made of but also how to use them during ritual. To do this, I investigate two scholarly discussions of mantra to critique the categories scholars use to describe mantra. First, I address whether mantras should be considered "magic" and how such a categorization impacts the academic approach to the study of mantra. Second, I examine the discourse surrounding mantras as speech acts. These definitions of mantra inform one of the function of mantras within their ritual context.

Illness and Immortality. Patricia Sauthoff, Oxford University Press. © Oxford University Press 2022.
DOI: 10.1093/oso/9780197553268.003.0003

Mantras as Magic

The main focus for both practitioners and scholars has been the soteriological function of mantra. However, mantras also have non-redemptive outcomes, such as those found in the six acts (*ṣaṭkarmāni*): appeasement (*śānti*), subjugation (*vaśya*), immobilization (*stambha*), enmity (*dveṣa*), eradication (*uccāṭa*), and liquidation (*māraṇa*).[10] Dundas describes the *ṣaṭkarmāni* as part of a system of "black magic" found in medieval India.[11] Though this phrase exists mainly as a pejorative in English,[12] he points out that the thirteenth-century Jain monks who chronicled such activities did not find moral struggles when it came to engaging with black magic.[13] The *Netra Tantra* prescribes mantric recitation of appeasement, the only one of the *ṣaṭkarāni* not to be considered malevolent (*abhicāra*) by the sixteenth-century *Mantramahodadhi*.[14] Consequently, questions regarding the relationship between mantra and magic arise.

Ritual language typically differs from ordinary language. As Burchett points out, academic descriptions of magic focus on the claim that magic comes from a belief that words have inherent efficacy.[15] Early academic work that examines magic describes it as an act in which people do not distinguish between word and object. Cassierer says magical belief occurs when one concludes that "word and name do not merely have a function of describing or portraying but contain within them the object and its real powers."[16] By considering mantras as objects that contain the salvific nature of Śiva, one could say that Cassierer's definition applies to mantra. However, definitions of magic tend to focus on the worldly, pragmatic outcomes of rites rather than the spiritual and redemptive.[17] Mantras, especially within the Tantric tradition, "can be used to different ends—ends that, though different, are not necessarily incompatible. . . . [L]iberation, supernatural powers, and even destructive magical abilities can not only be taught in the same text, but even be bestowed to an adept through the performance of one ritual only."[18] In other words, Tantra does not see a contradiction or distinction between rites for liberation (*mukti*) and those for worldly enjoyment (*bhukti*). This means the categories of religion and magic cannot apply to mantras as the categories themselves are faulty.[19] However, Timalsina explains that "some Tantras relegate audible chanting to the performance of black magic [which] suggests again that audible repetition is considered by Tāntrikas to be a lesser form of mantra practice."[20] Burchett is correct that the categories are imperfect. However, Tantric texts do make a distinction between higher and lower mantric practice. Such a definition of magic focuses on the form the rite takes rather than the results. Mantras then can provisionally be described as religious language that contains magical characteristics.

Mantras as Speech Acts

This definition of mantra leads to an important question: Are mantras actually language? Understanding both sides of this theoretical argument helps us to ascertain the *Netra Tantra*'s own description of mantra and allows analysis of the text. Though the nature of mantra given in the *Netra Tantra* does not directly speak to this issue, it does shed light on its theoretical stance.

Austin recognized that language goes beyond the communicative and that words or utterances are themselves action.[21] Staal argues that while mantras and language share phonological and pragmatic properties, the use of mantra in ritual and meditation brings about effects that are "ineffable" and "beyond language."[22] Further, he does not believe that mantras have the power of transformation or the ability to bring about new existences because mantras only allow their users to access what already exists.[23] Staal does concede that mantras—and in fact, most utterances—are speech but not speech acts, which he defines as "language utterances by which an act is performed"[24] and that "depend on context and on the speaker, and are therefore indexicals."[25] As indexicals, that which they reference shifts from one context to another. They also contain two kinds of meaning: linguistic meaning or character and content.[26] In this way, he likens mantras to bird calls, the "babblings and pre-sleep monologues" of children, and glossolalia, all of which give access to a pre-linguistic state of mind.[27]

Wheelock also points to a pre-linguistic state of mantras. However, he shares the view of Eliade and Padoux that mantras do not signify an outside referent in the objective world but instead point to the source of language, which is itself the source of all creation.[28] As such, he says that mantras need not adhere to communicative function and that the most essential feature of ritual utterances is that they "are speech acts that convey little or no information."[29]

Using Staal's rubric, Tantric mantras cannot be considered speech. One cannot use the mantra *oṃ juṃ saḥ* to call forth any deity other than Amṛteśa because the mantra *is* the deity it summons. However, a practitioner can visualize the body of different deities using this mantra. Ultimately this worship is one in which he honors Amṛteśa through the deity's multifaceted nature. Any perceived difference in reference simply comes from the user of the mantra misunderstanding its nature. The meaning and content of a mantra is also not variable nor does it fluctuate with context. Staal also claims that "in Sanskrit, a mantra is *never* called an act (i.e., *karman* or *kriyā*)."[30] We do find *japa kriyā*, the act of reciting the mantra, in a handful of Tantric texts[31] as well as *japa karman*.[32] This indicates that medieval Sanskritists were at least open to considering the recitation of mantras as speech acts. These writers emphasize the activity of mantric recitation through the addition of verbal elements.

Alper points out that in the *Śiva Sūtra Vimarśinī*, Kṣemarāja argues that mantra is something one does.[33] Quoting the *Svacchanda Tantra*,[34] Kṣemarāja says

> *ātmano bhairavaṃ rūpam bhāvayed yas tu puruṣaḥ |*
> *tasya mantrāḥ prasiddhyanti nityayuktasya sundari ||*
> [Only] the mantras of a man who is united with the eternal, that is, one who has realized he is Bhairava, are successful, O Goddess.[35]

Kṣemarāja explains that the verb "to become" or "to realize (√*bhū*)" refers to cognition, which itself is the inner emergence of Bhairava.[36] Alper is correct that Kṣemarāja believes mantras to be effective redemptive personal activities for those who understand that they are tools for recognition of the divine.[37] For those who do not comprehend mantras in this way, mantras appear to be magic spells that offer their users the ability to impose the user's own will upon the world rather than call forth and rely on the will of the deity.[38] Further, both the *Svacchanda Tantra* and Kṣemarāja's *Netra Tantra Uddyota* use *mantra karaṇa* to denote mantra as action.[39] Kṣemarāja asks, "In what manner do [the users of mantras] perform the [act of] practicing mantras?"[40] The answer to this question is less important here than the fact that it has been asked at all. The question refers to mantric procedure, while Kṣemarāja finds nothing extraordinary about mantra as an action. A *mantrin* must perform mantra in the same way that he performs ritual observances, yoga, etc., in order for the mantras to be effective. Similarly, the *Svacchanda Tantra* says, "From the efforts of mantric actions (*mantrakaraṇa*), ritual observances (*kriyā*), yoga, etc., [he finds results] in highest Śiva."[41] Again, the text emphasizes that mantras, like other religious behaviors, have a performative, active quality. This example is important because, while the *Tantrāloka* includes the phrase *mantrakriyā* in several places,[42] Abhinavagupta uses it in a compound to refer to mantra and ritual observance tied to yoga and knowledge (*jñāna*). However, the *Svacchanda Tantra* is clear when it applies *karaṇa* to mantra as a way to refer to the act of doing.

Staal may be correct that *some* mantras are not speech acts. These mantras do not involve intention[43] or express thought,[44] or possess meaning,[45] and only occasionally accompany acts.[46] Many other mantras do in fact have these qualities. The *Netra Tantra* shows that mantras are made of unbounded energy, contain all thirty-six principles or realities (*tattvas*), have meaning, and are synonymous with Śiva and Śakti. Further, mantras are intimately tied to Śiva's will and therefore have intentionality. For Staal, it is the user whose speech must contain intention, thought, and meaning to qualify as a speech act. However, when the practitioner focuses on the deity invoked by and equivalent to the mantra, he finds these qualities present. Further, it is irrelevant whether mantras accompany other acts. Mantric recitation (*japa*) and the placing (*nyāsa*) of mantras are actions in the same way that shouting and gesturing are acts. Such acts characterize and accompany ordinary speech without changing the nature of that speech. They help to accentuate and focus speech, and they tell us something about the intention and meaning of the speech, but they are not synonymous with that intention or meaning.

Vedic mantras come directly from verses of Vedic texts while Tantric mantras are often series of phonemes that do not adhere to ordinary grammar or vocabulary. This makes them appear nonsensical to those untrained in their semantic technicalities. Taber describes mantras as "indicators not strictly as assertions but in the most general sense; not only can they take on various syntactic forms, they often depend on mythologic and symbolic associations."[47] It is these associations that, for the initiated practitioner, provide the mantra's meaning in the form of mantric technicalities. As we saw above, the text discloses the components of the mantra by associating them with objects. The phonemes of the *mṛtyuñjaya* mantra are connected to life, sacrifice, and Śiva. These mythological and symbolic links not only provide meaning to the individual units of the mantra but also convey its outcome.

Staal argues that Vedic mantras do not convey information despite the fact that those taken directly from texts are syntactically capable of doing so. He says that prose mantras, chanted interjections (*stobha*), and "the numerous sounds and noises that pervade the other ritual uses of the Vedas" are not used like ordinary language.[48] Further, he argues that even those mantras that do come directly from texts are not treated like verse by their users and therefore it is impossible to try to attain any syntactical meaning from them.[49] Mīmāṃsān philosophers, who emphasize the importance of Vedic ritual, addressed this idea and adopted the viewpoint that the meanings of words found in the Vedas are the same as those used in ordinary language. In other words, whether in ritual or daily life, syntactical meaning remains the same. Were Vedic and ordinary language not the same, men would be unable to understand Vedic injunctions and therefore could not follow them.[50] In this Mīmāṃsān interpretation, the intentionality of the Vedic injunction is a speech act even without the injunction itself being articulated, because inherent in these dictums is a promise.[51] Mantras, however, do not have this inherent illocution but express their intended meanings by using the language of injunctions. Therefore, in the Mīmāṃsān view, mantras too are utterances with intention as well as speech acts, because speech acts involve actions in which intention is expressed and realized.[52]

Padoux says that while Tantric mantras have no semantics, their connection to ritual gives them structure and syntax. This means that while mantras do not themselves have meaning in an ordinary linguistic manner, they are used in a meaningful way in rites with intention and purpose.[53] Further, Staal's argument relies on the notion that mantras accompany other actions and therefore are not acts on their own. Padoux uses the example of purification (*mantraśuddhi* or *mantraśodhana*) rites. Here the *mantrin* purifies mantras by writing the *mātṛkā* mantra[54] on a lotus. This demonstrates that mantras are in fact speech acts as they are the focal point of the practice that puts mantras into an active state.[55] If one simply utters the mantra—without intention or without putting it into action first through purification and activation—the mantra will not be effective. Through bodily action, whether that be reciting the mantra, writing it on the drawing of a lotus, or touching the written mantra with flowers or leaves,[56] the practitioner imbues the mantra with the divine, its meaning, and its objective.

Questioning the Nature of Mantra: NT 21.1–19

Having touched on the functionality of mantra, I now turn to what constitutes mantras. The *Netra Tantra* presents a dialogue between Śiva and Pārvatī in which she enquires about the nature of mantra. Additionally, she asks Śiva to explain what gives mantras their vitality. Her question is a query into the cosmological nature of mantras.

> O Deva, of what are mantras composed? What are their characteristics? What are they like? What power [do they] possess? What makes them powerful? How are they able [to be effective] and who impels them [to be productive]? (NT 21.1)[57]

Pārvatī's line of inquiry indicates mantric physicality. As such, she speculates that mantras must have components and characteristics. They are things that can be seen and experienced through the senses. This means that mantras are more than simply a sum of their vocalized phonemes. Padoux says, "Mantra is sound (*śabda*) or word (*vāc*); it is never, at least in its nature, written,"[58] and though the practices of the *Netra Tantra* do contain the written form of the mantra, the text generally focuses on the act of writing the mantra, not the written form itself. This written mantra acts as an extension of sound, which is inseparable from the mind of its user and also consciousness itself.[59] Pārvatī's question does not contradict Padoux but instead offers another framework through which one can think about the form of mantras. By asking "What are the characteristics of mantras, and what are they like?," Pārvatī acknowledges that there are circumstances in which mantras have an embodied form as part of their essential nature.

It is important here to remember that in the medieval Indian worldview, the Cartesian dualism between mind and body, spirit and matter, etc., does not exist. Instead, the human body contains both corporeal (*sthūla*) and subtle (*sūkṣma*) elements that encompass the mental and physical. Additionally, the highest (*para*) body is the body as inseparable from Śiva. The Tantric body exists in a spectrum, from corporeal to subtle to highest, in which the outermost bodily sheath (*kośa*) is the material (*anna*) and the innermost is bliss (*ānanda*).[60] Sāṃkhya philosophy describes the psychophysical body through twenty-five *tattvas*. The corporeal *sthūla* body consists of the five gross elements (*mahābhūta*), while the *sūkṣma* body consists of five subtle elements (*tanmātra*), five organs of action (*karmendriya*), five sense organs (*buddhīndriya*), the mind (*manas*), ego (*ahaṃkāra*), and intellect (*buddhi*).[61] Here the mind has the capacity for both sense and action. Tantra builds on Sāṃkhya's twenty-five *tattva*s for a total of thirty-six.[62] For now we need only focus on those directly associated with the *sthūla* and *sūkṣma* bodies. Here, sound (*śabda*) is included in the five subtle elements. This indicates that the text wants to call the *tattva*s to attention when Pārvatī asks about the nature of mantras. Her questions include those about the agency of mantras. That Pārvatī's question asks about mantric agency means this

Tantra allows for an agent—someone or something—who impels mantras and makes them active.

If the human body exists on a spectrum of *sthūla* to *sūkṣma* to *para*, then mantras must as well. The ritual officiant utters or visualizes mantras in rites. Like bodies, mantras are intimately tied to the *tattva*s, which make their use effective. Both the *Vijñāna Bhairava*[63] and Somānanda's *Śivadṛṣṭi*[64] define recitation (*japa*) as contemplation and ceaseless awareness of one's identification with Śiva. Thus, *japa* expresses the spontaneous and internal repetition of the primordial sound (*nāda*). This means that true concentration during recitation requires the practitioner to focus on an abstraction rather than a particular name or mantra. The primordial sound itself is the form of everything.[65] The *Vijñāna Bhairava* and *Śivadṛsti* view mantras from a more esoteric perspective than the *Netra Tantra*. Their heterodox position is fully aniconic, whereas texts such as the *Siddhayogeśvarīmata*, *Svacchanda Tantra*, and *Netra Tantra* rely on physical representations of deities. This includes the installation of mantras onto idols, where one installs the mantras of the deity onto the appropriate material object, which has been bathed and purified in the same way as the disciple.[66] In the *Tantrāloka*, Abhinavagupta seeks to explain this contradiction, saying that installation onto an idol does not apply the essential nature of Bhairava to the material. Instead, officiants should only perform mantric installation on idols that do not come from Bhairava texts and to mantras of the Siddhānta system.[67] In other words, Abhinavagupta proposes that the *Netra Tantra* refers to an icon that is only a physical representation of the deity and not one that is embodied with the essential nature of Bhairava.[68] In noting Abhinavagupta's effort to refute this inconsistency, I wish to highlight that the *Netra Tantra* does allow for the essential Bhairava to physically manifest and it is only in the Trika interpretation of Abhinavagupta where this view becomes problematic.

> O Deva, if [mantras] consist of the nature of Śiva, [which is] ubiquitous, formless (*śūnyarūpin*), and [if he] does not perform action, how can [mantras] be agents of action? And how do they create a state [in which one] performs them [when they are] formless (*amūrtatva*)? Who does [that performance] without an individual body? Speak, O Lord. An action of [one who is] bodiless cannot be seen, O Parameśvara. When having a body [results in a condition] in all living beings of [being] bound, how does the agency of the bound [individual] contradict those agents [who are] devoid

of power? Thus, [because] mantras consist of the nature of Śiva, how do they actually accomplish [anything]? (NT 21.2–5)[69]

The *Netra Tantra* describes a Śiva who is all-pervading and formless. This Śiva does not act as the performer of action. In other words, Pārvatī understands Śiva as unconstrained by the *tattvas* and yet able to impact the *sthūla* and *sūkṣma*. Pārvatī describes the nature of Śiva as formless (*śūnyarūpin*) or immaterial (*amūratva*).[70] In other words, not only is Śiva amorphous, but he is, in fact, disembodied altogether. The text enquires as to whether something that is disembodied, and therefore something that one cannot experience through the sense organs, is capable of being an agent of action. Somānanda offers the clearest refutation of this conception. In his *Śivadṛṣṭi*, Somānanda argues that consciousness does not appear to have material form[71] and that consciousness does not operate in the same way as the physical body.[72] Instead, like the *mantrin* in meditation, Śiva creates by means of his will. "Omnipresence and multiplicity of nature exist by means of will. It is not the case here that [Śiva] produces the universe by transforming himself, since his nature is as it is in immediate conformity with his will."[73] In other words, Śiva does not act as an agent of action in the same way that embodied beings do. What he creates is simply the product of his consciousness. Mantras then are both made of Śiva's nature and creations produced by the will of his formless consciousness. This creation is also a spontaneous by-product of his will.

The next set of questions suggest that mantras are made of Śakti. Where before the *Netra Tantra* questioned how the disembodied could act, it now focuses on a Śakti defined by motivated performance. The text takes for granted that Śakti is capable of performance and implies, through the use of the phrase *śaktirūpa*, that Śakti has an embodied form. This Śakti has substance and exists in a definable state.[74]

> But, if [mantras consist of] the forms of Śakti, whose Śakti and of what kind? O Deva, what [does] Śakti cause, what is her purpose, and of what kind is she? If [mantras] do not possess Śakti, what is worshipped with Śakti? Independence (*svatantra*) cannot be accomplished by anyone without perfection (*siddha*). What is conquerable [by one who is] imperfect (*asiddha*)? One supposes that [which is] imperfect. Somewhere Śakti exists. In this sense she is not empty of substance. The incorrect perception (*viparyaya*) [is] that the pure form of Śakti [constitutes] the mantras. (NT 21.6–9ab)[75]

The ninth century *Śiva Sūtra*, contemporary with the *Netra Tantra*,[76] explicates the nature of Śakti. The *Śiva Sūtra* describes "the production of a body in unification with Śakti."[77] In the *Netra Tantra*, one aims for a body free from illness and death. This is, of course, accomplished through the use of mantra. If the mantra does in fact consist of Śakti, unification with the mantra is fusion with Śakti, which in turn gives rise to this healthy body. This newly created body does not depend on the will of Śakti but, according to Kṣemarāja's commentary on this verse, the will of the practitioner. Kṣemarāja then quotes the *Lakṣmīkaulārṇava*,[78] which says that, without unification (*saṃdhāna*), initiation and the attainment of *siddhi*s are not effective, nor is mantra, the application of mantra, and the practice of yoga.[79] Though the *Netra Tantra* does not always conform to the non-dual view of its commentator, this passage is still useful. The non-dual texts focus on unification with Śakti while the *Netra Tantra* describes a state in which the mantra is possessed of Śakti. Both agree that it is the coupling of Śakti and mantra that impacts the mantra's effectiveness.

Whereas Śiva lacks agency, the second sentence of this passage assumes that Śakti is that which causes, i.e., acts. Elsewhere, the *Netra Tantra*, which Kṣemarāja cites in his commentary on *Śiva Sūtra* verse 19, says, "he is the source of all the gods and Śaktis in various ways. She has the characteristic of the source of *agni* and *soma*. All originates from her."[80] For Kṣemarāja, this demonstrates the non-duality of Śiva and Śakti. But it can also be read through a non-dualistic view that says as separate entities, Śiva is the unmoving *puruṣa* while Śakti is the agent of action, the material world, and *prakṛti*. The thirteenth-century Tamil Śaiva Siddhānta *Śivajñānabodha*[81] describes the independence of Śakti as a sunbeam, inseparable from Śiva, the sun, and yet distinct. In this metaphor, the text says the sun "is called 'sunbeams' when shining on those objects [that it illuminates] but 'sun' when shining on itself."[82] The *Netra Tantra* also uses the metaphor of the sun, saying that the highest Śakti is made of Śiva because the beams of the sun, fire, and heat are inherent and situated in the sun.[83] The *Netra Tantra* does not say if those beams are distinct from the sun. However, it does say that, following the will of Śiva, those who obey become free of passion and transform so that they are no different from Śakti.[84] At minimum, the practitioner can become identical with Śakti, if not with Śiva.

It is easy enough then to understand Śiva as unmanifest potential and Śakti as Śiva's potential in its inextricable but embodied form. If read from a non-dualistic viewpoint, the sunbeam or rays of the sun are an emanation of the sun that is wholly dependent upon it in order to shine. Consequently, Śiva is the unmanifest mantra and Śakti the manifest. The *Netra Tantra* itself is ambiguous about the independence of Śakti but, as I demonstrated using the above metaphor, it is not contradictory to the text's analysis of mantra. It is important to consider both views. Though Kṣemarāja comments upon and interprets the text through his own non-dualistic (*advaita*) beliefs, the text itself does not always conform to his point of view.

Finally, Pārvatī questions how imperfection influences one's independence. If Śakti is the manifestation of Śiva, she must be prone to the imperfections found in the manifest world. A *siddha* attains independence because he has become perfected. Therefore, one who is not yet a *siddha* can only conquer the imperfect. He can reach the state of Śakti but not that of Śiva. To truly become independent or self-dependent (*svatantra*), he must go beyond the imperfect. This is why even the purest form of Śakti cannot form the mantras. Were Śakti alone sufficient, no one would be able to go beyond the imperfect. Śakti's will is limited. Only the will of Śiva is truly independent.

Pārvatī then considers a third possibility: that mantras are *aṇu*.[85] Generally, "*aṇu* means fine" or "minute." More specifically it refers to an atomic unit. Here *aṇu* denotes something that is embodied and therefore limited. That which is *aṇu* has an individual soul. Though Śakti has the potential for embodiment and contains substance, she is still embodied in the most abstract of ways. In the metaphor of the sunbeam, Śakti is embodied and therefore visible but never so fully embodied that one is able to grasp Śakti in his hands. Something that is *aṇu*, no matter how small, exists in the limited, gross world. That which is *aṇu* lacks the potential for embodiment because it is already material. When speaking about the individual's relationship to aṇu, texts often connect it to impurity (*mala*). Singh says:

> The bondage of the individual is due to the innate ignorance or *āṇava mala*. It is this primary limiting condition which reduces the universal consciousness to an *aṇu* or a limited creature. It comes about by the limitation of the *Icchā Śakti* of the Supreme. It is owing to this that the *jīva* considers himself to be a separate entity cut off from the universal stream of consciousness. It is consciousness of self-limitation and imperfection.[86]

In Singh's assertion, the limited creature (*aṇu*) is that which creates the impression of individuality since it acts as a barrier for the practitioner. This keeps the practitioner from realizing the purity and indistinguishability of himself and the divine. Where Śakti is susceptible to the imperfections of the manifest world, the limited creature is innately imperfect. Can this mean that mantras in their most gross form are imperfect? I return to this question later in the chapter. First, it is important to understand how a mantra manifests in the gross world.

The *Kiraṇa Tantra* describes the relationship between Śiva and mantra as follows,

> He is in primal unvoiced sound [*nāda*], in almost gross sound [*bindu*], in (the sound of) ether, in (the gross sound of) mantras (that express Śiva Himself), in (the coarser mantra-souls called) *aṇus* in the power (which controls those), in the seed(-syllables such as Oṃ that precede the enunciation of mantras) [*bija*], in the sound units (of the seeds) [*kalā*], and in the end(-sounds such as the final nasalization of the seed syllable Oṃ).[87]

Here, Śiva manifests himself in all moments, those just before utterance, those of utterance, and those in which sound reaches its final resting place. Through this process Śiva controls everything through sound.

The *Mālinīvijayottara* touches on the limited condition (*aṇu*) in its teachings about a threefold yogic practice, which is similar to that found in the *Netra Tantra*. The *Netra Tantra* teaches the corporeal, subtle, and highest yogas. It emphasizes the manipulation of the physical world. The yoga of the *Mālinīvijayottara* emphasizes three types of absorptions (*samāveśa*) that allow the practitioner to realize his identity. The three are *āṇava*, *śākta*, and *śambhava*. The first, *āṇava*, includes bodily and breath practices such as mantra, *mudrā*, *maṇḍala*, and *nyāsa*.[88] *Śākta* yoga focuses on the mind. It contains meditation on visualized objects. Finally, pure consciousness, the state of being reconciled with Śiva through *śāmbhava* yoga, allows the devotee to reach inner awakening.[89]

If mantras are *aṇu*, they are limited objects of the gross world. They are both physical and finite. This means that mantras can contain impurities. This leads Pārvatī to question how something limited by impurity can cause someone to become pure. The gods view mantras as Śiva rather than *aṇu*, because mantras have the ability to confer benefits on those who use them. This apparent contradiction is at the heart of the *Netra Tantra*'s query into the nature of mantra.

> But if mantras were limited (*aṇu*) [they] would have embodied forms. [They would] possess their own essential selves (*ātmasvarūpa*) and be known as impure not power. Whose impurity does the impure remove? Limited mantras [and] those who use them are not perfected, O Parameśvara. Without existence, the three kinds of *tattva*s are kept from a multitude of objects. There, union is declared to be the desire for another living being's welfare. The gods and *āsura*s view mantras as powerful and invincible. [Mantras] confer benefits [because they are] all-favoring, all-bestowing, all-pervading, and Śiva. Briefly, O Mahadeva, speak to my question. There is not anyone higher than yourself, O Lord of the World. Please tell all, O Great Śiva, if I please you, O Lord. (NT 21.9cd–14)[90]

To utter a mantra, the disciple requires that it be limited and embodied. But, because mantras are limited, Pārvatī questions how they can remove impurity. She also provides the answer. Just as mantras are threefold, there are three kinds of *tattva*s: pure (*śuddha*), pure-impure (*śuddhāśudha*), and impure (*aśuddha*). The *tattva*s from *śiva* to *śuddhavidyā* belong to the first category, those from *māyā* to *puruṣa* to the second, and from *manas* to *pṛthivī* to the last. They move from the most etherial to abstraction to gross physical objects. This mirrors the *Netra Tantra*'s description of mantra.

In Śiva's response, the text evinces that the nature of mantra contains all three aspects simultaneously. They have the nature of Śiva from which the form of Śakti emerges. This makes them limited. Mantras, like everything else, exist in all three states.

> Ah! The question [you have] asked me is not answered elsewhere, [although] I declare it in all teachings. The foolish, [those] always concealed with illusion, do not know. It is not worship [if] you speak the mantra [devoid of] the three kinds of *tattva*s. Meanwhile, let it be. A world lacking the *tattva*s does not accomplish [anything]. Everything that is seen is made out of the three *tattva*s. O Devī, without three kinds of *tattva*s, no meaning of a word [can be] known. From this are all three kinds of *tattva*s, [from] highest to lowest. Mantras possess the nature of Śiva, are to be known as the form of Śakti, [and] in that manner [are] *aṇu*. Unbounded energies proceed [through] the distribution of the three kinds of *tattva*s. (NT 21.15–19)[91]

The remainder of the chapter continues to describe Śiva, Śakti, and *aṇu* but does not add much to our understanding of mantras. It characterizes Śakti as will (*icchā*), knowledge (*jñāna*), and action (*kriyā*),[92] as it is in many other texts of the Śaiva tradition. The *Netra Tantra* also reiterates that impurities suppress *ātmans* and a practitioner can only be saved through the will of the highest deity, Parameśvara or Śiva.[93] It tells of a Śiva who is disembodied potential while Śakti plays the role of material cause.[94] The practitioner draws on mantras in their threefold pronounced (recited and/or written), mental (*dhyāna*), and bodily (*mudrā*) forms to approach Śiva and seek his divine grace.[95]

Exposition on the Components of the *Mṛtyuñjaya* Mantra: NT 22.5–18

The *Netra Tantra*'s twenty-second chapter returns once more to the *mṛtyuñjaya* mantra. It reveals the components of this mantra without encoding. Śiva explains that there are countless mantras, all of which comprise Śiva and are made manifest by Śakti. They bring about earthly enjoyments (*bhoga*), including health, wealth, and power as well as spiritual liberation (*mokṣa*).

> Listen! I will speak to the question that remains in your heart. All the innumerable mantras, on all occasions, have the majesty of Śiva and Śakti, all are endowed with Śakti, all grant rewards (*bhoga*) and liberation (*mokṣa*), and [all] are nourished by one's own Śakti. However, the highest *deva* is tranquil, in possession of imperceptible *guṇa*s, [namely,] Śiva who consists of all, who is pure, and who is to be understood as unsurpassed. This Parameśvara is the ultimate substrate of [the mantras]. They have arisen through his will [i.e., they are self-arisen or self-illuminated consciousness (*bhāvagrāhyaś cidghanatvena svaprakāśaḥ*)] and [the mantras are] impelled [to act] through his Śakti. [Therefore,] all [mantras] become successful because they have authority everywhere. That which is the supreme abode is Śiva, the receptacle (*ālaya*) of all beings. Mantras are fruitful [because their] power arises from him. (NT 22.5–10ab)[96]

Of the countless mantras, the *Netra Tantra* says the *mṛtyuñjaya* mantra, which it calls Parameśvara, is the highest. Its power springs from Śiva's will (*icchā*), becomes active through Śakti, and leads to dissolution into the divine. The concept of dissolution (*ālaya*) refers to absorption (*laya*).[97] The practitioner achieves this dissolution and absorption when he becomes undifferentiated from the divine.

The *mṛtyuñjaya* mantra can be used for a variety of outcomes, unlike some other mantras that have very narrow and specific usages.[98] Most of the rites described in the *Netra Tantra* are occasional (*kāmya*), those performed in order to gain an object or a personal advantage (such as wealth, children, driving out of enemies, or the alleviation of disease). Kṣemarāja explains that the *mṛtyuñjaya* mantra brings about the spoils of war, offers freedom from disaster, casts out impurities,[99] and conquers death. As a universal mantra (*mahāsāmānyā*), *oṃ juṃ saḥ* is less impacted by the impurities of improper use than other mantras. The text does give very precise instructions on how to interlock the mantra with the person on whose behalf it is used in order to maximize its effectiveness. Like many mantras, the *mṛtyuñjaya is* activated spontaneously by the power of Śiva. It relies on his autonomy, which makes it successful in all its various tasks.[100] However, despite its universality and immunity from certain impurities, correct usage is still an important factor in mantric ritual performance.

The *Netra Tantra* describes eleven types of interlocking, in which the mantra (A) and the name of the person on whose behalf the rite is performed (*nāman*), or the action or goal of the ritual (*abhidheya, sādhya*) (B) follow particular patterns.[101] The sequences found in the *Netra Tantra* sometimes differ slightly from those found in texts such as the *Agnipurāṇa*, *Phetkāriṇī Tantra*, or *Tantrarāja Tantra*, among others,[102] though just as often the texts give the same definitions as those found in the *Netra Tantra*. Padoux also notes that the *Netra Tantra* is unique in its eleven types of practices as most texts include only six.[103] A brief description of these eleven varieties is given here:

saṃpuṭa: when spoken, the pattern follows BAB[104] with the mantra enclosed by the other mantric elements when written it appears as the mantra written above, below, to the left, and to the right of the *sādhya*
grathita: wherein the syllables of A and B are alternated in order to bind them together in written form and appear as the letters of the alphabet inscribed to make a border around the diagram
grasta: writing the mantra on all four sides of the *nāman* or *sādhya*
samasta: writing or uttering the *nāman* before the mantra with one repetition, BABA
vidarbhita: *nāman* before mantra[105]

ākrānta: placing the mantra around the name, which is at the center, ABA
ādyanta: usually meaning "beginning and end"; here Kṣemarāja says that the *nāma* follows the mantra, which is then followed by three more mantra repetitions,[106] ABAAA
garbhastha: the reverse of the written *saṃpuṭa*, with the *sādhya* surrounding the mantra above, below, and to the left and right
sarvatoṛta: BAB, though the pattern is the same as in *saṃpuṭa*, here the *mantrin* places the *sādhya* or *nāma* before and after the mantra
yuktividarbha: BABBB (the opposite of *ādyanta*)
vidarbhagrathita: repeating the mantra three times after the *nāman* for the pattern BAAA[107]

Though described in the text, the *Netra Tantra*'s rites do not call for the use of all eleven varieties. The *saṃpuṭa*, *samasta*, *ākrānta*, and *ādyanta* kinds appear most often in the *Netra Tantra* and *yuktividarbha* and *vidarbhagrathita* appear only in the section of the text and commentary that describe the different mantric patterns. Of all eleven types, only *saṃpuṭa* and *grathita* have distinct written and spoken forms. Though mantras are intrinsically an acoustic phenomenon, within the ritual context they have power in their written manifestation because they are imbued with the power of the spoken form.[108]

Whether they are written or spoken, mantras arise by the will of the deity. As such, the act of enveloping mantras emulates the cycle of creation and destruction or that of birth and death.[109] I return to this discussion shortly. Suffice to say for now that this cycle instantly removes impurities, thus leading to the attainment of earthly enjoyments or liberation.

Finally, the *Netra Tantra* describes the deity and how he protects the practitioner. Kṣemarāja expands on this through a rhetorical analysis (*nirvacana*)[110] that explains why it uses the word *netra* to name the *mṛtyuñjaya* mantra. This analysis plays with the root √*nī*, including its forms of *netra* and *netṛ*, focusing on the root's association with leadership and protection. Śiva is the leader who brings one away from fear and toward liberation. By doing so, he protects, and the mantra is the weapon he uses to safeguard those who follow him.

> The leader [Śiva] of these [mantras] is eternal, restraining, untroubled, unexpanding (*niṣprapañca*), without appearance (*nirābhāsa*), and causes protection (*trāyaka*). He does all, he protects the trembling minds [of those

> who are afraid of *saṃsāra*]. He leads. From [Śiva's] leading, [the practitioner] shall attain liberation from great fear. Thus, [the mantra] is called "*netra*" because [it] protects. It is called *netra* [because] it leads to *mokṣa*. It shall save [the disciple] from the great terror. It is called *netra* from the roots leading and saving. [Moreover,] it is said to be *netra*, being that which gives life to all creatures. [Just as *netra* in the sense of the eye makes everything clear because it illuminates everything, it is also referred to as *netrabhūta*, from this [comes] all life].[111] Parameśvara is like the Lord [i.e., the owner or controller] of the entire multitude of all mantras. (NT 22.10bc–13)[112]

The narrative Kṣemarāja offers in his commentary on this passage demonstrates his non-dual perspective on the nature of Śiva. This differs greatly from the original text, in which the deity can clearly be read as separate from that which he protects.

> [Śiva is] he who exists in a fixed condition, who brings about all conditions [in all] time[s] and direction[s] but is not touched by [those conditions]. He controls them. He is their leader, [he leads] quickly,[113] he wishes it, and he quickly brings [that which is wished for into being. He] projects [all conditions] outward and he also causes them to be made one with himself [internally, inside his consciousness]. And for this reason, he can also be understood as their leader. Untainted, transcending the impurities (*mala*), beginning with minuteness (*āṇava*),[114] and free of afflictions (*upaplavas*). In the same way, one should construe *nisprapañca* and *nirābhāsa*. The diversity of the world has passed away from him, [as have] contracted manifestations [such as persons or things]. He is called the threefold protector (*trāyaka netrā*) because he protects all and he is the liberating (*tāraṇa*) because he is the savior. Śiva is Mṛtyujit, whose nature is Paramaśiva, which is salvation. He protects those whose minds are terrified. And this is the *nirvacana* of *netranātha* on the basis of similarity of syllables and vowels (NTU 22.11).[115]

Where the *Netra Tantra* says that Parameśvara controls the mantras, it does not indicate that mantras emanate from him. In fact, aside from leading and protection, the Śiva of the *Netra Tantra*'s verses does not perform any creative actions. Conversely, Kṣemarāja declares that in his role as protector, the deity projects his wishes outward and therefore causes things to be both internally and externally part of his own divine consciousness. For Kṣemarāja, the deity does not liberate another that needs saving but instead frees the other of its impurities and afflictions in order to eradicate the distinction between the afflicted and himself. To justify this reading, Kṣemarāja takes the words in the original verse, *nitya*, *niyāmaka*, *netṛ*, *nirupaplava*, *nisprañca*, and *nirābhāsa* and makes the claim that because all begin with the root √*nī* (meaning "to protect" or "to lead"), all protect. This proves to Kṣemarāja that his understanding of the nature of the divine is correct because the protective quality is inherent. *Nirvacana*s of this type are common in Tantric literature.[116] They allow exegetes to analyze literature to bring about deeper scriptural revelations. In the case of Tantric literature, this often means the commentators's goal is to "enforce or modify beliefs by encoding meaning into already existing terms."[117] This allows for an overlap in meaning where Kṣemarāja does not adjust the text itself but encodes meanings that logically adhere to his system of thought. In doing so, Kṣemarāja has not undermined the divine revelation found in the *Netra* and other Tantras. Instead, he has uncovered further revelations hidden in the text.

Kṣemarāja's use of *nirvacana* offers inherent justification for the name of the text.[118] The *Netra Tantra*, because of the very nature of its name, actively leads. Like Śiva, it protects and guides its reader away from physical affliction, demonic possession, and the terror of *saṃsāra*.

Once the text has revealed Śiva as the leader and protector, it explains each element of the *mṛtuñjaya mantra* without any encoding whatsoever, beginning with *oṃ*.[119]

> *Oṃ* (*praṇava*) exists as the vital energy [i.e., life] (*prāṇa*) of living beings. It is established as that which keeps [living beings] alive. *Praṇava* enables [those beings] with all [their] parts. He [who knows this] shall know Śiva. (NT 22.14)[120]
>
> [*Praṇava* is the universal pulse or throb that is unstruck, active ideation (verbalization that is not the result of contact with organs) which is like *kalpa*, the first acceptance of the cognition and action of all that is to be known and done for all living beings, because there could be no knowing and no doing without [*praṇava*]. For when [*praṇava*] is present, life becomes fully established. The life [of living beings], which is the flow of the in-breath (*prāṇa*) and out-breath (*apāṇa*), etc., is *ātman*. Otherwise, that life would be unestablished, like the wind that drives a bellows. [*Praṇava*] grasps everything with its constituent parts (*kalā*). [*Praṇava*] is unestablished, has become manifest by means of [Śiva's] internalized autonomy, is

> without [anything] remnant, [and composed of] the constituent elements that will be taught. [*Praṇava*] begins with the letter *a* (*akāra*) and *u* (*ukāra*), etc. In the same way [i.e., because he is made of the same constituent parts], [the *mantrin* is able] to grasp everything up to *samanā*[121] (he internalizes all levels of the sound). [*Praṇava*] also brings about [in the *mantrin* an] awareness of Śiva. And by means of that, [the *mantrin*] will become aware of Śiva [not in the usual way of knowing] but through the power of *paravāk*[122] in its highest non-dual nature.][123]
>
> [*Praṇava* enables him to grasp] the great sixfold path [of emanation and reabsorption].[124] [This path is] established by the six causes[125] [of the great sounds]. [The *mantrin*] makes sacrifices [into fire] with all knowledge (*vidyā*), which has been propelled by the sound *juṃ*. (NT 22.15)[126]
>
> [The middle syllable (*juṃ*) is the middle *tattva* (*vidyā*). [By the word] propelled [the text means to] say, [the *mantrin*] offers into fire by the method of ascending and descending the central domain. That is to say, by this means he casts everything (i.e., the entire universe) into the great fire.][127]

Descriptions of *praṇava* can be found throughout Sanskrit literature. It is central to Brahmanical and Buddhist ritual and yogic practices and commands a wide variety of interpretation and usage.[128] In the *Netra Tantra Uddyota*, Kṣemarāja associates it with the breath, saying *oṃ* is itself to be interpreted as the breath exercise (*prāṇayāma*). In his commentary on the *Svacchanda Tantra*, Kṣemarāja provides a more detailed description of the power of *praṇava*:

> Having recited the *praṇava* constantly, one should burn three fires in the extraction of caste of the limited soul's body, while reciting, "I perform the extraction of caste of such and such a person *svāhā*." Then also while reciting, "I perform the effecting of the state of being a twice-born, *svāhā*" one should burn the three fires for the purpose of effecting the state of being a [true] twice-born that has as it essential function the production of abode of the *śuddhavidya*[129] [*sic*] with mantras which have an unfathomable power, for the purpose of the suitability of effecting a portion of the manifesting of Rudra.[130]

Kṣemarāja sees *praṇava* as a purifier. It leads its users to the knowledge of non-distinction. When the text focuses on non-distinction in the world it teaches *praṇava*'s ability to remove caste from a practitioners' physical body.

Thus, the caste impurities that separate people from one another disappear. The body is then reborn in a purified, twice-born state in which a practitioner rests in knowledge of the divine. Though the *Netra Tantra*'s focus is largely on a king and the *mantrin* in his employ, the mantra and the rites, even when performed on behalf of a monarch, have an effect on society at large, regardless of caste distinctions.

Next, the text offers a semantic analysis (*nirvacana*) of the mantra's final component, *saḥ*. The *Netra Tantra* associates the phoneme *sa* with various characteristics. These words, *svarūpa*, *samyak*, *savisarga*, etc., describe *sa* and begin with the sibilant *s*. Kṣemarāja then adds that *sa* and *visarga* (*saḥ*) fuse to reveal the truth that Śakti's true nature is undifferentiated from Śiva's nature. According to the *Netra Tantra*, the full oblation (*pūrṇāhuti*) occurs when the *mantrin* utters *saḥ* at the end of the *mṛtyuñjaya* mantra. Here he realizes Śakti's fusion with Śiva. Kṣemarāja interprets full oblation as the fusion between Parameśvara and Śakti, and adds that it is through this union that the universe achieves completion.[131]

> [*Sa*] is that which is self-perceived (*svarūpa*), true (*samyak*), possesses the attribute of gratification (*saṃtṛptilakṣaṇa*),[132] the receptacle of all *amṛta* (*sarvāmṛtapadādhāra*), together with *visarga* (*savisarga*), and the highest auspicious thing (i.e., Śiva), which is full and uninterrupted, without any breaks. (NT. 22.16–17ab)[133]
>
> [Then, that which is Śiva, that domain that consists of nothing but consciousness and is named Paramaśiva, which is denoted by such terms as *svarūpa*, which has been previously explained. Together with *visarga*, fused with highest truth (*samarasa*) together with [the highest level of mantra] *unmanāśakti*,[134] which is the highest autonomy. By means of that bliss of the nectar of Śiva, which has been obtained by firmly settling oneself in the practice of the third seed (*sa*).][135]
>
> By means of that [*saḥ*], she [*śakti*] is constantly full, [she is] the full oblation (*pūrṇāhutyā tu pūrṇayā*). He is known as Śiva, the holder of power, who acts through her. Namely, [she is] the one supreme Śakti, whose nature is will (*icchā*), knowledge, (*jñāna*), and action (*kriyā*). [She] arises spontaneously [and her] utterance is automatic. [She] exists in one's very nature, is one's very nature, and is self-arisen. (NT 22.17cd–18)[136]
>
> [The *mantrin* who has achieved the highest practice through the internal recitation of the mantra, is manifestly Śiva himself, the holder of power. This is [how everything that appears] separate, connects.][137]

It is unclear what exactly the text means here by *pūrṇaṃ nirantaraṃ tena pūrṇāhutyā tu pūrṇayā*. Descriptions of *pūrṇāhuti* occur through Śaiva literature. It is usually connected to a *mūlamantra* and may be performed at the conclusion of oblations, rites of atonement, before the dismissal of a deity during fire rites, and others.[138] In his commentary on the *Netra Tantra*, Kṣemarāja describes *pūrṇaṃ nirantaraṃ* as the moment in which "the *ātman* consists of all essences, contains Paraśakti, and is the *ātman* of all immortals."[139] Further, he says, "in the perfect *pūrṇāhuti* she brings about Paramaśiva. [*Pūrṇāhuti*] is called all-pervading (*viśva*) because she brings the Śakti of all immortals."[140] In other words, through the utterance of the syllable *saḥ*, which here is the final oblation, everything becomes Paramaśiva.

Kṣemarāja next reintroduces the *mantrin*. The individual who performs the rites is largely absent from the main text, but Kṣemarāja takes the opportunity to introduce a non-dualistic idea, namely, that the *mantrin* himself is Śiva. Practically, this means that the person for whom the rites are performed understands that the *mantrin* should be treated as the deity. This, of course, gives the *mantrin* significant social power. The *Kulārṇava Tantra* says,

> Whoever regards the guru as a human being, the mantra as mere letters, and the images [of deities] as stone, goes to hell. . . . The guru is the father, the guru is the mother, the guru is God, the supreme Lord. When Siva is angry, the guru saves [from his wrath]. When the guru is angry, nobody [can help].[141]

Though the *Kulārṇava Tantra*[142] is more esoteric and transgressive in outlook than the *Netra Tantra*, Kṣemarāja appears to share its viewpoint. The idea of guru as God is so common throughout Indian traditions that there is no need to make such a belief explicit. What is relevant here is that the *Kulārṇava Tantra* equates the *mantrin* with the mantra. This means that the will of Śiva is identical to that of the *mantrin* and the mantra.[143] The *Kulārṇava Tantra* allows the guru to retain his human characteristics, such as anger, and at the same time identifies him with the divine. Though it may seem contradictory, this recognizes that the guru attains his divinity during ritual. He is inherently divine but only recognizes such during initiation (*dīkṣā*) and consecration (*abhiṣeka*). During these two events, divinity is conferred upon him.[144] Even when he officiates the *dīkṣā* of another, the guru must first purify himself with mantras. Only then can he perform *dīkṣā* for the initiand.[145]

Abhinavagupta takes the idea of guru even further, saying that those gurus who are self-arisen or have attained spontaneous liberation (*svayambhu*) are higher than those for whom *dīkṣā* is performed (*kalpita*). The former guru attains his initiation through the goddesses within his own consciousness while the latter attains initiation by means of his own human teacher.[146] Regardless of the manner in which a guru obtains his *dīkṣā*, that initiation is intimately tied to the power of the mantra. This mantra permeates the various bodies of the initiand in order to bring him into the Tantric fold and thereby change him at the corporeal, subtle, and highest levels.

3

Iconography

Forms of Amṛteśa and Mṛtyujit

Visual Representations

The medieval period in Kashmir proved transformative for religious thought. The composition of the Tantras, the commentaries on them, and the original works by writers such as Somānanda, Utpaladeva, Abhinavagupta, and Kṣemarāja offered an ever-evolving system of religious practice. Though many texts alluded to by these writers and commentators have been lost, there remains a rich corpus of material. The physical history of medieval Tantric practice is much more difficult to access.

Much of the academic focus on Tantric temple architecture concentrates on areas outside of Kashmir. The approximately eleventh-century Orissan *Śilpa Prakāśa* remains the only surviving text to focus on Hindu temple architecture from a Tantric viewpoint.[1] White has catalogued medieval Tantric temples in the Deccan plateau and in modern-day Tamil Nadu, Andhra Pradesh, Uttar Pradesh, and Odisha.[2] He cites no examples from Kashmir save for a reference to the *Rājataraṅgiṇī*, which mentions a site containing "circles of mothers," surrounded by an image of either Śiva or Bhairava.[3]

Several museums house examples of Tantric images from Kashmir.[4] The British Museum holds a stone standing image of Śiva Maheśamurti that dates from approximately the ninth century. One of its three faces appears to be Bhairava, with fanged teeth and a headpiece that bears skull images and severed arms.[5] The Metropolitan Museum of Art houses a late sixth- or seventh-century copper alloy or brass ritual mask from the region that has been identified as Bhairava because of the small fangs that protrude from the mask's mouth and its exposed upper teeth. The earlobes of the mask are stretched in a style often found in Buddhist statuary and has facial features that recall the Greco-Roman influenced Gandhara style.[6] Though only two examples, these images demonstrate the diversity found within representations of Bhairava. The older image, that of the mask, is rather benign in appearance compared

Illness and Immortality. Patricia Sauthoff, Oxford University Press. © Oxford University Press 2022.
DOI: 10.1093/oso/9780197553268.003.0004

to the statue, which looks like the more common fierce Nepalese depictions of Bhairava.

Sanderson[7] has identified three representations of Amṛteśa and his consort Amṛtalakṣmī from the Himalayan region that correspond to descriptions of the deities in the *Netra Tantra*. These small bronzes, which were most likely used in shrine room *pūjās*,[8] are all assigned to the tenth or eleventh century and have been previously labeled Umā-Maheśvara or Viṣṇu and Lakṣmī. Bühnemann adds to this a fourth bronze sculpture from the eleventh century also originally identified as Umā-Maheśvara or Umā-Maheśvara as Kumbheśvara.[9] The characteristics of these images are shared among the icons of Nepal's Tusā Hiti (Royal Bath), which dates to approximately the seventeenth century. Like the bronzes, these images closely correspond to descriptions of the deity as found in *Netra Tantra*, especially at 3.17–23b and 18.63–69ab. Though manuscripts of the *Netra Tantra* made their way to Nepal as early as the thirteenth century,[10] Bühnemann demonstrates that the images of Mṛtyuñjaya[11] do not begin to appear until the seventeenth century in Nepal. Therefore, she argues that the Tusā Hiti sculpture is more likely based on descriptions of the deity from manuals that follow the *Netra*'s tradition rather than from the *Netra Tantra* itself.[12] This statue, and a presumed second statue at Mohancok Hiti in Kathmandu,[13] are thus far the only images of Mṛtyuñjaya found in Nepal that correspond to the description of the deity in the *Netra Tantra*.[14] Similarities between text and object demonstrate the influence of the text and the descriptions of the deities within.[15]

Bühnemann traces a very different iconographical representation of Mṛtyuñjaya outside of Kashmir and the Kathmandu Valley. Found today in Odisha, Kerala, Tamil Nadu, and Bihar as well as available for purchase online, this Mṛtyuñjaya bathes himself in nectar (*amṛta*) that flows from pots that he holds above his own head or from the moon. According to Bühnemann, these images likely come from descriptions in the twelfth-century *Prapañcasāra* and begin to appear in the thirteenth or fourteenth centuries. Such images commonly appear in popular figurines as well as calendar art.[16]

The Mythology of Śiva

There are echoes of Śiva's mythology in the iconography of the *Netra Tantra*. I first explore traditional representations of Śiva in order to contextualize the varying forms—from Amṛteśa, Netra, Mṛtyujit, Bhairava, Tumburu, Kuleśvara, and so forth—found in the *Netra Tantra*. I also examine a Purānic story from the medieval period that includes several elements typically found in Tantric representations of the deity. This helps to place Tantric worship in the medieval period and shows that its heterodoxy found roots in orthodox depictions of Śiva.

There is no mention of Śiva in Vedic literature.[17] The word first appears in the *Śvetāśvatara Upaniṣad*[18] as an adjective meaning auspicious.[19] Michaels warns against the common assumption that Śiva originated in the Vedic deity Rudra. He notes that the association between the two only begins in the fifth or fourth century BCE.[20] In the *Śvetāśvatara Upaniṣad*, Rudra is the supreme deity who dwells alone in the mountains and though a master archer, does not use his arrows to harm.[21] Later works describe him as having the characteristics of an ascetic, such as matted hair and body smeared with ash.[22] Eventually, the myths of Śiva and Rudra became conflated, with Rudra becoming one of the many names of Śiva. In their mythology, both are excluded from Vedic rites, Rudra for being a foreign deity[23] and Śiva because of his asceticism.[24] This exclusion defines both gods as outside the Veda (*vedabāhya*). Śiva/Rudra's outsider status carries through into the Tantric tradition. The earliest recorded Śaivas are the Pāśupatas, who first appeared in approximately the second century CE.[25] The group worshipped Rudra as the cause of the world and flourished from about the fourth to seventh centuries, spreading beyond the Indian subcontinent.[26]

A second narrative that relates to the ancientness of Śiva deserves attention if only to dispel its widespread misidentification of Śiva as an ancient native deity. In the 1920s, archaeologists found an early seal from the Indus Valley Civilization[27] at Mohenjo-Daro. Sir John Marshall claimed the seal was "recognizable at once as a prototype of the historic Śiva."[28] Marshall describes the figure has having three-faces, seated in a yoga-like position, arms and neck adorned with jewelry, a headdress featuring a pair of horns and a tail, and surrounded by an elephant, tiger, rhinoceros, and buffalo. He then compares this image to medieval representations of Śiva to justify his identification.[29] Marshall's identification of the seal as a representation of Śiva requires that Śiva be a pre-Aryan, Dravidian deity who was appropriated into the Vedic pantheon.[30] Bryant points out that scholars have also interpreted the seal as the buffalo demon Mahiṣa, a goddess, or a servant of the deity.[31] Others identify the seal as proof of the Indo-Aryan identity of the Indus Valley Civilization, interpreting the seal as representing Agni,

Indra, Rudra, the sage Ṛṣyaśṛṅga, or Śiva as an Indo-Aryan deity, rather than pre-Aryan.[32] Suffice to say, the evidence does not favor the identification of the seal as a representation of a proto-Śiva. However, this misidentification persists.[33]

The fourth- to sixth-century *Vāyu Purāṇa*[34] tells one of the earliest versions of the story of Śiva's exclusion from the Vedic sacrifice. In the *Vāyu Purāṇa*, Śiva learns about the deity Dakṣa's plan to hold a sacrifice without him and sets out to destroy it. From his mouth, Śiva creates Vīrabhadra, who has a thousand heads, feet, and eyes. Vīrabhadra also holds a thousand clubs and arrows as well as a conch, discus, mace, bow, axe, and sword. The association with Śiva is clear from the tiger skin that drips with blood, the elephant skin, and the serpents that adorn Vīrabhadra. The *Netra Tantra* (9.19ab–26) describes an iconographic form of Sadāśiva who wears a tiger skin and holds a bow and a Bhairava (10.1–7) covered with an elephant skin and bearing a sword. At the command of Śiva, Vīrabhadra destroys the sacrificial vessels and he and his army, which Vīrabhadra creates from his pores, devour the sacrificial offerings of meat and medicinal liquids.[35] Vīrabhadra's destruction of the sacrificial vessels subverts the Vedic order and brings him into control of the rites.

Vīrabhadra announces that his sole purpose is to destroy the sacrifice on behalf of the fury of Śiva. Dakṣa then acquiesces to Śiva and begins to worship him with a thousand and eight names. Dakṣa calls Śiva the protector of children, master of Sāṃkya and yoga, source of *sattva guṇa*, the *oṃkāra*, one who is celebrated by members of all castes, the ocean of milk, the wielder of the skull-staff (*khaṭvāṅga*), reciter of the *gāyatrī* and *oṃkāra* mantras, the vital airs, destroyer of death (*kāla)*, preserver of living beings, protector of worlds, one who is unconquerable, the remover of ailments and diseases, and drinker of wine. Of these names we find many parallels in Tantric Śaiva practice. The main purpose of the *Netra Tantra*'s rites is the protection of the monarch, including his children and his kingdom.[36] He does this by both protecting children and removing ailments and disease. Tantric worshippers shed their caste through the initiatory rites and Bhairava carries the *khaṭvāṅga* as he wanders in penance.[37] Further, the name Mṛtyujit is a *tatpuruṣa* compound (formed from *mṛtyu* "death" and √*ji* "to conquer") making him the conquerer of death.

Finally, Dakṣa tells Śiva that Śiva pervades all and is the inner soul of all beings. Therefore, Śiva did not need to be invited to the sacrifice as he was already present.[38] In the tenth to twelfth century *Śiva Purāṇa*,[39] the sage

Dadhīci says that Śiva makes everything holy and without him the sacrificial sphere would be nothing more than a cremation ground.[40] However, even the cremation ground is a place for the worship of Śiva, who presides over it in much of the mythological canon. For example, in the *Mahābhārata*, Śiva tells Umā that after searching for a pure place in which to dwell he became frustrated and created two types of demons: *piśācas* and *rākṣasas*. To protect people from his creations, Śiva keeps them in the cemetery and chooses to live with them. Further, he says that only heroes can live in such a place and those who seek liberation can find him there.[41] As such, this location is not exceptionally transgressive. In addition to being the place for seekers of liberation, the *Mahābhārata*'s Śiva says that the charnel ground is not for those in search of long life or the impure.[42] This means that even in an orthodox text like the *Mahābhārata*, purity within an impure place exists. When Śiva's practitioners move to the cemetery grounds, they deliberately choose a transgressive lifestyle that puts them at odds with the *mores* of larger society.[43] This recasts the charnel ground as a place for literal and active defiance of standard religious rules. However, the Tantric does not go so far in his heterodoxy as to ignore the precedent set in the orthodox literary tradition. Śiva's traditional home is the cemetery ground, which makes it a natural place for his followers to perform rites. A truly transgressive act would be to chant the Vedas within the charnel grounds. The *Dharmasūtras* of Āpastamba, Gautama, Baudhāyana, and Vasiṣṭha all forbid Vedic recitation in cemeteries.[44] This again demonstrates that Śiva exists outside of Vedic orthodoxy. Not only do the Vedas not mention him but they cannot be recited in his dwelling place.

Cheating Death

The concept of conquering or cheating death appears in a wide variety of Sanskrit texts. It is unclear when exactly the idea became associated with the form of Śiva as Mṛtyujit, Mṛtyuñjaya, or Amṛteśa. Though a hymn called *mṛtyuñjaya* appears in the *Ṛg Veda*, Witzel notes that there is no word-for-word rendering (*padapātha*)[45] for the verse,[46] which indicates that it is a later addition to the text. Further, texts often refer to this hymn as *tryambaka* rather than *mṛtyuñjaya*.[47] The *Śiva Purāṇa* refers to it as the *mṛtyuñjaya* mantra in several places and attributes its composition to Śiva.[48] Rocher notes that the *Śiva Purāṇa* is more composite than many other *Purāṇas*, therefore making it difficult to date. Rocher dates some parts to as early as the ninth century and others to as late as the fourteenth.[49] This makes early parts of the text concurrent with the *Netra Tantra* and others contemporary with or later than Kṣemarāja's eleventh-century commentary. The *Padma Purāṇa*, parts of which date to the eighth to eleventh century,[50] tells the story of a brahman called Karuṇamuni who gathers by a river with other sages to make offerings. When Karuṇamuni sniffs a lime meant as an offering, another brahmin curses him and turns him into a fly for a hundred years. One of Karuṇamuni's brothers kills the fly and a passing goddess, Arundhatīdevī, sprinkles ashes on the dead body of the fly while reciting the *mṛtyuñjaya* mantra. The mantra brings the fly back to life.[51] Though this story does not involve Mṛtyujit as the deity, the goddess's use of the mantra demonstrates a similarity with Mṛtyujit as he appears in the *Netra Tantra*.

Einoo notes that texts as early as the *Atharva Veda* refer to death-conquering rituals.[52] Later texts, such as the *Garuda Purāṇa*, the *Netra Tantra*, and *Skanda Purāṇa* began to call Śiva Mṛtyuñjaya, Amṛteśa and related variations.[53] All three texts date to roughly the same time period. The *Skanda* is probably the oldest, with parts dating to the sixth century.[54] Dalal dates the *Garuḍa Purāṇa* to around the ninth to eleventh centuries.[55] Hazra and others claim the text dates to no earlier than the tenth or eleventh century.[56] Dating issues aside, it is clear that the association of Śiva with a deity called Mṛtyujit, etc., became common during the ninth century. While it is beyond the scope of this study to pinpoint exactly when Mṛtyujit and Śiva merged, it remains an important question. What matters most here is that the *Skanda* and *Garuḍa Purāṇas* use both the name Mṛtyuñjaya for the deity and the *mṛtyuñjaya* mantra.[57] There is no doubt that the *Garuḍa Purāṇa* refers to the same mantra found in the *Netra Tantra* as it gives the mantra in its entirety: *oṃkāraṃ pūrvam uddhṛtya juṃkāram tadanantaram | savisargaṃ tṛtīyaṃ syān mṛtyudāridryam ardanam*.[58] This demonstrates a familiarity with the mantra outside of the *Netra Tantra*.

The fourth- to tenth-century *Mārkaṇḍeya Purāṇa*[59] contains the most explicit story of how Śiva came to be known as Mṛtyuñjaya. A man named Mṛkaṇḍu performs penance to Śiva in order to please him and to obtain a son. Śiva gives Mṛkaṇḍu the choice between a wise, pious, and virtuous son who would live only sixteen years or a dull, evil son who would live a long life. Mṛkaṇḍu chooses the former. His wife gives birth to a son, Mārkaṇḍeya. Upon telling Mārkaṇḍeya that he will not live long, the boy becomes an ascetic who performs penance, wears clothes made of tree bark, and allows his hair to mat. On the day of his death, Mārkaṇḍeya is deep in meditation which creates a radiant heat that keeps Yama's servants from approaching him. Eventually, Yama himself comes for Mārkaṇḍeya. Seeing Yama, Mārkaṇḍeya embraces a statue of Śiva and Yama encircles both with his rope. Śiva angrily emerges from the statue, killing Yama and saving Mārkaṇḍeya's life. Mṛkaṇḍu praises Śiva, and calls him Mṛtyuñjaya and Kālakāla when Śiva gives Yama his life back and makes Mārkaṇḍeya sixteen years old forever.[60] The *Netra Tantra* does not use the name Kālakāla to describe its main deity but the name appears in the *Vāyu Purāṇa* as an epithet for Śiva when he drinks the poison (*kālanāla*) that emerges from the Ocean of Milk.[61] The *Mārkaṇḍeya Purāṇa* does not describe Mṛtyuñjaya in detail. The only text I am aware of other than the *Netra Tantra* dedicated mostly to Mṛtyujit is the *Mṛtyuñjaya Purāṇa*. The *Ekāmra Purāna*, which may date from as early as the fifteenth century,[62] mentions the *Mṛtyuñjaya Purāṇa* in its list of secondary Purāṇas (*upapurāṇas)*. Unfortunately, this is the only reference to the *Mṛtyuñjaya Purāṇa*, which has not survived.[63]

Worshipping Amṛteśa

The Śiva of the *Netra Tantra* bears several names: Bhairava, Amṛteśa, and Mṛtyujit or Mṛtyuñjaya.[64] One can worship him by these names or in the form of a host of medieval deities. The *Netra Tantra* devotes several chapters to descriptions of the many forms in which one can worship Amṛteśvara. These illustrations demonstrate that the *mantrin* can perform worship to any deity using the mantra *oṃ juṃ saḥ*. Sanderson argues that the Śaiva officiant is to worship Amṛteśa as whichever deity the calendrical occasion requires. This demonstrates what he calls the "universality of Amṛteśvara."[65] In other words, when the *mantrin* worships Indra, he actually worships Amṛteśa in the form of Indra (*indrarūpa*).[66] Further, Sanderson notes that though these calendrical requirements center on brahmanical worship, in the Kashmirian *Nīlamatapurāṇa*[67] such worship includes the days of Buddha's birth and attainment of *nirvāṇa*.[68] That worship of the Buddha falls within the brahmanical sphere demonstrates that the distinctions between what we now call Hinduism and Buddhism were more fluid than they are today. Certainly, at the time of the *Netra Tantra*, differences in philosophy and practice were known and acknowledged. Both Utpaladeva and Abhinavagupta actively defend their points of view against Buddhist ideas in dialogic treatises. Through these dialogues, Utpaladeva and Abhinavagupta acknowledge that their own system of thought has appropriated and been influenced by Buddhist philosophical concepts.[69]

The *Netra Tantra* does not go into great depth about how to perform such calendrical worship. It assumes that its *mantrin* is versed in such practice and so focuses on colorful descriptions of how one should visualize the deities. Most important, it emphasizes that these deities are different aspects of Amṛteśa.

> Now I shall explain the protection of the king (*rājarakṣā*) [with the mantra]. [The *mantrin*] should write the name [of the king] enveloped in the middle of the mantra. Above this, O Beautiful, he should worship Bhairava, Deva and Amṛteśa. The *devī*s and *dūti*s are joined with him at the end [of the mantra] on the petals. Thus, the servants [become] bound to the root mantra. Outside of the lotus, [the *mantrin*] should draw the very white moon maṇḍala (*śaśimaṇḍala*), and outside of that, a square endowed with the mark of a *vajra*. Thus, having written [all this] with saffron, bile, and white milk, he should worship in peace with an all white [offering]. In this way, he [gives] ediblc offerings and liquor to the appropriate, voracious form [of the deity]. He worships with a mixture of white sandalwood, dust-colored powdered camphor, seeds, grain, and sesame, [mixed together] with white sugar [that has been] combined with ghee and milk. All meditation done with effort and volition is the highest, etc. [and] causes one to thrive, etc. If, while [performing the agreed mediation], worshiping with Mṛtyujit [in mind, the king] obtains great peace [*mahāśānti*] instantly. (NT 10.39–45)[70]

At 21.72–73, the *Netra Tantra* reiterates that Śiva appears in the form of Amṛteśa, Mṛtyujit, and Bhairava. Amṛteśa produces a non-death (*amṛta*) of unparalleled strength, Mṛtyujit offers escape from death, and Bhairava creates the universe. The mantra associated with these different versions of the deity produces boundless glory, successful authority in governmental matters, release from *saṃsāra*, and union with Śiva.[71] That the mantra is associated specifically with governmental authority demonstrates the strong connection between religious and political power. The *mantrin* gains social currency by his ability to produce successful results in the public sphere. Though the popular credit for such success lies with the ruler and not the *mantrin*, the monarch on whose behalf the *mantrin* performs the rite will continue to employ him. Likewise, if his rites begin to fail and the ruler flounders in governmental matters, the *mantrin* may find himself replaced in the king's favor. By worshipping Amṛteśa in the form of other deities during their established festivals, the *mantrin* ensures the continued protection of the king and kingdom while adhering to mainstream brahmanical practice.

Deities in the *Netra Tantra*

In its first chapter, the *Netra Tantra* introduces Mṛtyujit (1.34–36) as the conqueror of death. It focuses on the outcomes of his worship rather than his physical description. Chapter 2 of the *Netra Tantra* charts the visual and aural elements of the *mṛtyuñjaya* mantra but does not anthropomorphize the deity. Only when the text begins to describe the daily ritual, which requires meditation on the deity, does the *Netra Tantra* begin to explain Mrtyujit's appearance. The order of the rites in Chapter 2 closely mirrors those in the *Svacchanda Tantra*'s second chapter. In the *Netra Tantra*, deity visualization occurs after the practitioner has performed the purificatory bath (*snāna*) and ritual oblations to the deities (*tarpaṇa*). After this, the *mantrin* enters the ritual space, burns up the impurities of the body, and replaces them with a divine body made of the three *tattvas*. This new body consists of the conceptualized mantra. The *mantrin* prepares for ritual offerings to the deity (*mūrti*) and his thoughts turn to meditation and yoga.[72]

After the creation of a Tantric space and body, and once the practitioner is about to present his offerings, the *Netra Tantra* introduces a meditation on Amṛteśa in his form as Mṛtyujit.

> And so now, having constructed the *amṛta mudrā*[73] or the *padma mudrā*,[74] [the *mantrin*] should meditate on the *ātman*. The deity is equal in splendor [to that] of ten million moons, as bright as pellucid pearls, and as magnificent as quartz stone. He resembles a drop of cow's milk, jasmine, or mountain snow, and is everywhere. One should think of him [dressed in] white clothes and ornaments, [draped in] a radiant garland of pearls, bulbs like moonlight, etc. His body is anointed with white sandalwood and dust-colored powdered camphor. In the middle of the *somamaṇḍala*, [he is] bathed in thick, abundant waves of nectar (*amṛta*) [that make the] moon quiver. [He is] one-faced, three-eyed, seated on a white lotus, fixed in the

> bound lotus seat (*baddhapadmāsana*). [He is] four-armed, large-eyed, the hand [fixed in the position] of granting wishes and safety, [holding] a full moon, radiant, filled with *amṛta*, holding a water pot, [and] completely full of the world, the moon in his lovely hand. [The *mantrin*] should remember him adorned with a reverence that is all white. (NT 3.17–23)[75]

This is the Mṛtyujit of the bronzes and stone statues mentioned earlier, whose right hands take the position of the wish-granting gesture and hold a water pot, while the single visible left hand cradles the full moon.[76] When the *Netra Tantra* returns to the iconography of Mṛtyujit in Chapter 18 it adds the image of the consort Amṛtalakṣmī, and says nothing more about Mrtyujit's appearance.[77]

> After [the *mantrin*] has meditated on the beautiful form as indicated earlier, he should worship Mṛtyujit and Śrī Devī [Amṛtalakṣmī], seated on his lap in the middle [of the *somamaṇḍala*. She is] as clear as pure crystal, she possesses the same luster as mountain snow or a drop of jasmine. [She] resembles the swelling moon [and] shines forth like cow's milk. [She is as] white as pearls, covered in white clothes, adorned and resplendent with jewels, white garlands of pearls, moonstone, etc. [Amṭralaksṃī is] beautifully adorned with white garlands, wreathes, *mālā*s, [and] lotuses. [She] laughs, has beautiful limbs [and] a bright white smile. She is charming [and] wears a pure white crown. [She has] one face, three eyes, [and is] seated in the *baddhapadmāsana*, adorned with a yoga strap (*yogapaṭṭa*), a conch and lotus in [her] hand, the hands [forming the gestures of] wish-granting and protection.[78] Four armed, Mahādevī is marked with all auspicious signs. (NT 18.63–68)[79]

Images of Mṛtyujit and Amṛtlakṣmī that correspond to those in the text appear in at least one of the royal baths in the Kathmandu Valley. This, along with the distribution of manuscripts of the *Netra Tantra* in Nepal, underline the impact of the text within the Himalayan region.

Neither Mṛtyujit nor Amṛtalakṣmī possess any of the frightful characteristics of Tantric deities such as Bhairava. Bhairava is defined by his fanged teeth and adornments of skulls and severed arms. Mṛtyujit and Amṛtalakṣmī are delicate, pure, and unmoving. The only movement found is their constant bath of nectar. The *Netra Tantra* describes an extension of Amṛtalakṣmī called Maheśanī, who has eight arms. Her four additional hands hold a bright gem that yields all desires (*cintāratna*), a water pot that is constantly full of *amṛta*, and the sun and moon. She stands on a white lotus that itself is above treasures. Auspicious elephants adorn her.[80] Those who worship this goddess in their homes receive as rewards life (*āyus*), power (*bala*), honor (*yaśa*), fame or glory (*kīrti*), wisdom (*medhā*), and beauty (*kānti*).[81] Such worldly desires would surely be appealing to a monarch hoping to maintain or legitimize his rule.

After the initial illustration of Mṛtyujit, the *Netra Tantra* spends Chapters 4 through 8 on initiation and yogic practice. It then returns to iconography in Chapters 9 through 13. What follows is a partial translation of these chapters that focuses on the main deity described therein. Most of the deities are accompanied by goddesses and other attendants, many of whom share their characteristics.[82]

Chapter 9 begins with Pārvatī enquiring about the universality of Amṛteśa. She asks how he is able to confer *siddhi*s on practitioners who follow other philosophical or textual traditions. This allows Śiva to explain that Amṛteśa himself is formless. When a disciple meditates on Amṛteśa he can do so using the image of any deity. Ultimately, the worship of all deities is the worship of Amṛteśa.

> Amṛteśa is supreme. He is free of disease. His nature is inherent, fully enumerated, constant, eternal, and immovable. [He has] no form or color, and is the highest truth. Because of that, he is omnipresent. The splendid Deva delights in all *āgama*s, pervades all mantras, and grants all *siddhi*s. In this way, he is like a transparent crystal sewn onto a colored thread, always reflected with its color, [and] seeking [to] look like this and that. Thus, in this way, Deveśa [is found in all] *āgama*s. He gives of all *sādhaka*s the benefits [of worship] from all directions [i.e., no matter what their tradition]. Because of him, splendid gems light up [differently] under different conditions, giving the fruits of all *āgama*s in all streams. Thus, he is Śiva, Sadāśiva, Bhairava, Tumburu, Soma, and Sūrya, with his own form arising bearing no form. (NT 9.5–11)[83]

Even Mṛtyuñjaya, described in the earlier passage, is only a specific form of the ultimate deity of the *Netra Tantra*, Amṛteśa. As this passage indicates, Amṛteśa takes the form of Śiva and Bhairava, themselves often characterized as omniscient, omnipresent, and omnipotent. As the *mantrin* visualizes these different deities, he is required to worship them according to the traditions of their followers. Not only does this allow for the *mantrin* to perform calendrical rites in accordance with tradition but it also allows for the worship of Amṛteśa to continue unabated. Sanderson notes that the attributes of Sadāśiva and Viṣṇu are unique to Kashmir, which demonstrates almost certainly that the text was written there.[84] This also helps to explain the addition of Buddha, who, at the time, was worshipped in Kashmiri orthodox brahminical circles.

Again, the *Netra Tantra* offers a *nirvacana* to explain the variety of names attributed to the deity.

> He is called Netra because he protects the restrained and bound. He who escapes death is called Mṛtyujit. Thus, he [who] grants immortality is called Amṛteśa. (NT 9.12b–13)[85]

The name Netra derives from √*nī*, the verbal root meaning "to protect"; Mṛtyujit stems from *mṛtyu*, with the verbal root √*mṛ*, "to die," combined with √*ji*, "to conquer"; and Amṛteśa from *amṛta*, again from the root √*mṛ* with the negative prefix *a*, meaning "non-death." This is combined with the word "god," *īśa*. Though all are the same deity, these names demonstrate the different aims for worship. Some seek relief from worldly ailments, others to overcome death, and still others seek liberation (*mokṣa*). One attains immortality or non-death (*amṛta*) through a variety of means, including living one's full life or living to the age of one hundred.[86] Further, one can have the rites of *amṛta* performed for one who is already dead. This demonstrates that the rite is not just for earthly immortality but also for enjoyments in subsequent lives and for liberation.

After the *nirvacana*, the text then describes Sadāśiva, on whose form the initiate (*sādhaka*) can choose to meditate. The illustration of Sadāśiva here is not extraordinary. The *Netra Tantra* instructs the initiate to meditate on the form of Sadāśiva, which it describes as made of Sadyojāta, Vāmadeva, Aghora, [Tat]Puruṣa, and Īśāna. These five *brahmamantras* also make up Sadāśiva's five faces. The *Tantrāloka* describes Sadāśiva as *pancamantratanu*: one whose body consists of the five mantras.[87] These mantras connect to five of the six *aṅgamantras*, namely, *hṛd*, *śiras*, *śikhā*, *kavaca*, and *astra*,[88] which we encountered in the discussion of *nyāsa* in chapter 3. Further, the mantras also correspond to elements and cardinal directions and activities (see Chart 1).

Chart 1: *Brahmamantras* and their correspondences

brahmamantra	direction	*aṅgamantra*	element	activity
Sadyojāta	west	*hṛd*	earth	emission
Vāmadeva	north	*ś + iras*	water	maintenance
Aghora	south	*śikhā*	fire	reabsorption
Tatpuruṣa	east	*kavaca*	wind	veiling
Īśāna	zenith	*astra*	ether	grace

Source: Modified from lists and illustrations found in Davis 2000: 48–51.

After this cursory description of Sadāśiva's body, the *Netra Tantra* then instructs the *mantrin* to utilize the mantra to perform his rites. In other words, the practitioner is to visualize Sadāśiva in order to worship the formless Amṛteśa. To do this, the *mantrin* must use the *mṛtyuñjaya* mantra. The text then describes the image of the deity.

> [He] resembles the swelling moon, a heap of mountain snow. Five-faced, large-eyed, ten-armed, [and] three-eyed, [he] has a serpent as a sacred thread. He is covered in a garment made of tiger skin. [He] sits in the bound lotus pose atop a white lotus, [holding] a trident, blue lotus, arrow, *rudrākṣa*, [and] a mallet. The highest is done in the right and heard in the left. [Sadāśiva has] a shield, a mirror, a bow, a citron tree, and a water jar. On his head is a half moon. [He who meditates on Sadāśiva] should perceive the Eastern face as yellow; the Southern a wrathful, terrible black [that has] an unnatural, tusked mouth. [The Southern Sadāśiva] bears a skull rosary and makes the world tremble. [Sadāśiva's] Western [face] resembles snowy jasmine and the North a beautiful red lotus. The face above the [other] Śiva [faces] resembles a crystal [i.e., colorless]. Thus, having meditated, [the *mantrin*] should worship Deveśa according to the rule [stated in the canon]. He should revere Īśāna, etc., and Sadyojāta, etc., in each's own form, on open, unoccupied ground, on a *liṅga*, in water, above a lotus, and in each's own direction. (NT 9.19ab–26)[89]

As Sanderson notes,[90] the objects Sadāśiva holds here are unique to the Kashmirian tradition, with a more typical collection being a trident, axe, sword, thunderbolt, and fire in the right hand, a snake, noose, bell, *mudrā* of protection.[91] Other deities described in the *Netra Tantra* also deviate somewhat from their more familiar forms. Even the related *Svacchanda Tantra* differs in its description of gods such as Bhairava, demonstrating the lack of continuity in early Tantric literature. Törzsök has mapped some of these iconographical shifts in which some deities gain extra heads or faces in order to concur with the mantric technicalities required for worship.[92] What remains consistent in the iconographic descriptions are the repeated characteristics that indicate a Śaiva affiliation for visualization. For example, many of the deities wear a *rudrākṣa*. This indicates their devotion to and being forms of Śiva. Others hold their hands in the *mudrās* of wish-granting and protection, as does Mṛtyuñjaya.

Following Sadāśiva, the *Netra Tantra* describes Bhairava and Bhairavī, a terrifying couple that the text reminds us should be kept secret. Though the text describes Sadāśiva before Bhairava, it gives much more attention to Amṛteśa as Bhairava. Like Amṛteśa and Sadāśiva, Bhairava appears in various colors. His frightening and screaming mouth is matched by his assortment of dangerous and deathly ornaments. Like many of the goddesses, Bhairavī has the same ornamentation and weaponry as her male counterpart. Due to this repetition I have often not translated descriptions of the goddess, though I do include Bhairavī here to demonstrate how the text presents female deities. Though I have not translated their descriptions in full, it is important to note the appearance of goddesses, *dūtī*s, and servants alongside and surrounding the deities. One must visualize these characters alongside the male deities as it is often these personalities who actually grant *siddhi*s to the practitioners. In the *Sāradatilaka Tantra*, Bhairavī appears not as a fierce deity, nor as a consort of Bhairava, but as a smiling goddess with a beautiful face who is the source of both speech and the universe. She holds a jar of nectar and is herself bathed in nectar.[93] In the *Netra Tantra*, Bhairavī holds the medicinal *śatavārī* (*Asparagus racemosus*), a plant grown in the Himalayan region and used in Āyurveda to delay aging, improve mental faculties, and help fight disease.[94] Worship of her, then, is preventative and suppresses that which brings about disease rather than simply curing an illness once it has manifested. Again, this makes worship of Amṛteśa, throughout the calendrical cycle, vital for the continued health and prosperity of the king and kingdom.

> Now, at this moment, I shall explain the distinct appearance of Bhairava, [who] resembles an ointment [that clears the eye]. He has a nature that burns up and dissolves all things. Five-faced, atop a corpse, ten-armed [and] terrible, he resembles troops with demon mouths. He rumbles,

> [producing] a terrible noise, speaks with a gaping mouth [adorned with] with large tusks, [his face] bent in a frown. He is mounted on a lion, wears a snake garland, and bears a *mālā* and begging bowl. [He has] a torn mouth from [which he emits] a great roar. [His body is] covered by a cloth of elephant skin, a flower crown, [and] the moon. [Bhairava] holds a skull-topped staff (*khaṭvāṅga*) and skull bowl. [He] bears a sword and shield, holds a hook and noose. [His] hand[s posed] in the wish-fulfilling and protection [*mudrā*s. He] holds the thunderbolt of a great hero. [He also] holds an axe and a hatchet. Having worshipped Bhairava, [the *mantrin*] remembers being joined in union [with] him, [in the same way as] dissolution in fire. (NT 10.1–7ab)[95]

This reference to dissolution in fire mirrors the moment in initiation (*dīkṣā*) in which the bound soul becomes purified. By calling attention to this moment, the *Netra Tantra* reminds its reader that worship of any deity can bring about this same state of purification.

Like Sadāśiva, Bhairava has five faces. However, these faces are not described in the same depth as those of Sadāśiva. This indicates that all of Bhairava's five faces are tusked and gaping. It is difficult to trace the emergence of Bhairava within the Tantric pantheon. Törzsök notes that deities bearing the name Bhairava and male deities accompanied by *yoginī*s, who she says are often called Rudras, appear in early Tantric Śaiva texts, such as the *Siddhayogeśvarīmata*, *Timirodghāṭana*,[96] and the *Niśvāsa*'s *Nayasūtra*.[97] The earliest of these texts, the *Nayasūtra* does not describe Sadāśiva but instead discusses the four-faced deity Īśvara. It describes the southern face of Īśvara as "like a dark cloud, with tawny brows, mustache and eyes, with a face terrible by its wrinkled brow, skull-bearing and adorned with snakes; one should visualize the southern face as Bhairava/many-formed (?*bahurūpam*), bearing matted locks."[98] Similarly, the passage earlier in this chapter that describes the *Netra Tantra*'s Bhairava describes him as bearing a dark southern face, called Aghora, who wears skulls. The similarities between Aghora and Bhairava have been pointed out by Hatley.[99] The *Netra Tantra*'s Bhairava does appear to expand upon the characteristics of Aghora in its description of Bhairava. Further, it gives the goddess who accompanies him the name Aghoreśī. After a brief description of Bhairavī/Aghoreśī, the *Netra Tantra* returns to its description of Bhairava.

> [Bhairavī][100] has the appearance of vermillion or *lac*. [She has] erect hair, a large body and is dreadful and very terrifying. [She has the medicinal

plant] *śatavārī*, is five-faced, and adorned with three eyes.[101] [Her hands bear] curved talons. [She has] eyes like the hollow of a tree and wears a garland of severed heads. [Ten-]armed, like Bhairava [she also] bears Bhairava's weapons [of an axe and hatchet]. [She is] called *icchā śakti* [and she] moves toward union with one's own will. Having celebrated this form, [the *mantrin*] thinks of her as Aghoreśī. In all Tantras [this] is taught and secret. It is not made clear. My abode is visible by anyone on earth, [but] difficult to obtain. One should always worship [in times of] peace and prosperity, to suppress sickness and vice, [which are] the root cause of wasting away, [and] for the protection of cows, brahmins, and men. One meditates on [Bhairava] as having equal radiance to snow, jasmine, the moon, or pearls. [He is] as clear as the curved moon and similar to immovable quartz. [He is] clear like the burning of the end of time, resembles a flower on the sacred tree,[102] and appears red like innumerable suns or, rather, red like a lotus. [He is] equal in radiance to yellow orpiment. The *sādhaka* remembers Deva, who has the form of *icchā*, with whatever beautiful [form of the deity the *sādhaka* chooses]. [Thus, the deva] gives [the *sādhaka*] the fruits of *icchāsiddhi*. Any one [of the deity's] forms bestows, any one [of his] beautiful [forms] grants *siddhis*. [The *sādhaka*] may meditate [on the deity] in the middle of a lotus. He should worship there with the corresponding offerings [for the form of the deity he has chosen to visualize], such as foods, flowers, perfume, and nectar.[103] (NT 10.7cd–17ab)[104]

The *Netra Tantra* does not give much in the way of a description of the goddess, but it is clear that she shares many of Bhairava's attributes. The *Netra Tantra* mentions her here because she is to be meditated on in conjunction with Bhairava. Kinsley notes that there appear to be no myths that explain the origin of Bhairavī.[105] He discusses several different descriptions of the goddess, one of which varies greatly from that found in the *Netra Tantra*. The *Śāradā Tilaka Tantra* describes Bhairavī as beautiful. She has a single, white face with three eyes, and holds a book, a rosary, and a jar of nectar.[106] This example is notable as it is unique among descriptions of Bhairavī and yet belongs to the literary tradition of medieval Kashmir, though certainly after the writing of the *Netra Tantra*.

As the *Netra Tantra*'s iconography continues, it describes Bhairava and Bhairavī as surrounded by four *devīs* and four *dūtis*. Here it gives attributes to the *devīs* who sit at the four cardinal directions. All have four arms and one face. Siddhā stands in the East. She is peaceful, all white, and rides an antelope. Raktā resembles Bhairava with her red body. She wears a garland of skulls, holds a head, stands upon a corpse, and wears an elephant skin around her shoulders, a tiger skin around her hips. Like Raktā and Bhairavī, Śuṣkā has a terrifying form. She is red, surrounded by a rope of nerves, and her hair stands erect. She wears a necklace of skulls, a tiger on her shoulders and a man's skin on her hips. She sits atop the demon Kumbhāra, who has the neck of a camel, the shoulders of an elephant, the ears of a horse, the face of a ram, snakes for legs, turtle claws, and a fish taịl. Finally, in the North sits Utpalahastā, dressed in blue, blue skin, and riding atop a lion. The *dūtī*s sit at the inter-cardinal directions, beginning in the Southeast. The text gives little description of the *dūti*s Kālī, Karālī, Mahākālī, and Bhadrakālī.[107] The grinning servants Krodhana, Vṛntaka, Karṣaṇa, and Gajāna merit even less attention.[108] Nevertheless, they are an important part of the meditation and this passage shows the detail of the visualization.

Again, the text reiterates that a practitioner may choose the form of the deity he wishes to worship. In making this choice, the *mantrin* must be sure to use the correct offerings for the chosen deity. Most important, worship is to take place regardless of circumstance. This is why it is so vital that the *mantrin* worship Amṛteśa in various forms. Amṛteśa provides the benefits of protection by preventing ills in addition to removing them once they have presented themselves.

Another form of Amṛteśa, Tumburu, dominates Chapter 11 of the *Netra Tantra*. Törzsök notes that earlier Tantric representations of Tumburu give him four heads, one facing in each of the cardinal directions.[109] This allows him to look at the goddesses and recalls a tale in the *Mahābhārata* in which a goddess circumambulates Śiva. So that he may see her uninterrupted, he creates three additional heads.[110] The *Netra Tantra* gives him a fifth head, saying that he must appear like Sadāśiva.[111] In many Tantric descriptions of Tumburu, he is called upon for his healing properties as well as his ability to bestow powers of seduction, destruction through sorcery, subjugation, and the eradication of enemy armies. He can also protect a person and his or her health and offers other semi-magical results.[112]

A Khmer inscription that dates to the reign of Khmer king Jayavarman II in the ninth century describes special rites of Tumburu.[113] In the Khmer inscription, four scriptures that increase the kingdom's prosperity issue from each of Tumburu's faces. It is unclear why the *Netra Tantra* insists on a correlation between Tumburu and Sadāśiva, but Tumburu's four lower heads may still face the *devī*s at the cardinal directions with the fifth atop these four.

The *devīs* appear in the colors that belong to *maṇḍala* worship: white, red, yellow, and black. These colors agree with the facial colors of Sadāśiva, again establishing the connection between the two deities and Tumburu's retinue.

> Now, at this moment, I will tell the most high teaching to be worshipped with this mantra, for the sake of peace from all calamities, resulting in the fruits of all *siddhis*. [He worships] Deva as Tumburu in the middle of an eight petaled lotus, in the *maṇḍala*, [starting] in the East, O Devī. [The *sādhaka*] honors the Lord who is ten-armed, five-faced, and three eyed, with the form and faces like Sadāśiva. He [has] a half-moon in his topknot, sits in the blue lotus *āsana*. [Tumburu is] white like a drop of frosty jasmine, similar to mountain snow. [He wears] a serpent as a sacred thread and is adorned with snake ornaments. [Tumburu is] adorned with all jewels, a tiger skin on the ground [below his] hips, a garment of elephant skin, mounted on a very strong bull, and wears a rhino hide. Adorning Deva is a white flower and a spade. [He] holds an elephant hook and noose. Deva holds a wheel and a rosary, hands [held in the] wish-granting and protective [*mudrās*]. *Devīs* and *dūtis* stand in all directions, beginning in the East, etc. Thus, the female servants are in their proper places at the entries [of the *maṇḍala*]. The *dūtis* are called Jambhanī, Mohanī, Subhagā, and Durbhagā. The servants are called Krodhana, Vṛntaka, Gajakarṇa, and Mahābala. He installs Gāyatrī and Sāvitrī to the left and the right. [The *sādhaka*] installs a hook above and immediately after, *māyā* below. All this is always to be joined with the root mantra. The *devīs* are white, red, yellow, and black, four-faced, four armed, three eyed, and in [their] hands bear golden hatchets, sticks and rosaries. Mounted on a corpse, Jayā *devī* shines forth [in white]. Four-armed, four-faced, three-eyed, red Vijayā holds grass, a bow, a shield and a sword, [while] standing upon an owl, O Devī. Ajitā [is yellow, like] the calyx of a lotus. Four-faced and four-armed, [she] bears a spear and a bell and rests on a flat hide. Seated on horseback, the Great Devī [Aparājitā] is adorned with many ornaments and resembles a broken sapphire [i.e., black]. [She is] adorned with four faces, four arms, three eyes, and holds a grass noose, a jewel, a bowl, and a mace. [She] stands firmly on a divine seat, clothed in gold clothes and gold ornaments. [When one] worships and meditates on [the *devīs*, as they] stand in the cardinal directions, [the *devīs* grant the practitioner] the fruits of *siddhi*. However, those who are *dūtis* bear a form adorned with one face, two arms, and three eyes. Adorning [them is] hair, shorn with scissors. They sit on a fish, a turtle, a *makara*,[114] and a frog.

> The servants are two-armed and hold a sword and a hide, [faces bent] in a crooked frown [on their] single faces, [which is adorned with] three eyes. [When] meditated on, [they] burst forth with white, etc., colors, giving the fruits of *siddhis*. Gāyatrī is a beautiful red color, adorned with one face, sitting in the bound lotus seat, the eye opened in meditation. Sāvitrī is the color white, eyes gone to inward meditation. The *devī* Māyā is dark and four armed. [One of her] pairs [of arms] holds a great cloth that conceals the world. (NT 11.1–24a)[115]

Within the *mantramārga* textual tradition, five streams of revelation emit from the mouths of Sadāśiva. From the upward facing, top head, Īśāna, comes the Siddhānta scriptures. The Vāma Tantras emerge from the North-facing, mild Vāma face. These texts focus on Tumburu and his sisters. The Dakṣiṇa Tantras focus on Bhairava and emerge from the Southern Aghora face. Finally, the Gāruḍa Tantras come from Tatpuruṣa's Eastern-facing mouth, and the Bhūta Tantras from Sadyojāta's face at the West.[116] Sanderson notes that the works of the Vāma Tantras made some impact in Kashmir but do not appear to have taken hold in the same manner as texts of the Dakṣiṇa Tantra stream.[117] Both the Vāma Tantras and Dakṣiṇa Tantras focus on goddesses, a characteristic that is reinforced in the earlier description of Tumburu. The Buddhist philosopher Dharmakīrti[118] commented critically about texts he refers to as the Ḍākinī Tantras and Bhaginī Tantras.[119] Dharmakīrti's commentator Karṇakogomin associates the Ḍākinī Tantras with the taking of life and identifies them, among others, as "Tantras of the Four Sisters." Sanderson identifies the sisters as Jayā, Vijayā, Ajitā/Jayantī, and Aparājitā.[120] These, of course, are the *devī*s described earlier in the chapter and associated with Tumburu. Further, Sanderson notes that in the *Netra Tantra*, Kṣemarāja refers to the Ḍākinī Tantras in reference to a method in which *yoginī*s kill their victims.[121]

Goudriaan has published the only known Vāma Tantra, based on a single extant Nepalese manuscript.[122] This text, the *Vīṇāśikha Tantra* focuses on magic and describes rituals to subjugate kings and queens.[123] Unusually for a text focused on *yoginī*s, the *Vīṇāśikha Tantra* does not include deity possession and indicates that such practice was not part of early goddess worship.[124] The *Vīṇāśikha Tantra*'s description of Tumburu differs from that of the *Netra Tantra*. As noted earlier, only in the *Netra Tantra* does Tumburu have five faces. In the *Vīṇāśikha Tantra*, Tumburu has only four faces and the goddesses who surround him have different attributes, though their colors and mounts are the same.[125] The *Vīṇāśikha Tantra* describes the worship of its goddesses as mantric recitation that stems from a square *maṇḍala* that contains all the letters of the alphabet.[126] The practitioner extracts the *bījas* from this *maṇḍala* and each *bīja* is associated with either the deity or one of the goddesses that surround him.[127]

The deity Māyā found in the *Vīṇāśikha Tantra* provides further evidence that the Vāma Tantras and Ḍākinī Tantras likely refer to the same set of texts. In the *Netra Tantra,* Māyā wields a large cloth that she uses to conceal the world. In the *Vīṇāśikha Tantra,* one gains power over another by locating the five *bījas* within the victim's heart. The *yogin* uses Māyā to cover the victim internally and externally to render him powerless.[128]

After the *Netra Tantra* describes Tumburu and his attendants in detail, it affords less attention to the remaining deities. Viṣṇu, in the form of Nārāyaṇa, appears twice: in his first form he sits atop a lotus and in the other he is mounted on Garuḍa. These variations appear consistent with the physical record, as the sculptural tradition of Nārāyaṇa in medieval Kashmir shows great variety.[129]

> Thus, [I have] spoken the *kaulika* rule of the *mantrarāṭ*. I again shall tell another method by which [the deity] grants fruits. He should always think of the four-armed Nārāyaṇa arising. [Nārāyaṇa has] two, long, lotus petal eyes, one face, has the appearance of a [blue] linseed flower, [and is] adorned with all [of his] instruments: a conch, discus, mace, and lotus. Deva bears divine garments [and] sits atop a divine flower [i.e., a lotus]. [He is] decorated with a gleaming crown of rubies, a small bell, and a net. [He] wears heavenly earrings. Or, he should meditate [on Nārāyaṇa] atop Garuḍa, Śrī at his side. [He should visualize Viṣṇu] very white and beautiful [with] three faces [that] resemble the moon, six arms, decorated like Varāha Hari, [his hands] endowed with [the shapes of] wish-granting and protection. Śrī is of the same color and holds the same weapons, suitably beautiful and charming before the eyes of Devadeva. [The *mantrin*] places *devīs* at the four cardinal directions and members (*aṅga*) at the intermediate compass-points. Thus, he worships [the *devīs*] Jayā, Lakṣmī, Kīrti, and Māyā at the cardinal directions, [where they] hold a noose and hook, hands [in the *mudrās* of] granting wishes and protection. He meditates [on them] before the eyes of the Deva, assuming the shape of [whichever] goddess is chosen. The members are similar to the Deva, [with] his color and hold [his same] weapons. (NT 13.1–9)[130]

The goddesses Jayā, Lakṣmī, Kīrti, and Māyā appear in the Pāñcarātra *Jayākhya Saṃhitā*,[131] though there they have no cosmological function.[132] Bhattacharyya notes "a perfectly Tāntric atmosphere permeates through the whole work."[133] By this, he means rites of anointment (*abhiṣeka*) and a focus on *mudrā* and *maṇḍala* appear throughout the text.

The text continues with its visualization of forms of Viṣṇu—first, in the form of a young boy and then in whichever of his avatars one chooses. Such flexibility allows the Śaiva to participate in Vaiṣṇava rites without imposing upon them a distinct Śaiva interpretation. Thus, the Śaiva practitioner co-opts brahmanical deities as manifestations of Amṛteśa. Meditation on the forms of Viṣṇu, or any deity, is then actually meditation on Bhairava and henceforth, on Amṛteśa.

> Or, [the *mantrin*] worships a very handsome, eight-armed, yellow Deva. He is naked, sits on a ram, and is unadorned. He rests on one horn [of a sheep and] offers up a pile of wheel spokes, the hand . . .[134] having the shape of a boy. [He is] constantly at play with a flock of beautiful, naked women. The goddesses Karpūrī, Candanī, Kastūrī, and Kuṅkumī stand at the cardinal directions, and have a similar form as the Deva. The *devīs* grant the fruits of the desired *siddhis*. What more should be said here? He remembers [Viṣṇu's] many forms. Thus, he thinks [of him] with a collection of many faces, many weapons and [many] arms [i.e., the cosmic Viṣṇu], reclining, taking a wife, joined with Lakṣmī,[135] alone, [as] Narasiṃha, Varāha, or Vāmana, Kapila, or an honorable man, unadorned, or even without parts. With whatever his nature, one should recall him with any state of being. It is said Bhairava is made up of him. Pārameśvarī is called order. [This then is the abode of Mṛtyujit.] (NT 13.10–16)[136]

Sanderson points out that this version of Viṣṇu, who rides a ram is likely an iconographic representation that is unique to Kashmir.[137] Kṣemarāja says it comes from the *Māyāvāmanasaṃhita*, a text that has not survived.[138] A thirteenth-century Kashmiri text composed by Rājānaka Jayadratha called the *Haracaritacintāmani* is the only other known appearance of the deity in this form.[139] The goddesses, whose names mean camphor, sandalwood, musk, and saffron, also do not appear as goddesses elsewhere.

The text next moves to a depiction of Sūrya, the sun deity. A ninth-century sculpture of Sūrya, housed in the Sri Pratap Singh Museum in Srinagar, depicts Sūrya seated atop a chariot with seven horses.[140] Ruins of an eighth-century sun temple in Kashmir, about fifty kilometers from Srinagar, remain understudied. Historical descriptions by early archaeologists fail to describe statuary in detail,[141] while modern studies show that those sculptures that do remain are worn down.[142] This means the *Netra Tantra* offers a unique illustration of Sūrya as imagined in medieval Kashmir. The size and location of this temple, which appears to have been in use until the fifteenth century, demonstrates its importance during the medieval period. Four of six temples that Kalhaṇa cites in the *Rājataraṅgiṇī*, described by Stein and others, appear to have been smaller than the Martand sun temple.[143] Of these other temples, all ascribed to the reign of Lalitāditya (c. 725–761/2),[144] three are Buddhist and three Vaiṣṇava.[145] Kalhaṇa praises Lalitāditya for building these and many other shrines, including those dedicated to Śiva and Jain saints.[146]

Unlike the previous deities, the *Netra Tantra*'s description of Sūrya does not report a retinue of goddesses. Instead, the eight planets, Nakṣatras, and Lokapālas[147] surround Sūrya, each on its own lotus. The Nakṣastras vary in number.[148] They are either heavenly bodies, stars, constellations, or lunar mansions through which the moon moves.[149] The Lokapālas are associated with the consecration of temples,[150] the installation of deities, and consecration rites.[151] They appear again in the *Netra Tantra*'s nineteenth chapter, where they offer protection to the sleeping king.

> Now, I explain that which consists of light [i.e., Sūrya]. He manifests the *siddhi* of man. [Sūrya] resembles a red flower, and is equal in splendor to red juice. [He is] the color of a heap of vermillion, as beautiful as a ruby, appears as the color of safflower. [He] looks like the flower of a pomegranate [and] resembles Soma at the end of time. [Sūrya has] one face, three eyes, four arms, possesses a noble nature, and [holds his] hands in the shape of the wish-granting and protection [*mudrās*]. [The *mantrin*] should imagine [Sūrya] with one hand [holding] a *vajra* [and] one a bridle. [He is] mounted on a chariot [on which are yoked] seven horses. [He] wears a serpent as a sacred thread, a garland of red flowers [and is] anointed with red perfume. Or [the *mantrin* should visualize him with] eight arms, bearing the weapons of the Lokapālas. [Here Sūrya is endowed with] three terrible faces, [each with] three eyes, [and he is] disfigured. One should worship him [visualized as] mounted on a horse in the middle of a lotus. [The worshipper]

> honors [his] heart, head, and topknot, enveloped with the weapon of sight. [The *mantrin*] is to worship Deva [in a lotus] the eight planets in the middle of a second lotus, the Nakṣatras in a third, and the Lokapālas in a fourth. [The *mantrin*] worships the eight weapons [of the Lokapālas which] stand in a fifth lotus. (NT 13.17–25ab)[152]

This image differs greatly from an eighth-century brass Kashmiri figure of Sūrya currently housed at the Cleveland Museum of Art.[153] This figure has one head, two arms, and holds lotus flowers in both hands. He has two eyes and an inlaid sacred mark between his eyebrows that has been lost, his face is adorned with a mustache, and he wears a crown decorated with flowers. Most strikingly different from the Sūrya described in the *Netra Tantra* is that the bronze figure stands rather than sits mounted on a chariot or horse. Lee notes that the long, belted robe and boots is similar in style to those worn by Buddha statues from Afghanistan. The boots of the Cleveland image are identical in style to those found on a seventh-century marble statue of Sūrya in the National Museum of Afghanistan.[154] Like the description in the *Netra Tantra*, the Kabul Sūrya rides a chariot, though he has only four attendants.[155] The Kabul Sūrya is also notable for its European style of sitting.[156] A tenth- or eleventh-century Nepali relief found near Pātan also depicts Sūrya in this European sitting position. Shimkhada notes this figure shares other attributes with the Afghanistan Sūrya and may be based on Kushāṇa dynasty royal statues.[157]

Unlike the Kashmir and Kabul Sūryas, the Nepal relief finds its Sūrya surrounded by eight figures, likely the planets.[158] The *Netra Tantra*'s Sūrya remains unique. This is the only example of Sūrya I have been able to locate whose hands form *mudrā*s and hold a *vajra* and bridle. Several of the attributes of the *Netra Tantra*'s Sūrya echo those of Mṛtyujit, namely, the wish-granting and protective *mudrā*s and the sacred thread made of a serpent. Through worship of Mṛtyujit as Sūrya, the *mantrin* uses the *Netra Tantra*'s mantra to honor the entire astronomical world.

The *Netra Tantra* then describes Viśvakarman, who gave form to the universe. Though the *Purāṇa*s include many stories about Viśvakarman, he plays almost no role in Śaiva Tantric ritual. His inclusion here simply acknowledges his existence and role as divine architect. The *Netra Tantra* says very little about his appearance. This allows the practitioner to pay him homage through whatever means he feels necessary. Viśvakarman's body exists solely as a focal point for visualization.

> Furthermore, [I shall describe] Viśvakarman, the Lord of the world. [He] is bright as a ray of light, risen alone [i.e., from itself]. [Viśvakarman] has [either] two or four ams. [When he has four hands he] bears a stone cutter's chisel and a book with [his] beautiful right hand. [In the left he holds] a clamp and a cord. [The *mantrin*] must honor [him] by praising Devas, Siddhas, and Gandharvas. [The *mantrin* can choose to] worship [him] in a heap of [ritual] fire, or in water, or at mountains. In whatever place he thinks [of Viśvakarman], [the deity] grants the fruits of desire. (NT 13.25cd–28)[159]

Finally, the *Netra Tantra* describes Rudra, Brahmā, and Buddha. Here Umā accompanies Rudra, Brahmā rides his goose Haṃsa, and the Buddha, fixed in meditation, offers his protection, especially to women. In several places, the *Rājataraṅgiṇī* points out that royal women constructed many Buddhist temples, *stūpa*s, and monasteries.[160] Such royal patronage of Buddhism appears to have peaked during the reign of Lalitāditya.[161] By the mid-ninth century, royal patronage appears to have come to an end. If Sanderson's dating of the *Netra Tantra* is correct, the practice would have nearly disappeared by the time of its composition.

> Assuming the form of Rudra, [Amṛteśa holds] a dazzling white conch shell bowl. [Rudra has the] form of Sadāśiva [and the *mantrin*] visualizes [him] with four arms, mounted on a man. [Rudra] has noble nature [and holds] a spike for safety. Carrying a citrus tree, mighty Deva [also] has a rosary. Now, [the *mantrin*] should think [so that] Deva appears, his many arms posed in a dance [position]. [The *mantrin* meditates on Rudra] who holds Umā at [his] side. Or [the mantrin visualizes Rudra] as half of Viṣṇu. [Or finally, the *mantrin* visualizes Rudra as] taking a bride. [The *mantrin*] worships him nearby.
>
> The auspicious Brahmā [has] four faces, four arms, beautiful eyes, and a red complexion. [He holds] a bundle of very sharp grass [that] hangs down [from his hands]. [Brahmā is] mounted on Haṃsa, holds a stick and *rudrākṣa*, carries a water jar for protection, [and] the four Vedas. [He] gives the fruits of all *siddhi*s.
>
> The Buddha, the great yogi, sits on a lotus, [head] bent, listening, and wearing mendicant's rags. [He possesses] beautiful lotus eyes, has a lotus[-shaped] mark, and is fixed with a jewel. [He is] established in the world, positioned in *samādhi*, his hands [making the] wish-granting and protection

> [*mudrās*]. Deva holds a *rudrākṣa* and a lotus. Thus, [the *mantrin*] should worship and meditate upon Buddha, [who] grants the fruits of *mokṣa* to women. (NT 13.29–36)[162]

After it provides this detailed iconography of the different deities, the text lists various deities and schools of thought. To worship according to each school's particular rules with the *mṛtyuñjaya* mantra allows the practitioner to obtain the benefits of the ritual. This takes place because Amṛteśa is present in all physical forms and also in all philosophical systems.[163] This allows the king's officiant to worship Amṛteśa during all calendrical festivals. The *mantrin* honors the deity of each particular festival and simultaneously performs rites in honor of Amṛteśa that ultimately protect and prolong the life of the monarch.

The descriptions of deities in the *Netra Tantra* can be read as genuine embodiments of the *mṛtyuñjaya* mantra itself. Each iconography depicts a different god but in fact each is a reflection of the colored thread, which shines forth through the crystalline nature of Amṛteśa. The more iconographies the text offers, the more it proves to its practitioner that the nature of the divine is in fact formless. It also allows for the continued protection of the king throughout the year, as all worship becomes worship of Mṛtyujit.

4
Identity and Purity

Creating the Tantric Identity

The practices and objects deployed in non-dual Śaiva Tantric ritual have roots in orthodox Vedic rites. Ritual objects such as butter, milk, sesame seeds, etc., feature in both. Animal sacrifice, which fell out of favor in Brahmanic Hinduism, appears in Śākta and Tantric practice; in fact, before that it survived at the margins of medieval[1] India for centuries.[2]

Most scholars believe that the origins of Tantra stem from Vedic or folk/tribal practices.[3] Wedmeyer follows Woodroffe[4] in arguing that Tantra had its roots in orthodox Brahmanical practice. Wedemeyer rejects the view that links Tantra to tribal or lower caste foundations: "What very little evidence we have for the direction of transmission of Tantric culture suggests unmistakably that the tribal or marginal communities were in fact *targets* of Tantric transmission, not the source."[5] Following Sanderson,[6] he believes that Buddhist monks initiated untouchable communities.[7] Urban argues, following Davidson,[8] that Tantric development drew on interaction and mutual transmission between Vedic and non-Hindu traditions and practitioners.[9]

I am inclined to agree with Urban and Davidson. The links between these communities were probably complex, and in the transmission of ideas and practices, they were probably bi-directional. This is clearly the case for Tantric Buddhist and Śaiva practices, which were in constant conversation.[10] Wedemeyer argues that the literature in which transgressive practices are described required institutional support for composition, transmission, and preservation.[11] This, no doubt, is true.[12] Yet it must be considered that social communities also support a variety of religious institutions and sects. Furthermore, not all religious practitioners stem from the upper classes or castes.[13] Sanderson points out that Śaivism, in particular, and Tantra, in general, were not completely dependent on royal patronage. Their popularity remained steady through dynastic changes. In short, institutional support came from various structures across all levels of society.[14]

Illness and Immortality. Patricia Sauthoff, Oxford University Press. © Oxford University Press 2022.
DOI: 10.1093/oso/9780197553268.003.0005

The *Svacchanda Tantra* allows for the initiation of members of many castes. An initiate sheds his social caste to become a member of the caste of Śiva. This new identity eclipses the caste status of the non-Tantric society. While this could, in theory, indicate the erasure of hierarchy within a society, these new Śaiva identities create new hierarchical categories. The first replaces caste distinction with initiatory status. The second involves power exchanges between Tantric and non-Tantric practitioners. The Tantric simultaneously maintains multiple identities. His status as a Tantric would normally be concealed from the non-Tantric; therefore, he is in sole possession of knowledge that shapes interactions with non-Tantrics. Secrets are the property of those who know them. This allows the bearers of secrets to control the exchange of secrets within ritual. It also empowers them to compose their own histories by controlling access to information about themselves.[15] The difference between Tantric and non-Tantric practitioners is more pronounced than these categories suggest.[16] Simmel postulates that secret societies institute a system of graduated secrecy.[17] Within this community, a practitioner receives more knowledge over time. This, in turn, imbues the practitioner with increasing levels of insider knowledge. The greater the knowledge a practitioner holds, the farther removed he is from the outsider.[18] However, this view requires a concept of progress that does not exist within the Tantric perspective. During calendrical rites that use the *mṛtyuñjaya* mantra, the *mantrin* worships the deity appropriate for the seasonal festival. He does so with the mantra that honors Amṛteśa. Thus, he appears to conform to orthodox practice but is, in fact, engaged in a Tantric sphere of worship. While one might expect that this practitioner has gained more knowledge through practice, the final outcome of initiation is liberation, regardless of initiatory status. What differs for initiates is the final reality (*tattva*) in which a practitioner rests after initiation. This is determined by the level of initiation received. For the Tantric practitioner, the continued practice of daily rites keeps him in the good graces of the deity. He need not learn the entire metaphysics of Tantra in order to achieve salvation.

Where Simmel's point applies is in his argument that secrecy affects individual interaction.[19] The person with the secret—here the Tantric initiate—is at a social and spiritual advantage. This is because he is aware of his Tantric affiliation and conceals that information from the non-initiate. This advantage changes if the non-Tantric becomes aware that there is a secret. Awareness of secrecy impacts the exchange. Gibson calls this "leakage."[20] In the case of leakage, one or both parties may be aware of the status of the other.

For example, a Tantric initiate may be aware that he is interacting with another initiate who does not know about the status of the first mentioned initiate. How each individual responds depends upon the ways in which that knowledge colors their interaction. It is also contingent upon whether the parties wish to retain their secrets. In the *Rājataraṅgiṇī*, Kalhaṇa is aware of, or at least believes himself to be aware of, the Tantric allegiances of others. However, he does not directly reveal those religious affiliations. Instead, he implies the Tantric initiatory status of various individuals.[21] For example, he attributes the ability to transmute metals into gold by means of magic to a King Jalauka in order to associate him with Tantric practice.[22] In making these implications, Kalhaṇa contributes to the leakage of secrecy. For readers savvy enough to understand his implications, Tantric practices appear throughout the text. For those who are unaware of Tantric attributes, Kalhaṇa preserves the secret and does not openly disclose anyone's initiatory status.[23]

The relationship between Tantric practitioners, transgressive practice, and the monarchy is problematic for Kalhaṇa. As Törzsök demonstrates, Kalhaṇa disapproved of monarchs' involvement in transgressive Tantric rites.[24] However, Kalhaṇa does not object to a king's use of mantras to obtain supernatural powers or to indirectly come into contact during ritual with an impure practitioner.[25] Kalhaṇa hints that the Kashmiri king Harṣa's[26] downfall is due to his participation in transgressive behaviors.[27] However, Kalhaṇa does not directly place blame on the king or openly expose him as a Tantric initiate.[28] Instead, Kalhaṇa attributes the king's downfall to those around him. Historically, scholars have linked Harṣa's behavior to extravagance and insanity rather than Tantric affiliation.[29] Kalhaṇa also indicates the Tantric affiliation of another king, Kalaśa (ruled 1063–1089 CE), more directly. Kalhaṇa focuses on Kalaśa's disregard for caste rules and predisposition for sensual pleasures and overindulgence.[30] Kalhaṇa indicates that these behaviors caused the king's downfall and attributes his Tantric involvement to his bad character.[31] For non-Tantrics, such as Kalhaṇa, a king's affiliation with transgressive Tantric practice diminishes his power. He often blames exposure to Tantric teachers as the cause of royal misfortune, disease, and death.

However, the *Rājataraṅgiṇī* reveals that Tantra and even transgressive Tantric practices were publicly tolerated at the Kashmiri court. Kalhaṇa's allusions to Tantric practice indicates that both he and his readers would have had enough knowledge about such practices to decipher his indications.

Törzsök has painstakingly documented some fifty examples from the *Rājataraṅgiṇī* that suggest transgressive Tantric practices.[32] This partial openness extends well beyond Kashmir. Sanderson has charted the spread of non-dual Śaiva Tantra throughout North India, the Himalayan regions, and beyond.[33] He notes three factors in the successful spread of Śaiva practice and philosophy: community support of initiates by the uninitiated, the cultivation of practices that accommodated brahmanical religion while claiming to transcend it, and alliances between Śaiva practice and kingship to assure royal patronage.[34]

Caste: Initiation and Purity

The *Rājataraṅgiṇī* describes caste distinctions as an ordinary part of Kashmiri society.[35] In some regions of India, caste differences could lead to varying punishments for one and the same crime. This does not appear to have been the case in medieval Kashmir. This does not mean that caste was not an important part of Kashmiri society. The account of Harṣa's interaction with low caste women places purity as central to inter-caste sexual activity. The *Rājataraṅgiṇī* also focuses on lesser types of physical contact, such as the ingestion of food prepared by a member of a lower caste.[36] Such contact again leads to physical pollution. For Kalhaṇa then, religious practitioners must make clear distinctions between what is pure and what is impure. This agrees with the Siddhānta view in which one distinguishes between pure and impure substances and rejects the latter. This dualistic (*dvaitācāra*) perspective of purity differs from the non-dual (*advaitācārā*), in which practitioners mix pure and impure substances. The latter approach appears in Bhairava Tantras, such as the *Netra Tantra*, despite the text itself teaching a dualistic epistemology.[37] The relationship between purity and impurity, from the *dvaitācāra* perspective, results in the belief that the pure is antithetical to the impure.

Marglin's study of purity demonstrates that the opposition between pure and impure is asymmetric. For the pure to remain so, the impure must be kept separate. However, the impure benefits from commingling with the pure.[38] This adheres more to the *advaitācārā* perspective. Take, for example, milk and blood. If the pure substance (milk) becomes mixed with the impure (blood), the milk is no longer pure. However, if the impure substance (blood) becomes mixed with the pure substance (milk), the blood becomes diluted and less impure. This creates a hierarchical structure in which the pure becomes impure only through contact with the impure. Something that starts out impure corrupts as it comes into contact with that which is pure. For example, a high caste person may give food to someone of a lower caste. In this case the food does not purify nor does it pollute. However, when the inverse occurs and a low caste person gives food to a higher caste person, the food causes impurity.[39] The relationship between what is pure and what is impure depends on the initial status of the individual person or substance. The lower caste decreases its impurity and the higher becomes impure.[40] This means there is no longer a pure-impure binary in which only one or the other exists. Nor is there a state in which both exist simultaneously. Instead, what remains is a relational system in which levels of purity and impurity fluctuate in response to interaction with other levels of purity.[41]

The *Svacchanda Tantra* creates a new, relational category. Through initiation, practitioners abandon their caste distinction to become members of the caste of Śiva, i.e., Śaiva initiates. Members of all castes make up the Śaiva initiatory class. The new designation as a member of Śiva's caste supersedes the devotee's original caste. This new classification does not adhere to a pure-impure categorization. Instead the new caste is auspicious and eternal. Here, caste distinction only exists prior to initiation, as those rites purify and simultaneously remove caste identity.[42] After initiation, the *Svacchanda Tantra* allows only for differences in initiatory status:

> O fair-faced one, all those who have been initiated by this ritual are of equal nature, whether they be brahmins, Kṣatriyas, Vaiśyas, Śūdras, or others [of lower castes]. [For] they have been brought into a state of fusion with the nature of Śiva. All are said to be [Śivas,] wearers of [his] braids, their bodies dusted [like his] with ash. All Samayins should sit in a single row. Putrakas, Sādhakas, and Cumbakas [Ācāryas] should do the same. They may not sit according to the divisions of their former castes. [For] they are said to form but a single caste of Bhairava, auspicious and eternal. Once a person has taken up this Tantric system he may never mention his former caste. If any [initiate] mentions the former caste of any Putraka, Sādhaka, or Samayin he will have sinned and will be roasted in hell for three days of the life of Rudra, five of the life of Viṣṇu, and fifteen of the life of Brahmā. So, if he aspires to the highest Siddhi he must make no [such] discriminatory distinctions. O Empress of the Gods, it is [only] through [this] freedom

from discimination [*sic*] that one will certainly attain both Siddhi and liberation. (SvT 4.539c–545)[43]

The text mandates punishments for making reference to the previous caste of another, but this does not extend to the world outside of ritual where one expects regular caste-conformity.[44] Because membership in a Tantric circle is secret and not the societal norm, there is no evidence for exemptions to caste-based punishments for Tantrics.

Within Tantric practice itself we that find initiates of different ranks are sometimes subject to different rules and applications. For example, the *Svacchanda Tantra* prohibits the use of human bone rosaries (*mahāśaṅkhākṣasūtra*) by householders. Using such an object can cause agitation or anxiety (*udvega*).[45] What is pure for one is not necessarily so for another. Though the *Netra Tantra* describes all practitioners as members of the same spiritual caste, i.e., Śiva's caste, there are still divisions between practitioners of different initiatory levels. In spite of these divisions, the elimination of caste distinction by initiation subverts the social order and reinterprets and claims dominion over power. Rebellion against social distinction renders previous divisions less important than the new identities the *mantrin* confers through initiation. This process leads to a re-categorization of pure and impure. The lower castes become purer and the higher castes transcend their previous, purity-dependent, identities.[46] Such differentiation allows the social hierarchy to survive without contradicting the internal and segmented erasure of caste distinction.

Again, the *Rājataraṅgiṇī* explains why practices that transgress caste boundaries must remain secret. Kalhaṇa describes an incident in which King Yaśaskara (ruled 939–948 CE) punishes the brahmin ascetic, Cakrabhānu, for breaching the socially expected conduct of a member of his caste.[47] The king brands Cakrabhānu's forehead with a dog's foot. Cakrabhānu's uncle, a royal minister, performs a retaliatory rite against the king. This results in the death of the monarch seven days later.[48] Sanderson points out that Cakrabhānu's transgression occurred during a *cakramelaka*, a Kaula ritual that involves low caste *yoginī*s and male initiates.[49] Cakrabānu thus acted in accordance with his initiatory status, which supersedes that of his social rank. Further, though the king traditionally holds the highest place in the social order, the royal minister overrules the monarch and performs rites that implore the deities to remove the unjust king. The Cakrabānu episode demonstrates how the dangers of transgressive practice transcend ritual boundaries. These practices threaten participants in their ordinary lives if others discover their occurrence. In spite of this, Kalhaṇa demonstrates that many high-ranking members of the Kashmiri court engaged in such practice.[50] Marglin is thus correct when she says that the category of Śiva's caste offers purity to the lower castes but outside of the ritual space risks impurity for the higher castes.[51] Thus, public displays of Tantric rites, such as the *nīrājana*, cannot include heterodox elements. Only those rites that take place in secret can include the impure.

Purity and Interpretation: Auspicious and Inauspicious Dreams in the *Svacchanda Tantra*

Purity and impurity also play an active role in dream life. Brahmins have long been interpreters of the dreams of kings.[52] They look to dreams to uncover individualized symbols and desires and use predetermined cultural markers to assess dreams as auspicious (*śubha*) or inauspicious (*aśubha*).[53] Once categorized, rites can be performed to counter the negative effects of inauspicious dreams.

One such instance of dream interpretation occurs the night prior to initiation. The *mantrin* creates a sanctified space in which the initiand sleeps on a pile of *kuśa* grass. Upon waking on the day of initiation, the *mantrin* interprets the initand's dreams.[54]Before interpreting dreams, the *mantrin* undergoes purification rites. In order to bring another person into the secret Tantric fold, he himself must already be pure and unified with the divine. The student too becomes purified during the night as he witnesses the *mantrin*'s performance of rituals prior to sleep.[55] The *Svacchanda Tantra* tells us how the judgement of dreams begins:

> In the bright morning, at daybreak, after purification, etc., one by one as [explained in the previous chapter, the *ācārya*] should enter the house. The pupil, who has sipped pure water, holds a flower in his hand. After bowing to the guru, delighted, he should tell his dreams to the guru. (SvT 4.1–2)[56]

As with most Śaiva texts, the *Svacchanda Tantra* is a dialogue between Śiva and his consort. After it describes the actions of the student and *mantrin*, Śiva lists for Pārvatī the auspicious and then inauspicious symbols that appear in dreams. In both categories, symbols appear that are organized into thematic groups, such as colors or animals, or similar actions, or those that involve war.

> In [auspicious] dreams [the dreamer] drinks wine, eats raw flesh, smears insect feces and sprinkles blood. He eats food of sour milk and smears a white garment. [He holds] a white umbrella over his head, decorates [himself] with a white garland or ribbon. [He sees] a throne, chariot or vehicle, the flag of royal initiation. He decorates [these things] with a coral or betel leaf fruit. [He also] sees Śrī or Sarasvatī. (SvT 4.3–6)[57]

The auspicious symbols begin with red and white objects and items associated with state power. The red symbols of drinking wine and eating raw flesh immediately call to mind Tantric activity, as Śaiva practice sometimes contains the use of both wine and flesh. Fecal matter and blood are usually associated with filth and impurity. Here they are auspicious and indicate that the dreamer's initiation will be successful. This also forces an inversion of the dreamer's typical understanding of symbols. It reverses the usual associations and focuses on different rules and attitudes toward purity. White food, a garment, an umbrella, and a garland are juxtaposed with the red symbols. Sour milk, which would not be used in ritual, demonstrates that the dreamer is ready to cross into a state of purity and worship that transposes the ordinary. However, one cannot always assume such subversion. The text tells us that "[the disciple] achieves success after speaking in dreams with princes, *ṛsis*, gods, *siddhas*, *vidyāharas*, *gaṇas*, and teachers."[58] Unlike the objects that are typically categorized as impure, the hierarchy of society appears unchanged. The same people are powerful and auspicious in both realms.

As the *Svacchanda Tantra* continues with its list of auspicious dreams, it names typical symbols of good luck in the profane world. Among the auspicious symbols are celestial beings, places of power, animals, objects of worship, and medicines.

> [The dreamer] crosses over the ocean and river. Likewise, sunrise and indeed blazing fire [are auspicious. Also auspicious is when the dreamer] sees planets, constellations, stars and the disk of the moon. [When the dreamer] ascends the palace or a turret of the palace, climbs a mountain top, tree, elephant, young animal, bull, horse, or man. [In auspicious dreams, one] sees a chariot and also sees the *siddha* mantra,[59] obtains the perfected oblation and sees the gods, etc. [It is auspicious when one dreams of] a pill,

> wood for cleaning the teeth, yellow pigment on a sword or sandal, sacred thread, ointment, nectar, mercury, medicinal herbs, *śakti*, a water jar, lotus, rosary, red arsenic, or blazing objects of *siddha*s, which have red chalk as their ends. (SvT 4.8–13)[60]

The text then moves to the auspicious symbols of battle and worship. The *Svachanda Tantra* describes the disciple as a hero when he enters the charnel ground to perform his ritual duties.[61] The association with the charnel grounds demonstrates the connection of the Śaiva cults to the earlier *kāpālika* Śaiva ascetics.[62] Both the *kāpālika*s and later Tantric Śaivas, as well as Tantric Buddhist sects, use the charnel ground for practice in order to generate a transgressive atmosphere and guarantee privacy.[63] Cemetery grounds are not places into which the uninvited are likely to wander. Their danger and impurity are exactly what makes cremation grounds appealing and safe for transgressive practice.[64] Such locations entice practitioners with the confidence to overcome their fears. However, spiritual confidence does not necessarily mean the purview of initiated and high-level practitioners. Sanderson points out that "such is the power attributed to this contact with impurity that it is believed that it may take the place of the conventional process of initiation (*dīkṣā*) into the Kaula cult."[65] In other words, the uninitated practitioner with the confidence to enter the charnel ground for worship becomes initiated. This does not mean that all charnel ground practices took place within the physical space of an actual ground. Such rites appear in both symbolic manifestations, where they also work as a metaphor for internalized, mental visualizations, and as a very real setting for spiritual pursuits. The tenth-century writer Rājānaka Rāma[66] describes an internal practice in which he himself is the charnel ground, saying,

> Show [your Bhairava form] to me, who is a hero (*vīra*) moving in this [dark] night of existence (*bhavaniśā*), in a body that is nothing but a cremation ground replete with abundance of flesh, blood, serum, and bones.[67]

This passage demonstrates the trope of the hero, night, the body, and the charnel ground as a part of a coherent Tantric symbolism. Once the symbolic lexicon has been built, the practitioner then continues to view the whole world as a charnel ground "made frightful in virtue of the fact that whatever has come into being is subject to destruction."[68] Once in the charnel ground, the practitioner can then engage in transgressive practice with the female *yoginī*. The relationship between *yoginī* worship and charnel grounds is well established[69] Even though not a Kaula or Śākta text, the *Svacchanda Tantra* makes no secret of its own connection to the charnel grounds. Tantric texts such as the *Netra Tantra* use militaristic and battle motifs, especially in the *nīrājana* rite as described below. This martial aesthetic, alongside the imagery of the disciple as hero, demonstrates a clear metaphor between battle readiness and initiation. In dreams both are taken as auspicious symbols.

> After [the dreamer] has seen these [images listed in earlier paragraphs], he is successful. Likewise, [success comes to those who] obtain the Earth and a [battle] wound. Victory in battle and crossing the battle field, which is an ocean of blood and blazes like a place of the departed [are auspicious]. [Someone who] commands heroes and persons who rule [with] victory [are fortunate signs]. [A dreamer] sells costly meat and partitions the sacrificial victim for the gods out of respect. [The fortunate dreamer] worships the god with his own self and also recites mantras, meditates, and praises. Then he observes before his own eyes a beautiful honored blazing fire [i.e., he is prepared to take part in ritual]. (SvT 4.13–16)[70]

In this passage, costly meat is a euphemism for human flesh. The *Harṣa Carita* describes the penances undertaken by the populace to avert the death of King Pabhakaravatdhana. Young nobles burned their flesh with lamps to appease mother goddesses (*mātṛkā*), a Dravidian[71] offered a skull to solicit a vampire (*vetāla*), and servants held melting guggula on their heads to pacify Mahākāla. The king's relatives cut their skin to offer it as an oblation, and royal attendants openly sold human flesh.[72] The *Kathāsaritsāgara* mentions both the sale of human flesh in the cremation grounds[73] and flocks of *yoginīs* who meet in cremation grounds to kill and devour humans.[74] The seventh-century *Siddhayogeśvarīmata* says, "After accepting human flesh from the hand of a hero (i.e., a *sādhaka*), the hero is given the boon he desires."[75] While the imagery of war and human flesh trade may seem especially graphic to modern sensibilities, the above are just a few references from the literary tradition. This demonstrates that the imagery would not be out of the ordinary for the initiand.

The text then reveals its final auspicious sign. "After [the dreamer] sees Bhairava and Bhairavī, he accomplishes, there is no doubt."[76] It remains unclear from the text how many of these auspicious motifs the student must see in order for the initiation to take place. The text also does not indicate whether the *mantrin* prompts the initiand prior to sleep.

Here we have seen the hero climb from Earth to the divine. The inauspicious dreams that follow mirror the auspicious. The hero descends from Earth into hell.[77] As with the auspicious dreams, those deemed inauspicious appear in easily recognizable, multi-layered symbolic terms. Colors, meat, and war again play a large role in determining the unfortuitousness of a dream. The *Netra Tantra* offers far fewer inauspicious dream symbols than auspicious ones.

The inauspicious signs begin, "Thus, [in his dreams he] drinks the anointing oil and enters into hell."[78] This harkens back to the initial auspicious signs where the dreamer drinks wine and eats food of sour milk.[79] In the auspicious dream, the acolyte consumes things normally considered impure and in the inauspicious dream he ingests ritually pure substances, though they lead him to hell. The antithetical nature of this action alerts to us, and the dream interpreter, whether the student is mentally prepared for the unexpected and transgressive.

Next, where the text previously described imagery of ascension, it tells of a dreamer who descends. "[He] falls in a well, then sinks in the mud, falls from a tree, vehicle, or other transport. [He descends] from a palace or mountain."[80] After the body topples, various parts of the dreamer's body become mutilated as he dreams that he "cuts off [his][81] ear and nose or [his] hand or foot. [He] loses teeth or hair."[82]

Where auspicious dreams contain red and white images, the inauspicious focus on darkness, unlucky animals, and the activities of war,

> [The dreamer] sees a bear or monkey, demons, cruel beings, and dark men. [He sees those who] have erect hair, dirty ones, those who wear black garlands, clothes, and coverings. That man who, in his dream, embraces a red-eyed woman, he dies, there is no doubt, if he does not bring about peace. [He dreams of] the destruction of houses, palaces, beds, clothes, and seats; defeat of oneself in battle and theft of one's things. [He] ascends or is amongst donkeys, camels, dogs, jackals, and herons, vultures, and cranes. [He rides on] buffalos, owls, and crows, eats cooked meat, [wears a] red garland, and ointment for the body. [He] who sees black and red garments or an altered self [has inauspicious dreams]. In dreams [he] laughs and dances while [he] wears faded garlands, cuts up [his] own flesh.[83] [He dreams of]

> captivity, being eaten by a black snake, and [dreams of] a wedding. [If he] sees this in dreams, he is not successful. (SvT 4.21–27)[84]

Again, many of the auspicious symbols have inauspicious counterparts. The clothes that before were spotless and ready for worship are now dirty and impure. The enemy who was to be conquered is the self, and ritual objects are obtained instead of lost. Where the *Netra Tantra* describes raw meat and the self unaltered as auspicious, when it recounts the inauspicious, it details cooked meat and a transformed self. This final point is important because in the preparation for initiation, an activity that itself seeks to alter the individual, the initiand must not already be in the midst of change.

Upon the interpretation of inauspicious dreams, the *mantrin* performs various cleansing rituals to rid the initiand of the lingering impurities of bad luck.[85] These actions negate the relationship between the images and meaning, leaving the disciple purified and ready for entry into the Tantric space. By manipulating the signs in this way the *mantrin* replaces the signifiers and signifieds of the inauspicious signs. This helps prepare the initiand for the process of initiatory transformation by ensuring conditions are right for the adoption of his new Tantric body and identity.

5

Initiation

Dīkṣā: Building a New Identity Through Initiation

The *Netra Tantra* offers a concise outline of initiation. It explains how the initiand becomes fused with various cosmic elements, such as the *tattva*s, mantras, and in Kṣemarāja's non-dualistic reading, the highest reality, i.e., Śiva. From both the *Netra Tantra* and Kṣemarāja's commentary, it becomes clear how the process of initiation completely separates the initiand from both his physical body and his social self. This separation occurs at the various stages of initiation, from *samayin* to *ācārya*, wherein each level is associated with different *tattvas*. The change that the initiand goes through during the rites is not, "a mere development of preexisting seeds but . . . a transformation *totius substantiae*."[1] According to Durkheim, this change in one's entire essence stems from a literal death and rebirth wherein the newly initiated practitioner is instantly replaced by his new self.[2] As I demonstrate below, though neither the *Netra Tantra* nor Kṣemarāja uses the term "death," there is a clear rebirth as the individual adopts a new Tantric identity free from the bonds of his pre-initiated state and his place in the social caste hierarchy.

The text begins by stating that one takes initiation for experience or enjoyments (*bhukti*) and for liberation (*mukti*) in the same manner.[3] During the initiation process, the *mantrin* takes the initiand through the various *tattva*s, the number of which depends on the specificity and elaborateness of the rite. Such variations do not change the outcome. If we consider the *mantrin* to be a professional, we can conclude that the number of *tattva*s touched on during the initiation depends on the amount the initiand can afford. Kṣemarāja coordinates his list of *tattva*s with those found in the *Svacchanda Tantra*. The number found within the *Svacchanda Tantra*'s initiations include thirty-six, eighteen, nine, five, three, and one *tattva*.[4] Kṣemarāja closely ties the *Netra* and *Svacchanda Tantra*s' chapters on initiation together through his commentary, making it clear that the two were meant to be understood together.

Illness and Immortality. Patricia Sauthoff, Oxford University Press. © Oxford University Press 2022.
DOI: 10.1093/oso/9780197553268.003.0006

The *Svacchanda Tantra* spends much of its third, fourth, and fifth chapters on a discussion of the preliminary initiatory rites. The *mantrin* who performs the death conquering rites of the *Netra Tantra* would be well versed in initiatory rites. Thus, it is vital here for the *mantrin* to understand the micro- and macro-cosmic effects of his ritual performance.

> Now,[5] I will teach about initiation, [which] gives the fruits of experience (*bhukti*) and liberation (*mukti*). It may be done, for the expansion of the transcendent and immanent (*parāpara*), with thirty-six *tattva*s or with half that many [eighteen], half that [nine], or with five or three or one. (NT 4.1-2a)[6]
>
> [The thirty-six [are those] beginning with earth and ending with *śiva* [i.e., the complete set of thirty-six *tattvas*]. That halved, the eighteen elements [beginning with] the five elements [*pṛthvi*, *āpas*, *agni*, *vāyu*, *ākāśā*], *prakṛti*, *puruṣa*, *rāga*, *niyati*, *vidyā*, *kāla*, *kalā*, *māyā*, *śuddhavidyā*, *īśa*, *sadāśiva*, *śakti*, and *śiva*.[7] Or [again] halved, the nine [are] *prakṛti*, *puruṣa*, *niyati*, *kāla*, *māyā*, *vidyā*, *īśa*, *sadāśiva*, and *śiva*. The five are the gross elements, which like the five *kalā*s beginning with *nivṛtti* are seen as pervading everything. The three are *bhuvana*, *śakti*, and *śiva*,[8] pervaded by *māyā*, *sadāśiva*, and *śiva*.[9] The one is *śivatattva*, which pervades all.[10] For the expansion of both transcendent (*para*) and imminent (*apara*) power means, both liberation (*mokṣa*) and enjoyment (*bhoga*) may be accomplished in all these without difference.][11]

Once the text has expounded on *tattvadīkṣā*, it moves onto *kalādīkṣā*, the initiatory process that destroys the fetters that restrict the bound soul (*paśu*), and *padadīkṣā*, in which one draws the *maṇḍala* and its associated mantra. The text lists five additional paths for *dīkṣā*: the *kalā*s, *pada*s, speech sounds, mantras, or *bhuvana*s. Kṣemarāja explains each of these and rearranges the order so that the *pada*s follow the fifty speech sounds in the list order. He then clarifies the five *kalā*s and instructs one to repeat the *mātṛkā* mantra, which consists of all fifty phonemes in the inverse of their usual order, spelling out each individual phoneme to assure clarity. Kṣemarāja indirectly cites the *Mālinīvijayottara Tantra* as his source. His gloss on the *pada*s is somewhat unusual as one would normally expect nine total *pada*s, the eight consonantal[12] and one vocalic *pada* but here the text deviates and Kṣemarāja describes ten total *pada*s, presumably with *kṣa* standing alone as its own *pada.*[13] He explains that by using the eighty-one *pada* mantra found in the *Svacchanda Tantra* one can create the *navātman*. The *Svacchanda Tantra* teaches an unusual eighty-one *pada* mantra that utilizes the phonemes *oṃ, ha, ra, kṣa, ma, la, va, ya,* and *ū*. These are the same phonemes as those found in the *navātman* (with *oṃ* standing for *ṃ*) but with their attached vowels. The practitioner places *oṃ* at the eight compass points and the middle, with each of the other letters repeated throughout the mantra nine times to make an eighty-one-phoneme mantra.[14]

This is very different from the lengthy Śaiva Siddhānta mantra in which *padas* are measured in components rather than phonemes. For example, the Siddhāntan reads the six-syllable *oṃ namaḥ śivāyā*, traditionally the ending of the *vyomavāpin* mantra, as one *pada.*[15] The *Guhyasūtra* tells us that the *vyomavāpin* mantra should be used, in reverse order, during post-mortuary rites.[16] Dualistic *āgamas* teach that the *vyomavyāpin* mantra consists of *padas*, split into one, eleven, twenty, twenty-one, and twenty-eight groups to make a total of eighty-one.[17] Like the *mātṛkā* and *navātman*, the *vyomavyāpin* mantra contains all the letters of the alphabet. By pointing out the variations in form of this mantra, Kṣemarāja opens the *Netra Tantra* to varied readings and usages by practitioners of different schools. He does, however, clearly favor the reading of the most esoteric Kaula school that stems from the *Mālinīvijayottara Tantra*. Kṣemarāja both places it first in his commentary and refers to it covertly, so much so so that only one already versed in its contents would know the source. Regardless of the mantra used, Kṣemarāja shows the connection between the phonemes and the *tattvas*, with vowels that correlate to *śakti* and *śiva* while the consonants correspond to the remaining thirty-four *tattvas*. The *Mālinīvijayottara Tantra* then engages with sound theory as the practitioner utters the form, while the *Svacchanda Tantra* engages the body through the limbs and the paths that lead to the attainment of the *kalās*. Finally, Kṣemarāja emphasizes the numerical differences in the worlds (*bhuvana*) found within the three textual traditions he quotes. Through the commentary, Kṣemarāja assures that all six paths (*adhvan*), those of the word, *varṇa*, mantra, and *pada*, and those of what Padoux calls the "objective side,"[18] *kalā, tattva,* and *bhuvana*, are represented. The latter, those of the more experiential or empirical type, culminate in the *bhuvanas*. These are systematic subdivisions of the worlds or the cosmos, which vary greatly across texts and include everything from the divine world to various hells.[19]

[Now, after it has mentioned *tattvadīkṣā*, which has six varieties, the text now mentions the *dīkṣas*[20] of the *kalās*, etc.]

All *dīkṣā*s may be done using the five *kalā*s or the *pada*s or the fifty speech sounds or with the mantras or the worlds (*bhuvana*). (NT 4.2cd-3ab)

[The *kalās* are *nivṛtti*, *pratiṣṭhā*, *vidyā*, *śāntā*, and *śāntyatītā*.[21] The [*Mālinīvijayottara Tantra* instructs the practitioner to recite the] *mātṛka*, beginning with *kṣa*, etc.[22] These are the nine *pada*s. The tenth *pada* is the series of vowels beginning with *visarga* and ending with *a*. Following the teaching of the *Svacchanda Tantra* there are eighty-one *pada*s beginning with *ū*, taught in the layout called the *navātman*.[23] Or, following the hierarchical mantric system of the *Svāyambhuva* [*Sūtra Saṃgraha* and other texts of the Śaiva Siddānta school], then they are associated with the *vyomavyāpin* mantra. The fifty sounds that begin with *kṣa* [i.e., the consonants, are those that correspond to the] thirty-four *tattva*s that begin with earth and end with *sadāśiva*. The sixteen, which end with the sound *visarga* [i.e., the vowels, correspond to the *tattva*s, and are] considered the non-distinct *śakti* and *śiva tattva*s. In the [*Mālinīvijayottara Tantra*] the *pada*s [are the] form of uttered sound expressed in the middle [of the *maṇḍala*] engaged in seeing the mantra with regards to the bonds of dualism and non-dualism. The *Svacchanda Tantra* [says] the heart, the head, the topknot, the armor, the weapon, and the eye are the limbs. Simultaneously, the first *vaktramantra*s, in regard to being engaged in consideration of all *adhvan*s, do [*dīkṣā*] by attaining the five *kalā*s. The mantras are the limbs that produce existence from the non-existence of the *vaktramantras*. The *bhuvanas*, as observed in the [*Svāyambhuva Sūtra Saṃgraha*], are the subsequent one hundred eighteen. Additionally, [there] appear two-hundred-twenty-four forms in the *Svacchanda Tantra*, of this, other *āgama*s are in agreement, saying *dīkṣā* is composed of six *adhvas*.][24]

Kṣemarāja ends his commentary on this section with an explanation of his inclusion of different schools' interpretations. He says that the variations found within the text should not be seen as discrepancies or contradictions because the *Netra Tantra* summarizes the revelations found in various texts. This means the order and details of *dīkṣā* told in each *āgama* conform to what is taught within those *āgamas*. In other words, because each text is a revelation from the divine, they cannot be contradictory. Each practitioner should follow the rites for initiation that are detailed in the texts followed by his own school. This again demonstrates the universality of the *Netra Tantra*'s protective rites and allows practitioners from different schools to utilize them while continuing to worship their chosen deity.

Though the *Netra Tantra* only states that initiation brings about a state of potential (*śakti*) and manifestation (*vyakti*) for the initiand, Kṣemarāja uses his commentary to explain the remaining paths. Again, he quotes the *Svacchanda Tantra* to show that the practitioner needs to understand the teachings of the *Svacchanda Tantra* in order to understand those of the *Netra Tantra*. As White points out, the *Netra Tantra* is both derivative of, and less comprehensive and systematic than, the *Svacchanda Tantra*.[25] That it derives from the *Svacchanda Tantra* means that even though Kṣemarāja's commentary offers explanations that open the text up to practitioners of other schools of thought, the texts themselves are contextually tied together. However, this does not mean that Kṣemarāja's commentary necessarily captures the original meaning. Instead, he reads and comments on the two related texts to bring them into the non-dual Śaiva fold. Such a reading becomes clear in the following section of commentary, in which Kṣemarāja uses the *Svacchanda Tantra* to clarify his own understanding of the paths (*adhvan*), which do not occur anywhere in the original text's discussion of initiation.

> [Through initiation (*dīkṣā*), he is] prepared for all because through religious action [he becomes] the same [as the divine] in accordance with the nature of potential (*śakti*) and manifestation (*vyakti*). (NT 4.3cd–4ab)
>
> [This means, he should contemplate each of these paths [that has to be purified]. After [he] makes it the principle [path of worship he becomes the] pervader, [i.e., that which permeates the others] with the form of [potential or manifest] explicitness in the remaining five paths (*adhvan*). Included within [the path], as it has spread, is the form of potential. As has been said in the *Svacchanda Tantra*, "[he should] visualize the *adhvans* as pervaded by [the others and the others] pervaded by it.][26]

Once the text makes the purpose of initiation clear, it discusses the major points of initiatory performance. These begin with the guru, who must be highly trained. However, the spiritual status of the *mantrin* who performs the initiation does not determine his compensation for such performance. Instead, the initiand provides what he can afford. The *mantrin* demonstrates his dedication and generosity by taking whatever is offered to perform the initiation. Similarly, the amount of payment the initiand can provide to the *mantrin* determines the number of *tattvas* the *mantrin* will take him through during the initiation rite. An initiand who provides more opulent offerings will receive a longer and more exhaustive initiation. Additionally, the efficacy of the rite depends on the payment, often in the form of non-monetary gifts (*dakṣinā*) for the *mantrin*.[27] The level of initiation sought, *putraka*, *samayin*, *sādhaka*, or *ācārya*, may also require different amounts of *dakṣinā*,[28] though the *Netra Tantra* does not address this.

> [And this initiation,]
>
> [should] be set in motion by the highest teachers, in accordance with the best of the wealth [of the one for whom] the *mantrin* performs the *dīkṣā*. (NT 4.4cd)
>
> [People with wealth [should pay homage] with lavish ingredients; for others it may be done even with such meager ingredients as *dūrva* grass, water, and sprouts. For in this way there is a supremacy of our teachers [who] lack laziness and [are] free of greed].[29]

The *Netra Tantra* and Kṣemarāja then begin to explain how *dīkṣā* impacts the body. Again, we find a major difference between the commentary and the original text. Kṣemarāja elaborates on the preliminary details that must be done to the initiand's body. He also discusses visualization while the original text focuses on the presence of the goddess Vāgīśvarī, the goddess of speech.

> [First of all, [the *mantrin*] attaches the threads of the bonds to the disciple's body, then infuses the parts [of the body into that thread]. Then [the *mantrin*] respectfully approaches the path (*adhvan*), and [performs] worship and *homa* to the [six] *adhvans*. Then, [he] visualizes the three bonds [inside the *adhvans*]. Then, [the *mantrin* performs] such rituals as the installation [of] the *śakti*, which is the support of everything else.
>
> After he has done this,]
>
> He should worship Vāgīśvarī. (NT 4.5ab)
>
> [He should do that *pūjā*, [which] ends with offerings into the fire.]
>
> [The *mantrin*] should then install the bound soul (*paśu*) in her womb. (NT 4.5cd)
>
> [Namely, [the *paśu* is] the initiand (*śiṣya*), whom the [*mantrin*] has already sprinkled, beaten, and taken hold of his consciousness].
>
> [[Why should he put him in that womb?] Because he has been born in the fourteen diverse receptacles of experience [i.e., the first fourteen *saṃskāras*.]][30]

This passage begins with Kṣemarāja's elaboration on the threads of bondage. He clarifies that during the initiation process, the *mantrin* attaches a physical thread to the initiand's body. The *mantrin* then visualizes a fusion of the threads and the initiand's consciousness. The *mantrin* then places that consciousness into the womb of Vāgīśvarī, the speech goddess. From there, the *mantrin* brings the initiand's consciousness into his own body to purify it and connect it to Śiva. He then returns the Śiva-fused consciousness to the body of the disciple to complete the initiation. Through this process, the *mantrin* separates three bonds, impurity (*mala*), action (*karma*), and illusion (*māyā*), from the disciple. This offers the disciple liberation. However, the *mantrin* not only focuses on the fusion of the initiand's consciousness with Śiva. Through the initiation process the *mantrin* also transforms the initiand's physical body. Transformation and initiation are marked as complete through the removal of the disciple's topknot. When the *mantrin* severs the threads, he also cuts off the disciple's hair. He then throws both into the sacrificial fire. Thus, the *mantrin* marks both the soul and the body of the disciple transformed into a wholly other self, one that has fused with the divine. Through the initiatory process, the disciple is reborn.

Once the *mantrin* has placed the consciousness of the disciple into Vāgīśvarī's womb, the initiand proceeds through the purification process. This transforms him into a twice-born devotee of Rudra. It is important to note here that initiation into this sect supplants the devotee's former caste, at least according to Kṣemarāja and the *Svacchanda Tạntra*.[31] Through initiation, the practitioner sheds the bonds that fetter him to the cycle of rebirth in the world by replacing himself with a purified, reborn self that has been yoked to the divine. He has been purified and reconstructed in a new and perfected form, his bonds thrown into the sacrificial fire.

> [One goes through the *saṃskāras*:] conceived (*garbhādhāna*), born (*janana*), by virtue of taking up one's role (*adhikāra*), action (*laya*) and fruition (*bhoga*). Then [the initatiand] atones (*niṣkṛti*) and [proceeds through the remainder of the *saṃskāras* that] follow. All this should] be done with the *mūla* mantra. (NT 4.5–6ab)
>
> [Conceived (*garbhādhāna*) means taking root in various bodies, [*janana* is] to be born [out of that], *adhikāra* is the success of those who have grown to maturity and are suitable to experience *bhoga*. He's qualified to achieve karma, i.e., he can acquire its ability to bring about enjoyment matured by the great power of the mantras. It takes the form of being ready to perform

results. After that comes *bhoga*, which is the experiencing of pleasure, pain, and delusion. The process of action (*laya*) [is to] melt away any trace of fruition, which remains for a short period of time even though the *bhoga* has ceased. Then [comes] penance (*niṣkṛti*), which means the complete accomplishing of all *bhoga* that pertains to birth, life, and experiences. All this is to be done with sacrificial offerings into fire with the root mantra, three, etc., times. The penance should have a *homa* of one-hundred offerings. At the end of that, he should then meditate on the achievement of becoming twice-born and [his place as a] devotee of Rudra.

Once he has performed the *saṃskāra* [called] separation (*viśleṣākhya*), whose nature is the absence of being the agent of experience, once all *bhogas* have been completed].

Then, as proclaimed by tradition, [he should] cut the bonds with the *astra mantra*. (NT.4.6cd)

[Then, after [he has] cut the binding ties (*pāśasūtra*) with the *astra mantra*, which is taught to follow immediately after this separation, with the same [mantra] he should]

burn [that thread by casting it into the ritual fire].[32]

Next, the *Netra Tantra* explains in rather obtuse language how the bonds dissolve in fire. Kṣemarāja's commentary clarifies the passage, though even he struggles to make sense of the phrase *tatsthite*. This he takes to mean the place inside the heart of the initiand.

[And after that,]

[the bonds] have been reduced to ashes and reside there (*tatsthite*).

[He continues to use the same *astra* mantra [and] reduces to ashes the bonds, which completely cease and are without latent trace. [The locative of] *tatsthita* means he has visualized oneness of the consciousness of the disciple with the *mūla* [mantra]. The entirety [of the disciple's] body has ceased. [After that,] the place (*sthāna*) is established. [The *mantrin*] fuses the consciousness of his disciple with the mantra. Then, together with the disciple's consciousness, [the *mantrin*] causes [that consciousness] to enter into his own heart, raises it to *dvādaśānta*,[33] then projects it [back] into the heart of the initiand (*śiṣya*). *Tatsthitam* is to be analyzed as that standing (*sthāna*) [i.e., the *śiṣya*'s consciousness brought to rest in the initiand's heart]. (NTU 4.7)[34]

In other words, according to Kṣemarāja, once the bonds have been cut using the weapon (*astra*) mantra, thrown into fire, and reduced to ash, the *mantrin* fuses the consciousness of the now bodiless disciple with the mantra. He then brings the disciple's consciousness into his own heart and raises it up through his body and out of the top of his head in order to purify it. Finally, the *mantrin* projects the initiand's consciousness and the mantra back into the heart of the disciple, where it rests permanently. The initiand has cast aside his body for the rite and the initiand's cord (*pāśasūtra*) acts as a stand-in so that the physical body can be destroyed without harm to the initiand.[35] This does not mean that Tantric practitioners understand this as a symbolic act. The *mantrin* fuses very real bonds that tie the initiand to the world with the *pāśasūtra*. The process transforms the initiand's body through this process. The initiand then remains without fetters for the remainder of his life.

The *pāśasūtra* is one of the most important aspects of the initiation rite.[36] It consists of a cotton cord the same height as the initiand's body.[37] The *mantrin* purifies the *pāśasūtra* with both water and mantra before he hangs it from the disciple's topknot to his feet.[38] The *mantrin* then replaces the disciple's body with the cord by imposing the body's constituents onto the cord.[39] As Davis notes, the initiand remains passive throughout this process as the bonds stifle his innate powers of knowledge, action, and will.[40] This means that one cannot self-initiate and must utilize a *mantrin* who has himself been yoked to Śiva.

The initiand's subtle body ceases to exist. This body, made of eight parts (*puryaṣṭaka*) consists of the five primary elements of sense perception[41] and intellect (*buddhi*), self-consciousness (*ahaṃkāra*), and mind (*manas*). He must rid himself of this body in order to attain universal awareness. In Chapter 8, the *Netra Tantra* says that the initiand

> does not need to meditate on [that which is] rising upwards, nor practice [that which] goes downward, or [rests] in the middle (i.e., the breath). He does not need to concentrate on [that which is] in front, or anything to the side or in other directions. [He need not focus upon] that which is inside the body or outside of it. He does not have to see the sky or that which is below. He does not have to close the eyes, nor open them.
>
> He does not have to rest upon, lack support, or act as a support [for anything]. He need not concentrate on the five senses, what is real, sound, touch, essence, etc. Once he has abandoned all that he presides over, he becomes absorbed in *kevala*.[42] (NT 8.41–44)[43]

When he abandons everything, the practitioner loses his sense of individuation and becomes purified. Though the *Netra Tantra* does not define *puryaṣṭaka*, Kṣemarāja begins this purification process with the *kalātattva*. Often *puryaṣṭaka* is described as connected to the *tattvas*, from *pṛthivī* to *kalā* as in the *Tattvasaṃgraha*[44] or eight *tattvas* in the *Kallottara*.[45] Using either reading, the *puryaṣṭaka*, which is synonymous with the *sūkṣma śarīra*, contains some but not all of the *tattvas*. This helps to explain why the initiand sheds his body as he passes through the lower *tattvas* into the higher. According to Mīmāṃsaka thought, the *puryaṣṭaka* equates to a soul. This soul acts and experiences the fruits of those actions in both pleasure and pain. The *puryaṣṭaka* or soul is what reincarnates from one birth to the next.[46] For Kṣemarāja, the Mīmāṃsaka understanding does not go far enough. He adds that the *puryaṣṭaka* does not differ in substance from Śiva. Instead, a practitioner experiences the state of the *puryaṣṭaka*, in which he encounters the fruits of action, when he conceals his true nature, i.e., that of Śiva.[47] When one reaches the point where the *puryaṣṭaka* is completely dissolved, he then attains true enjoyment and assimilates himself into all *tattvas*, from *pṛthivī* to Śiva. In this moment, he attains Śivahood within his manifest body (*deha*).[48] Once the guru accomplishes this state in his disciple, he cuts off the disciple's topknot and places it into the sacrificial fire accompanied by the *mūla* mantra, which unites the disciple with Śiva.

> [Next, after [the *mantrin* has] caused the cessation, etc. [of differentiation], as taught of the eight-fold subtle body (*puryaṣṭaka*) through the offerings of inviting, reverence and oblation, [and] after he has purified all the paths, after he has first united [the initiand] with all the other *tattvas*, beginning with *kalā*, he should then]
>
> cut off of the topknot and perform *homa*.[49]
>
> [This means, after he cuts off the topknot, he should throw it into fire,
>
> and after [he has] cut [the topknot] with [that with which it] pervades (*vyāpti*) [i.e., he cuts the topknot and the *pāśasūtra*], he meditates on its correspondence to the flame [i.e., the fire consumes what is thrown into it and makes that which is thrown into it the same as fire], which has as its nature the power of vital energy, which is the basis of the cosmos.
>
> Such a teacher, who is richly endowed with expertise and yogic ability, who knows the reality of the fifteen topics that the *Svacchanda Tantra* teaches [and], "has understood the span of the breath and the circulation of the breath," should then,]

unite [the initiand] with that same *mūla* mantra. (NT 4.7)

[the disciple, whose bonds cease to exist, [and]

After he has let go of all mental activity, the [*mantrin*] should fuse [the disciple] with awareness. Then the bound soul attains Śivahood, rescued from the ocean of repeated incarnation. "As said in the *Svacchanda Tantra*, he should make [that disciple] one with Paramaśiva by causing him to enter into the highest *tattva*].[50]

Once the *mantrin* has fused the initiand with Śiva, he must ensure that the disciple remains in the *tattva* appropriate to the level of initiation he has received. These categories also explain the role of each initiatory level. For example, the *ācārya*, who has achieved the highest level of initiatory practitioner, reaches the highest *tattva* in the initiatory process but permanently resides in the *tattva* just below it. This means that he has experienced the highest *tattva*, but he must not remain there or he cannot perform *dīkṣā* for others.

[Then,]

After [the *mantrin* has] united [the disciple] with the highest reality, he should cause him to dwell there.

[In this way [the initiand] will become one with that [*tattva*]. Now, [let us turn to] the differentiation of union with the *tattvas* (*yojanika*),]

Thus, the [initiand] should know the *dīkṣā* in such a way that the *ācārya* is established [in the appropriate *tattva* so that he can perform] his duties in the Śivahood that embraces both highest (*para*) and final emancipation (*parapada*). For the *sādhaka* [the final *tattva* resting place is] in *sadāśiva*. For the *putraka* it is in the highest *tattva* [and] for the *samayin* in *īśvara tattva*. (NT 4.8–9)

[Śivahood [is that] whose level is *parāparapada*, "but Śiva, the ultimate cause, engages in action established in that." Stated in the *Svacchanda Tantra*, "[for the initiation of] *ācārya*s, the [*mantrin*] should perform fusion with lower *śiva* after he has fused them with higher *śiva*. For *sādhaka*s, immediately after fusion with *śiva*, the [*mantrin*] should perform unification with *sadāśiva*. For the *putraka*, [he should join him with] the highest *tattva*, [and for the] *samayin*, *īśvara tattva*. This is the distribution.][51]

The newly initiated become permanently fused into one of three *tattva*s. The highest *tattva*, *śiva*, is split into two: an impermanent state (*para*) and a permanent emancipatory one (*parapada*). The *puryaṣṭaka*, made up of the lower *tattva*s, then becomes permanently replaced and what remains of the individual resides in the appropriate *tattva* until death, unless he later becomes initiated into a higher level. Once the initiate sheds his physical body, he no longer differentiates himself from Śiva. In these highest states, the subtle (*sūkṣma*) body resembles the physical body.[52] But it is not subject to the limitations of spacial dimension or bound by time.[53] From *śiva*, the I-ness (*ahantā*) expands into that-ness (*idantā*),[54] subject becomes object. *Śiva tattva* is where one experiences pure thought (*cit*). It does not distinguish between subject and object. *Śakti* complements this the state of pure thought. Here, the initiate experiences pure bliss (*ānanda*). The forces of *cit* and *ānanda* contract and manifest the *tattva*s that follow them.

The brief chapter then ends,

> [To bring the matter to a close,]
>
> Thus, *dīkṣā* has been explained in brief, the full explanation is elsewhere. (NT 4.10)
>
> [[The text says,] briefly and elsewhere because this ritual of *dīkṣā* is extremely long and because it has been merely touched upon [here] in an extremely abridged form. He teaches that after the [*mantrin* has] first, correctly understood this expansive [rite] from the *Svacchanda Tantra*, [and other texts], he should put it into practice. The eye of Śiva is greater than all. It bestows on those rich in devotion, immersion in the highest abode, [and he] burns away of all the massive bonds.][55]

Ultimately, Kṣemarāja reiterates that the will of Śiva bestows liberation upon the newly initiated through the correct performance of the rites. This also garners the attention of the deity, who bestows liberation. Once purified and initiated, the practitioner can take part in the daily and occasional rites his tradition requires.

6

Religion of Monarchs

Tantric practice and symbolism often subvert the dominant distinction between purity and impurity. Though not the norm, transgressive practices do play a part in Tantric rites.[1] Such practices impact Tantra in both the sacred and profane realms. Transgressive actions require their performers to maintain a plurality of concurrent identities. The first within the orthodox world and the other as transgressor. Without some identification with the ordinary, the transgressive becomes the norm and is no longer capable of breaking taboo, therefore making it no longer transgressive. Where the practitioner's multiple identities come into conflict, transgression occurs. Taussig points out that secrecy (especially public secrecy) and transgression are intertwined.[2] Out of fear of punishment, the transgressor must not allow his act to be too widely known. At the same time, he must reveal the act for it to have any power. The revelation of the secret and transgressive action to trusted others leads to a shared secret.[3] This strengthens the bond between members of the secret community while keeping their activities hidden from outsiders, and thus safe from external retribution.

Douglas notes four types of social pollutions that lead to danger: crossing external boundaries, transgressing internal boundaries, the marginal spaces surrounding the boundaries, and contradiction within the system.[4] I focus primarily on the first: Tantric practice in conflict with external norms and rules. As a practice in opposition to the *mores* of larger society, Tantric activity must be clearly marked. Initiation rites help to delineate the boundaries between Tantric and non-Tantric membership. Once initiated, a Tantric practitioner may find himself exposed to transgressive behavior. This reinforces his position Tantric community while maintaining the protective shield of that community's shared secrecy. This allows him to reaffirm his Tantric identity in stages and does not force him to cross into the transgressive immediately on obtaining Tantric membership, though he is perfectly qualified to do so.

In Tantric practice, transgressive conduct often consists of three types of behavior: (1) the ritual consumption of, or contact with, forbidden and impure substances; (2) the designation of charnel grounds as sacred spaces; and

Illness and Immortality. Patricia Sauthoff, Oxford University Press. © Oxford University Press 2022.
DOI: 10.1093/oso/9780197553268.003.0007

(3) participation in sexual rites. During the ritual itself, practitioners use several types of sacred language to interact with deities. One such kind is an encoded pattern of speech called *chommakā*. In order to provide a protective cover for speech that describes ritual elements, the text gives a *chommakā* word that replaces an ordinary technical term. For example, the *Svacchanda Tantra* calls meat, "increasing power."[5] For a substance to be transgressive, the practitioner must first believe it to be impure. This means he adheres to the rules and *mores* of Brahmanical society. His second identity, as a Tantric practitioner, allows for the covert ritual consumption of meat within the Tantric sphere. During this ritual, practitioners eat meat in the presence of others who bear witness to their increase of power. Similarly, the charnel ground (called "tumult")[6] is the location at which all fear and afflictions of the mind are destroyed.[7] The place of burial and decay then becomes the place of worship because it inverts the ordinary associations of danger.[8]

Transgressive practice is not the main element of Tantric Śaiva ritual. However, such practice is the most socially dangerous. In her study of Tantra in the *Rājataraṅgiṇī*, Törzsök shows that Tantric practitioners were widely associated with prohibited sex,[9] meat eating, etc.[10] Such antinomian practices allow Kalhaṇa to paint a negative picture of Tantric practitioners. He correlates the downfall of several kings with their Tantric associations and transgressive conduct.[11]

Several early works describe punishments for specific behaviors. A comparison of the types of taboos found in Tantra with the punishments for prohibitions found in the *Arthaśāstra*[12] reveals many similarities. The consumption of forbidden foods and beverages results in exile. Those who cause another to consume the forbidden incur a monetary fine. The value of the fine varies with caste. Those who cause a brahmin to ingest the banned items receive the highest penalty.[13] The *Arthaśāstra* demands exile for those who consume the prohibited food and drinks of their own volition.[14] Sex with a person's aunt, daughter-in-law, daughter, sister, or the wife of his teacher requires castration,[15] to be followed by execution.[16] Cross-caste sexual relationships result in various punishments, from fines and the confiscation of property to loss of caste and execution.[17] These punishments are particular to the *Arthaśāstra*, though the prohibitions themselves are fairly consistent across dharmic texts. Not all Tantric texts prescribe the same types of transgressive behaviors. The *Mṛgendra Tantra*, an influential text in Śaiva Siddhānta circles, which influenced non-dual Śaiva texts,[18] prescribes very different punishments for transgressions. It calls for the performance of 10,000 recitations of eleven mantras for voluntary or involuntary sins, including the consumption of alcohol or sex with a master's wife.[19] This demonstrates that similar prohibitions existed across social and religious boundaries, but the response to such behaviors varied widely with tradition.

The *Rājataraṅgiṇī* does discuss specific penalties for transgressions. I highlight the punishments in the *Arthaśāstra* because of its widespread influence.[20] The *Rājataraṅgiṇī* implies that only brahmins were subject to caste-specific punishments.[21] As the *Mṛgendra Tantra* shows, punishments varied widely. However, killing a brahmin, drinking liquor, theft, sex with a teacher's wife, and criminal associations recur as crimes. Sex with a teacher's wife, a practice not unheard of in Tantric circles,[22] is often categorized as incest.[23] The *Arthaśāstra* does not give specific sanctions for kings, but the *Rājataraṅgiṇī* calls for kings to be punished for their transgressions. Kalhaṇa records that Harṣa worshipped low-caste slave girls as goddesses and had sex with them. He drank the magic potions they offered him[24] and had sex with his father's wives and his own sisters.[25] While the king escaped official punishment for this behavior, Kalhaṇa describes him as sullied and ties his downfall to his transgressive acts.[26] Though the punishments do not correspond to those of the *Arthaśāstra*, similar prohibitions existed in Kashmir, even for the king. Kalhaṇa does not find low-caste women posing as goddesses[27] particularly unusual. This demonstrates that he knew of such practices. If indeed the women he describes act as *yoginīs*, this open reference to Tantric practice demonstrates that the penalty for prohibited activities was not nearly as harsh as that laid out in the *Arthaśastra*. Clearly, transgressive Tantric practice occurred within courtly circles. In fact, Kalhaṇa himself did not object to Tantric practices such as mantric recitation to increase the monarch's pleasure or his acquisition of supernatural powers. Instead, he criticizes the transgressive rites that involve impure substances and sexual acts and ties them to the downfall of kings.[28] Törzsök hypothesizes that Kalhaṇa, himself a Śaiva, may have been particularly weary of such practices since they posed a risk to the reputation of Śaiva practitioners in general.[29] This would account for references to transgressive practice throughout the *Rājataraṅgiṇī*. Clearly, outsiders knew of such practices. If they were meant to be secret, they were not well guarded. This is demonstrated through the spread of Tantric practice throughout the region. Regardless of Kalhaṇa's personal opinion, the *Rājataraṅgiṇī*'s portrayal of Śaiva sexual practices suggests that they were an important part of Kashmiri religion. It contains several cautionary tales about the impact of transgressive practices on kings. This reveals a pattern of Tantric guru influence on the monarchy.

Evidence for Śaiva Tantric traditions begin to appear in approximately the sixth century.[30] Tantra quickly spread through South and Southeast Asia to become a fundamental part of religious life.[31] The Brahmanical Śaiva tradition continued to compose Purāṇic texts while its Tantric counterparts produced the corpus of texts called Tantras. In works such as the *Uttarabhāga*, *Kālikā Purāṇa*, *Devī Purāṇa*, and *Agni Purāṇa*, the distinction between Tantric and Brahmanical tradition is almost non-existent.[32] The spread of Śaiva practice occurred largely due to royal patronage. Sanderson argues that Śaiva success was largely due to the extension of "a body of rituals and theory that legitimated, empowered, or promoted key elements of the social, political, and economic process that characterizes the early medieval period."[33] Geertz describes the relationship between monarchs and Brahmins as one in which brahmins, especially priests, did not hold local political power. Instead, brahmins maintained a sense of spiritual superiority through their monopoly on scriptural tradition and esoteric knowledge.[34] Conversely, the political class maintained its own monopoly through governmental rulership.[35] The priest offered his services to the monarch and in exchange he received political favor and social protection.[36]

Kings, Poets, and Patronage

Royal patronage was important for many poets, playwrights, and philosophers in medieval Kashmir. Their families often possessed connections to the royal court. For example, the eleventh-century poet Kṣemendra was the son of an affluent and prominent Śaiva brahmin.[37] A contemporary of Kalhaṇa, Kṣemendra's work is often critical of Tantric priests and teachers.[38] Yet Kṣemendra studied literature with the great Tantric exegete and aesthetic philosopher Abhinavagupta.[39] Abhinavagupta's own connection to the monarchy is clear, as he traces his ancestry to the great scholar, Atrigupta, who King Lalitāditya invited to Kashmir in the eighth century.[40]

The twelfth-century author of the Śaiva poem *Śrīkaṇṭhacarita*, Maṅkha,[41] was the brother of a minister to Kashmir's King Jayasiṃha.[42] At the end of the *Śrīkaṇṭhacarita*, Maṅkha describes an assembly of scholars invited to hear his completed poem.[43] These men, Maṅkha assures his readers, praised the work.[44] He describes the assembly as made up of the most revered thinkers of his time. Among the scholars, Maṅkha lists Kalhaṇa and Jogarāja. The latter likely refers to Yogarāja, the commentator of Abhinavagupta's *Paramārthasāra*. Also present is Prakaṭa, who Maṅkha claims is better at religious matters than even Abhinavagupta. Maṅkha also describes the attendance of a celebrated philosopher named Suhala, and various poets, Vedantins, Mīmāṃsāns, Buddhists, Vaidikas, grammarians, and logicians.[45] Pollock describes the assembly as a demonstration of the vibrant and innovative literary culture of twelfth-century Kashmir.[46] However, according to Pollock, it also marks the end of the era of royal support of literature and subsequently the decline of Kashmir's literary tradition. No king is listed as present at the reading, and Maṅkha does not praise a royal benefactor in the poem.[47]

The *Śrīkaṇṭhacarita* displays clear Tantric affiliation in its devotion to the worship of Śiva. The poem can be read from a Tantric perspective[48] or as simply a poem of praise. Within the text, Maṅkha describes the different philosophical schools that were most influential in Kashmir at the time.[49] He maintains that the different schools merge into one, the non-dual Śaiva Tantra. This places non-dualism at the top of the philosophical hierarchy.[50] This view is similar to that of Abhinavagupta, who says the Indian philosophical systems are hierarchical. Hanneder organizes the various lineages of Śaiva Tantric schools according to an increasing heterodoxy which he sees a being defined by

> the degree to which female and ferocious deities come to the foreground. On the lower end of the scale, in the Siddhānta, only the consortless mild Sadāśiva is worshipped, his power being personified in his throne; in the Krama, the most heterodox of the Kashmirian cults of [Abhinavagupta's] time, the ritual centers on groups of female, ferocious deities. We arrive at the following sequence: the Siddhānta; the cult of Netranātha represented by the *Netratantra*; the cult of the Svacchandabhairava based on the authority of the *Svacchandatantra*; the Trika with its sub-levels; and finally, the Krama. The internal logic of this series is the notion that an increase of heterodoxy marks and increase of power and soteriological efficacy.[51]

This hierarchy culminates in Abhinavagupta's own school, the Trika. According to Abhinavagupta, practitioners attain incomplete liberation based on the limitations of the other schools. A practitioner can only realize the highest level of reality taught by each system. As Tantric Śaiva theology builds on the others and offers even a taxonomy of ever-higher possible levels of attainment, it must be, by this logic, the ultimate teaching.[52]

Protecting the King: NT 19.84–133

While the *Rājataraṅgiṇī* discusses certain transgressive acts by monarchs and makes clear reference to Tantric practitioners, it does so from an outsider's perspective. This means we have very little information on the actual ritual practice of monarchs. Instead, the *Netra Tantra* offers a look at rituals to be performed on behalf of kings. These rites protect the king and his kingdom—including the livestock, troops, and agriculture over which he rules. This chapter also focuses on demonic possession, from which the rites also protect.

The protective rite begins with the invocation of Mṛtyujit, the physical manifestation of the *Netra Tantra*'s Amṛteśvara. Mṛtyujit holds sway over the factors that bring about death (unhappiness, disease, inability to conceive, etc.) and offers protection from the demons that cause all afflictions.

> The tradition is secret and confers happiness and the best of all fortune. The pleased and pious adepts strive to obtain the favor of [Mṛtyujit].[53] They are liberated from all suffering. What I say is true, not false. (NT 19.84–85ab)[54]

After declaring its ability to alleviate all suffering, the text then says the *mantrin* will attain the benefits of the rite when he performs it on behalf of others. This includes the *mantrin*'s immediate family and pupils as well as kings and their progeny. The monarch's hired *mantrin* was a professional whose singular occupation was the performance of rites on behalf of the king.[55] His performances for members of his own immediate family ensure that the *mantrin* and those who surround him do not become afflicted by demons.

> This [*pūjā*] should prevent all suffering to arise in [the one who performs it]. [The *mantrin*] should perform [it] for his devoted wives, children, and his devoted pupils;[56] he should not practice it otherwise. [When he conducts the *pūjā*, he should do so] on behalf of kings and their offspring because, the king is always the head [of the family] of all stages of life [i.e., the king is

> always the head of all families in the kingdom, regardless of the status of his subjects]. (NT 19.85cd–87)[57]

The *mantrin* infuses white ash with the protective mantra and applies the ash to the body. This act renders the mantra visible and purificatory. He applies the forehead mark each time the king washes his face.

> One should always perform [the recitation of the mantra] for the sake of peace in obligatory rites, special rites, and for fulfillment of special wishes. [The *mantrin* should always] apply the forehead mark (*tilaka*) of white ash [infused] with seven recitations [of the Amṛteśa] mantra on [the king's] washed face. [This] removes the pollution caused by the mothers (*mātṛdoṣa*). (NT 19.88–89ab)[58]

The king also receives a consecrated flower. This bestows protection on him. The gestures of marking the forehead and presentation of a consecrated flower are physical indicators of mantric protection. These acts indicate to the gods and the king's subjects that the king is protected. Once the external marks of protection are complete, the king ingests food consecrated with the mantra. This brings the mantra into his body.

> Enemies[59] [i.e., harmful spirits] do [the king] no harm [when the *mantrin*] gives him a flower or betel-leaf that is consecrated by the mantra. The *mantravid*[60] should consecrate [the king's] food with this mantra. Eating [the food while imagining himself situated] in the middle of two moons,[61] he consumes the nectar (*amṛta*). The king stays on earth, liberated from all disease. (NT 19.89cd–91)[62]

The *mantrin* then proceeds to perform rituals to protect the king. The *mantrin* does not engage directly with the king, but instead venerates a water pot in the king's place. The use of a surrogate[63] is common in medieval religious practice.[64] The water pot is a common symbol of purity and here represents the purified king. The *mantrin* demonstrates his commitment to the king and his kingdom as a whole through rites that protect objects such as animals and weapons.

> When [the king] is at play with horses and elephants or in contests with weapons, [the *mantrin*] should venerate the water pot in order to protect

> him. [The *mantrin*] should perform this auspicious protection, which offers all benefits, whether [the king] is at play or for victory [in battle] in order to protect him from [the] many enemies that wish to destroy the king. (NT 19.92–94ab)[65]

The deity protects the sleeping king in the same way that the king protects his subjects, especially the sleeping troops in danger of attack, disease, and famine.[66] Sleep can also protect from evil despite that it also brings about risks.[67] In the *Netra Tantra*, the *mantrin* honors Mṛtyujit with pure substances that keep the king safe. He protects the king both in the waking world before sleep and in his dreams, where the king is exposed to various dangers.[68]

> Then [the *mantrin*] should venerate the water pot in order to protect the sleeping king. [The water pot is] made of silver and contains herbs, smeared with sandalwood and aloewood, filled with milk and water. He should worship Mṛtyujit with an all-white offering, with rice boiled in milk, guest water, incense, and flowers. Great sleep (Mahānidrā), who bewilders the world, is there. For the king's well-being at night and for his digestion when he eats, etc., this worship should continue [throughout the night] by the order of the God of Gods. Then [the king] should sleep the entire night. He should remain at ease, free of the dangers of *yakṣas*, *rakṣas*, *pisācas*, fear of disrupted sleep—which bring about *mātṛs*—and trembling from those afflictions. (NT 19.94cd–99ab)[69]

While the king sleeps, the *mantrin* turns his attention to the world protectors (Lokapālas).[70] These deities offer special protection to both the king and *mantrin*. Through his performance of the rites, the *mantrin* receives the same benefits of protection as the king. This keeps the *mantrin* pure and allows him to continue his rites. He must be pure to perform the rituals. Impurity would put the sleeping monarch at risk.

> Once [he has] venerated the water pot, [the *mantrin*] should worship the Lokapālas and their weapons with flowers, guest water, and [other ritual] offerings before the king. [The king] whose learned teachers constantly [perform these acts], [he] obtains what was said before [i.e., protection].[71] (NT 19.99cd–101ab)[72]

The mantrin perpetually exists in a ritual state. He always acts to maintain an active protective sphere. The singular focus of his ritual sets the *mantrin* apart from other Tantric practitioners. Such prophylaxis fends off distant and even imagined dangers. Even when rituals call for the king's subjects to worship other deities, his *mantrin* continues to worship Mṛtuyit.[73] This allows him to continue his rites aimed at royal protection.

> Thus says Lord Siva,
>
> The *mantrin* should worship Amṛteśa on all special occasions [and] on special dates in the form of *Kāma* [i.e., any deity that one wishes or is called for by a particular festival]. [He] shall always attain what he desires. He should worship [Amṛteśa] in the form of Indra[74] in order to achieve the protection of the population, to assure [an abundance of] grains of rice,[75] for the sake of protection in respect to wives and offspring, for the prosperity of his kingdom and for royal victory. [The *mantrin*] should worship [Amṛteśa] to benefit brahmins, cows, [for] his own protection, and [the king's] own people, offering abundant oblations at home[76] on the ninth day [of the light half of the month] *Mahānavamī*.[77] As said before, [this brings] long life, freedom from disease, and perfect health. (NT 19.101cd–105ab)[78]

The *Mahānavamī* celebrations give the king an opportunity to display his authority.[79] Descriptions of the ritual at Vijayanagara, near modern-day Hampi, from the fifteenth and sixteenth centuries record that lesser kings within the kingdom came to the capital to offer reverence to their royal overlord.[80] In return, the reigning monarch pledged to protect the kingdom after the deities their approval for the king to continue with his reign.[81] This royal ritual power reinforces the monarch's position in society. It demonstrates his wealth and royal fame, and it identifies the king with the deity.[82]

Geertz's notion of the "theatre state," says, "kings and princes were the impresarios, the priests the directors, and the peasants the supporting cast, stage, crew, and audience."[83] Applying this theory to medieval Kashmir raises the question of how the *mantrin*'s ability to protect the monarch demonstrates his spiritual power and how that power impacts him socially. It also shows that the *mantrin*'s relationship to the transgression found within Tantric practice impacts his role as royal officiant. Geertz's theater state is one in which temple dedications, public rites, mobilization of the masses, and the attainment of wealth were the driving force of politics itself.[84] Certainly, scriptures such as the *Netra Tantra*, *Svacchanda Tantra*, and many others advocate a genuine outcome rather than simply a public demonstration of power. However, the implementation of the rites catalogued by these texts can be read as a theater ritual. Ultimately, the outcome of all rites depends on the grace of Śiva if they are to be successful.[85]

Geertz's theory of the "theatre state" fails to capture the nuance and dynamics of Vijayanagara.[86] The lustration (*nīrājana*) and calendrical rites of *Mahānavamī* celebrations allow the monarch to participate in a grand expression of moral and cosmic unity.[87] However, these rites are temporary and not the primary function of the state. In addition to public rites, the kings of Vijayanagara built numerous and monumental temples[88] and encouraged pilgrimage.[89] For Geertz, court ceremonialism drives court politics and ritual does not reinforce the state but *is* the state.[90] But what about the Tantric practitioner who publicly participated in religious rites and celebrations?

For Geertz, the ritual life of court is paradigmatic of the social order.[91] This means the religion of court must also be more than a mere reflection of society. Appeasement rites gain the deity's attention so that his desire will be to fulfill the wishes of the *mantrin*. Rites, ritual objects, and holy places display the power of the divine in distinct forms.[92] Further, the supernatural powers of these objects, the monarch, and the *mantrin* grow "out of imagining the truth, not out of believing, obeying, possessing, organizing, utilizing, or even understanding it."[93] Clearly, the Tantric practitioner's supernatural power relies on the emic. He believes in the power of the deity, obeys textual authority, possesses *siddhi*s, organizes religious ceremony, utilizes his powers in those rites, and understands the technicalities of ritual elements. For the Tantric then, religion is not theater that drives more religion, but instead religion responds to and allows him to participate in the social order. The *mantrin* participates in ritual that drives society, not as an end itself.[94] Further, religious sovereignty existed outside of jurisdictional apparatuses.[95] With no centralized Tantric authority to uphold, teachers and exegetes were allowed to innovate, even when it came to their understanding of divine scripture.

This public demonstration of royal power and protection imparts victory to the king. This occurs when the *mantrin* honors the implements of battle. Mantric recitation infuses the weapons with magical powers (*siddhi*).[96] It is important to note that though the *mantrin* performs the rituals on behalf of the king, it is the king himself, by the grace of Amṛteśa, who possesses the power.[97] The *mantrin* is the vehicle through which the deity transfers power onto the king.

> The [*mantrin*] should take great pains to prepare the weapons for sacrifice [which brings about] *siddhis*. He obtains success with weapons [i.e., victory in battle]. He [who commissions the sacrifice] attains the fruit [of victory]. (NT 19.105cd–106ab)[98]

The text turns next to protection against internal woes. The *mantrin* first marks the king externally before he entextualises him internally through the consumption of consecrated food. The *mantrin* divinizes the weapons to protect the kingdom from external threats of war. He then protects the kingdom from internal strife and calamity.

> The [*mantrin*] is to perform the lustration (*nīrājana*) in order to secure prosperity of the king and in the kingdom when the king is touched by the power of death, when [the king], his sons, or his country are marked by signs of death, etc., when brahmins [and others] are [in danger] in all directions [i.e., in the capital and elsewhere], with the danger of loss of rice crops, grain, fruit, roots, and water, and in times of famine, disease, and great calamities.[99] After sacrificing as before, the [*mantrin*] should perform the water pot consecration. (NT 19.106–109)[100]

Several texts prescribe the *nīrājana* rite as an antidote to both external threats and internal calamities.[101] The *Arthaśāstra* says that the king "should have the lustration rite performed on the ninth day of *Āśvayuja* (September–October), at the beginning or end of an expedition, or during a sickness."[102] It also says, "In the case of disease or epidemic affecting farm animals, [the king] should have lustration rites of the stalls and equipment and the worship of their respective gods carried out."[103] Royal astronomers and *mantrin*s interpreted celestial, atmospheric, and terrestrial signs of danger. According to the *Viṣṇudharmottara Purāṇa*, the *nīrājana* should be performed at the sight of a double sun, a double moon, a red sun or moon at sunrise or at sunset when there are no clouds; when it rains blood, marrow, bones, fat, or flesh; when fires flare up without fuel or fuel that does not catch fire; when forest animals enter a village and village animals enter a forest; when water animals are on land; when dogs take sticks, fire-brands, bones, or cattle horns to cremation grounds; or when cows smack servants and wives with their tails.[104]

The *Bṛhat Saṃhitā* offers a glimpse of the complexity of the *nīrājana* ritual in the sixth century CE.[105] It required the construction of a large wooden arch and ceremonial house, made of *sarja* (Vatica Robusta/Sal tree), *udumbara* (Ficus Glomerata/Indian Fig tree), or *kakubha* (Terminalia Arjuna/Arjun tree) wood. The *mantrin* covers the inside of the house with *kuśa* grass and decorates the door with fish and banners. He brings horses to the house, adorns them with sacred plants, and worships them. After eight days, the king has a hermitage built to the south of the house, also covered with *kuśa* grass. In the hermitage, the *mantrin* builds a fire into which he offers sacred food and twigs. The king, a horse-physician, and an astrologer sit facing east on a tiger skin while the chaplains read and interpret omens. Consecrated animals are led through the arch while the sound of musical instruments fills the air. Horses or elephants, on their right legs or eating rice-balls consecrated with mantras, indicate victory. Fear or rejection of rice-balls signal defeat. At the end of the ceremony, a priest pierces the heart of a clay figure that represents an enemy in a mock military march.[106]

The *Netra Tantra* assumes the *mantrin* is already familiar with the *nīrājana*. Its description is simpler than those cited previously but does have its own distinctive elements. For example, in the *Netra Tantra*, the *mantrin* sacrifices a goat. This is a unique feature of the *Netra Tantra*. Like the *Bṛhatsaṃhitā*, it singles out white mustard as an important ritual element. The text gives different names for white mustard. These names, *siddhārtha* and *rakṣoghna*, contain double meanings that relate to the desired outcome. For example, white mustard, *siddhārtha*, plays on the compound *siddha* + *artha*, meaning the accomplishment of an objective or the achievement of magical power. Thus, the *mantrin* should use the name *siddhārtha* when he seeks accomplishment.

> [The *mantrin*] who is free from doubt should consecrate [the king] in a solitary place at night and on a day of auspicious protection. With auspicious cries like "victory!" and the sounds of the auspicious Veda, he should consecrate [the king] with water and make oblations of white mustard seeds (*siddhārtha*) [while he] proclaims the name [of the king]. When [he has] perfected [the king] through the *nīrājana* rite, O beloved, the *mantrin*, in order to protect and with an eager mind focused on the fire, anoints many [male] goats to satisfy the spirit community [such as the *mātṛ*s, *yoginī*s, and

> deities]. Once he knows the auspicious words and day, he then goes forth in three directions [north, northeast, and west], conferring *siddhi* to all. (NT 19.110–113)[107]

The king's consecration occurs at night and in a solitary place. The *Bṛhatsaṃhitā* prescribes that the *mantrin* build an arch and hermitage to the northeast of the city. Though it does not indicate how far from the city, this emphasizes the solitary aspect of the rites. The king arrives at the sanctum where the *mantrin* interprets omens. The *mantrin* then continues the ritual on the king's behalf. After the conclusion of the rites, the *mantrin* then proceeds to a more public[108] place. The *Netra Tantra* contains a similar description, in which the *mantrin* moves the rite into a house (*gṛhe*). Kṣemarāja assumes this to be the royal palace (*rājño gṛhe*). Sanderson believes that *gṛhe* refers here to the *śāntigṛha*. This is a temple for appeasement (*śānti*) rites that is often located in the northeast quarter of the palace or the residence of the Śaiva guru.[109]

> Then [the *mantrin*] should carry out the sacrifice—[which] confers *siddhi*—within the palace [*gṛha*] using the method described earlier with abundant oblation, for as long as seven days, O Devi. [The king] then acquires great royal fortune [and an] unconquerable kingdom, as [he] desires. And the king will obtain the *siddhis* of the earth and sky. Then, the [*mantrin* who performs] the *nīrājana* achieves [for himself] all the very best things, [and] destroys the aforementioned faults. O Devi, this is certain to take place. (NT 19.114–116)[110]

Finally, the ritual moves beyond the palace into the kingdom. In the *Netra Tantra*, the king's weapons and soldiers are not consecrated, only the king and his animals.[111] The solitary place (*nirjana*) is secret.[112] The ritual itself is also secret and calls for a separate, public *nīrājana*. The secondary rite enables the king to participate publicly in the ritual and allows for a concurrent Tantric version to take place. In the *Netra Tantra*, the *mantrin* focuses on Amṛteśa while in the center the *Bṛhatsaṃhitā* places the Sun, Varuṇa, the Viśvedevas, Prajāpati, and Indra, around Viṣṇu, in the center.[113]

The *mantrin* then performs further public rites. He places mantras on cows, horses, elephants, and goats. Using Amṛteśa's mantra, he consecrates these animals with red powder, mantra-infused water, and white mustard seeds. The protective *nyāsa* of the kingdom's animals gives them the same security as the king. Every symbol of royal authority calls for systematic protection to strengthen and maintain the king's position of power.

> The *mantrin* should honor [Amṛteśa] in the middle of the cows, from this the herd should increase. He applies vermillion (*sindūra*) or red chalk (*gairika*) infused with the mantra to the tips of the horns of the cow for [their] protection. He should perform the same rite to protect the horses. After he infuses the water jug with the mantra, he should pour it over their heads. White mustard seed (*siddhārtha*), empowered with the mantra [placed] on the throat or head protects the elephants, [so that they] are liberated from all disease. In this way, he should conduct [rites of] protection for all goats and cows, etc. (NT 19.117–120)[114]

Once the *mantrin* has protected the material symbols of royal power, he guards the kingdom against environmental calamities. Earthquakes, famine, and storms can all lead to the downfall of a ruler. The king cannot control natural events, yet they are a threat to his continued rule.[115] In order to prevent natural disasters, the king needs to form allegiances with the deities.

> [The *mantrin*] should [perform] rites and recitations to avert evil and famine, in times of great dangers, [such as] destructive earthquakes, meteors, massive rainfall and drought as well as threats of mice and other pests. He should conduct the ritual when flowers, etc., grow out of season, [when images of gods] are lost or break. [He performs the ritual when people are afflicted by] skin diseases, etc., fevers, untimely death or various sorts of pain, past faults or seizing spirits (*grahadoṣa*). Diseases from snake poison, etc., insect bites, etc., rheumatism, change in form, phlegm, hemorrhoids, eye diseases, skin diseases (*visarpaka*), etc., internal disease, and sickness caused by wounds, etc., by the thousands [can occur]; if various sorts of evils touch the *maṇḍala*, a defect arises from offense. When the deities curse brahmins, men, etc., interior diseases, anguish, and destructive thoughts[116] [occur], then, [the *mantrin* should] conduct the previous rite, for appeasement (*śānti*). (NT 19.121–128)[117]

The *Rājataraṅgiṇī* offers several examples of the sort of disasters described here. Kalhaṇa does not set out specific *nīrājana* rites but does place blame on monarchs for natural disasters. For example, during the reign of Sussala (c. early tenth century), Kalhaṇa says that relief from disaster did not even occur in dreams.[118] Kalhaṇa describes Sussula as a great warrior but whom the goddess of victory, Jayaśrī, abandoned when his troops were attacked by an enemy army.[119] During Sussala's second reign, in 1123, an earthquake struck Srinagar.[120] Sussula was not popular at the time and engaged in constant battle with his adversaries. Kalhaṇa says fire brought fear every day, brave soldiers died, and many other disasters overtook the kingdom. The fierce sun scorched the earth, repeated earthquakes destroyed the cities, and violent storms destroyed trees and rocks. Wind brought dust and severe storms.[121] He describes the fire storms that destroyed the city: The Vitastā[122] river was "lined on both banks with houses in flames, [and] looked like the sword of Death wetted with blood on both edges."[123] He writes that the devastation resembled the "dawn which brings the destruction of the world."[124] Only 100 men remained under Sussula's command and continued to fight until the end.

> Deceived by fate[,] the king bestowed upon his son merely the insignia of sovereignty, but did not hand over to him the government. As soon as the prince had been crowned, the blockade of the City, the drought, the plague, the robberies, and other troubles ceased And so the earth, too, bore rich produce, and in due course the scarcity ceased in the month of Śrāvans. [*sic*]. (RT 8.1234–1236)[125]

Kalhaṇa blames Sussula for these tragedies, though he does not identify religion or specific religious practices mandated during Sussula's reign.

In addition to *nīrājana*, the *mantrin* performs daily rituals to maintain the kingdom. His mere presence suffices to dispense evil. The daily fires provide the *mantrin* with a routine task that requires regular royal sponsorship.[126]

> [The *mantrin*] performs daily fire rites for the prosperity of the kingdom of kings. The [king] enjoys the kingdom happily, there is no doubt. [His] enemies, etc., disappear, even through one *pūjā*. Overcome, they escape into the ten directions like deer etc., from a lion. Poverty disappears from the [king's] family through the continual application of the rites. In whichever place and time the *mantravid* lives, none [of the following] will arise near him: plagues, diseases, *khārkhodas*, *grahas*, *śākinīs* of various sorts, *yakṣas*, *piśācas*, *rākṣasas*, seizers of children, *visphoṭas*, *vyantaras* or *asparas*. Any of the poisons that exist, famine and eclipses, none will arise because of the *mantrin* being there. (NT 19.129–133)[127]

The *mantrin* protects the king and the kingdom through worship. His presence acts as a conduit that connects the monarch with the deity; this turns him into a talismanic figure. His presence suffices to dispel many of the dangers that threaten a king.

Lustration (*Nīrājana*): NT 15.1–19a

In the previous section, I examined lustration (*nīrājana*) rites that protect the king and his kingdom through the enactment of bodily ritual. I now turn to an earlier chapter in the *Netra Tantra*, which explains how the *mantrin* deploys mantra and objects in *nīrājana*. The text constructs a symbolism for these objects and teaches the *mantrin* how best to apply the mantra. The symbolic association of white mustard with its various magical powers is particularly important. The text introduces several varieties of mustard seed[128] and utilizes *nirvacana* to link these names with their effects. Most rely on semantic wordplay and aim to construe the symbolic dialectic of the ritual and serve as mnemonic devices to assist in the performance.

> I shall now explain how the lord of mantra [Amṛteśa] provides all protection, [how] the protector of mantra is strong and great, and how white mustard (*rakṣoghna*) [becomes more effective] when infused with perfume. (NT 15.1)[129]

Many Buddhist and Hindu rituals use mustard seed to cure illness and drive away demons. Mantras render the seeds powerful. The *mantrin* then burns, tosses, or places the seeds on the head of the afflicted in order to chase off spirits.[130] To begin the rite, the *mantrin* infuses the mustard seed with the mantra. This simple action allows the *mantrin* to perform *nyāsa*, which protects the practitioner.

> A person who receives the white mustard seed, [over which the *mantrin*] has recited the mantra seven times, and who always keeps it on his head, he is freed of all faults. (NT 15.2)[131]

The text then explains why the *mantrin* draws on white mustard through what Yelle calls "fictitious (alliterative) etymologies."[132] Such etymologies, also known as *nirvacanas*, are quite common throughout Sanskrit literature.[133] Texts do not deploy them because their writers possess a poor command of Sanskrit. Instead, they serve to explain language and add depth and additional meaning to words used within the text.[134] Authors offer new ways to understand the words and their relationship to ritual objects through the invention of etymologies. While inaccurate from a historical linguistic point of view, they establish secondary associations between words and object. Such *nirvacanas* do not demonstrate misunderstanding or crude interpretation of language but signal a highly developed appreciation for language through plays on nuance and meaning.[135] They reduce the appearance of arbitrariness by naturalizing the way one speaks of events.[136] In other words, *nirvacanas* do not undermine the historical etymologies of words; instead, they deepen the symbolic associations of words and turn them into rhetorical devices that amplify their religious and philosophical meaning.

> [The *mantrin*] says the [Amṛteśa] mantra and performs exorcism to destroy all demons and also all [those] full of all envy. It protects, therefore he calls [white mustard] *sarṣapa*. It protects from all sides. (NT 15.3–4ab)[137]

While *sarṣapa* is the generic name for white mustard, the remaining etymologies use metonymy[138] to create links between the meanings of words and ritual function that serve to explain the natural attributes of the mustard seed.

> Since all *rakṣasas* run away and are killed, then O Devi, I call [white mustard seeds] *rakṣoghna*. They spread on Earth and in all battles between demons and the chiefs of gods. [Mustard seeds] are employed as killers of villains in order to accomplish (*siddhi*) the destruction of enemies. Since their purpose is accomplished then they are called white mustard (*siddhārthaka*) on Earth. They take away pride in evil-minded spirits. (NT 15.4cd–7ab)[139]

The passage introduces two compounds: *rakṣoghna* and *siddhārthaka*. When dissolved they mean "destroying of demons," *rakṣas* (demon) + *ghna* (destroying), and "whose purpose is perfection," *siddha* (perfection) + *arthaka* (*artha* [purpose] + *-ka* [an ending that denotes a doer, that which does]). These words, of course, also mean "white mustard." The etymology developed in the *Netra Tantra* gives white mustard as the primary meaning. It serves as an etymological explanation that describes the function of the mustard. The name given to the ritual object within the ceremony is important precisely because it denotes function. These are common names for white mustard, but the secondary, functional meanings given here require the reader to understand the grammatical and semantic analysis. Such *nirvacana*s also highlight the power of naming as ritual action.

> The *mantrin* who is present to achieve protection should offer the mark of the name (*nāmāṅka*)[140] to Agni in the fire. [He does this] through the performance of a *nīrājana* rite with a mind that is enraged, at a time when all beings everywhere [live in] fear and tremble. It is called *nīrājana* because it causes all good fortune. (NT 15.7cd–9ab)[141]

The noun *nīrājana* stems from the verb stem *nī-rāj* (*nis* +√*rāj* [to cause to illuminate, to shine upon], where √*rāj* also means to rule or to shine). Thus, the *nīrājana* illuminates like fire. It drives back evil, which causes radiance or good fortune.

The text continues to describe *nirvacana*s; its focus here turns to the colors white, red, yellow, and black.

> [When the *mantrin*] confers benefits [during] different ages (*yuga*s), [mustard seeds] appear in [different colors], bright white, etc.[142] When white they are called all-bestowing (*sarvaprada*), when red they are granting the kingdom (*rājyapradāyaka).* When they are yellow they are [said to] cause protection (*rakṣākara*), and when black they cause the destruction of the enemy (*śatruvināśakṛt*). In the four *yuga*s, [mustard seeds] always are bi-colored, yellow and black. That which is known as *rājasarṣapagaura*, O Beloved, this [other] bi-colored [seed] is not visible (NT 15.9cd–11).[143]

The names of the colors of mustard seeds derive from the outcome associated with their ritual use. The *mantrin* must use each color only for the symbolic purpose its name indicates. Such linguistic associations allow the different seeds to become the means to achieve what their names imply. Here a semiotic shift occurs. The signifier changes based on its signified. The mustard seeds themselves (the sign) remain unchanged on the surface level but achieve a new signification.

After it reveals the symbolic attributes of the colors of the mustard seeds, the text describes the rituals that deploy them:

> The *mantrin* should offer the oblation that grants all tranquility [with a] mixture of ghee, cow's milk, ground white sugar, and sesame seeds when one has come under the control of death [or has been] attacked by evil spirits. Indeed, he should offer the highest red mustard (*rājasarṣapa*) together with black sesame sprinkled with three kinds of oils.[144] Instantly, [this] produces the fruit of universal tranquility. (NT 15.12–14ab)[145]

This ritual is a truncated version of the death aversion rite found in the sixth chapter of the *Netra Tantra*. This rite does not serve as an alternative to medical treatment but protects against decay and evil spirits. The *mantrin* seeks to free the afflicted from all disease. He rids the body of evil spirits to bring about peace.

Once the *mantrin* has prepared the offering, he hands it over to the beneficiary. The *mantrin* cannot perform the ritual on behalf of the king without the king's active involvement, even though that participation can take place through a paid proxy. Once the *mantrin* places the mantra into the hand of the beneficiary, the recipient achieves unrivaled prosperity.

> If it is empowered by the [*mantrin*] and placed in his hand, that person shall attain unequalled prosperity (*saubhāgya*); there is no doubt. (NT 15.14cd–15ab)[146]

The *mantrin* protects against all things that might endanger a king's reign. The ritual offers specific benefits, such as safety for the kingdom's crops and livestock. It also bestows prosperity and freedom from faults (*doṣa*). *Saubhāgya* is here a vague sort of prosperity. It does not cover any one area of abundance but points to success, good luck, good fortune, and happiness. *Doṣa* too, which I translate throughout this work as fault, encompasses different kinds of shortcomings that include vice, deficiency, disadvantage, and disease.

> After [the *mantrin*] chants the mantra over [the mustard seed] seven times, he should drop it on the head of [the beneficiary], who then is released from all faults. (NT 15.15cd–16ab)[147]

The *mantrin* continues to infuse his surroundings with mantras. Verses 16 and 17 are incomplete but indicate that cloth may be used as medicine to disable enemies.[148] The text speaks of the importance of both the *mantrin* and the ruler. The *mantrin* pledges himself to the king through the resolve to chant the mantra perpetually, even while asleep. This displays both respect and dedication to the ritual. His participation in the ritual is constant. Withdrawal would prove disastrous as it would bring the protective shield of the Tantric realm to an end.

> The *mantrin* should chant the mantra for the benefit of the consecrated person [the king], in all directions day and night, whether [the consecrated person is] awake or asleep. The [consecrated] man then stays on Earth, evil spirits cannot kill him. (NT 15.18–19ab)[149]

The *mantrin* seeks to maintain his ritual purity so that he can perform these rites for the monarch at all times. The king himself avoids impurity as long as he does not participate in such practices.[150] This allows the *mantrin* to participate in transgressive rites without a king or his proxy. He prevents royal pollution through his ritual activities, even if performed on the king's behalf.

7
Conquering Death Through Ritual

Impurities, *Kāpālika*s, and Exorcism

Purity and impurity are key elements in Tantric ritual practice. Where the orthodox Brahmin performs the rituals in order to retain purity, the Tantric transgresses purity. The latter's participation in rituals that use substances deemed impure, such as meat, fish, human blood, or skulls, is an important characteristic of Tantric practice.[1] Törzsök notes an important difference in the way Siddhānta and Bhairava Tantras understand pure and impure substances. On the one hand, the dual (*dvaitācāra*) practices of the Siddhānta see purity and impurity as a binary. Practitioners determine what is pure and impure based on canonical and cultural expectations. They then make use of practices and substances deemed pure and reject the impure.[2] On the other hand, the Bhairava Tantras teach a non-dual (*advaitācāra*) practice. *Advaitācāra* rites involve the mixing of pure and impure substances.[3] In the commentarial tradition of Kṣemarāja, Bhairava Tantras, including the *Netra* and *Svacchanda Tantra*s, are read in a way that cancels binaries such as pure/impure, auspicious/inauspicious, and worshipped/sacrificed. Instead, these categories commingle. This leads to the creation of a new class that transcends binary classification.

The use of impure substances appears in the fifth century *Niśvāsatattvasaṃhitā*, the earliest extant Śaiva Tantra.[4] This demonstrates an early Tantric association with impure substances and raises the as yet unanswered question as to what or who inspired the use of polluting materials within the ritual context. Sanderson[5] and Wedemeyer[6] concur that Tantric practice stemmed from the cemetery ground rites of *kāpālika*s. Lorenzen traces the appearance of *kāpālika*s in the literary tradition to the Prakrit poem, *Gāthāsaptaśatī*. This text, traditionally attributed to the first century, likely dates to the third to fifth century.[7] In the *Gāthāsaptaśatī*, a woman incessantly covers herself with ashes from her lover's funeral pyre.[8] The approximately fourth-century Buddhist *Lalitavistara*[9] contains "fools" who smear their bodies with ashes in search of purification. Though not called

Illness and Immortality. Patricia Sauthoff, Oxford University Press. © Oxford University Press 2022.
DOI: 10.1093/oso/9780197553268.003.0008

*kāpālika*s, they also wear red garments, have shaved heads, carry triple staffs, pots, skulls, and *khaṭvāṅga*s.[10] These objects call to mind the *kāpālika*s, ascetics who cover themselves in ashes, carry human skulls as begging bowls, and call forth fierce deities such as Bhairava. By the sixth and seventh centuries, literary references to *kāpālika*s had become abundant.[11] During this same period, the *Niśvāsatattvasaṃhitā* was disseminated and came into its final form during the seventh century.[12] Wedemeyer contends that *kāpālika* practice could not have existed without institutional support. This support would have been available only to those of higher castes.[13] Further, Wedemeyer argues that *kāpālika* activities also would have made little impression on high-caste society if practiced by members of society's fringe or lower castes.[14] This appears to be the case, as very little extant textual evidence demonstrates a literary interest in the religious practices of low-caste or tribal people. However, this does not prove that *kāpālika* behavior was influenced solely by elites—simply that there is no existent record of their influence.

Sanderson explains how Kaula secret societies split from *kāpālika* cemetery groups. This shows that Kaulas reduced *kāpālika* ritual behaviors to their more erotic essentials.[15] This allowed the Kaulas to move almost entirely away from cremation ground activities. Kaulas turned to more internalized practices.[16] However, internalization still included orgiastic worship and casteless interactions.[17] These practices penetrated court and intelligentsia circles. The satirist Kṣemendra judged them to be one of the most significant social evils of his time.[18] The Kaula's apparent non-Vedic, heterodox rituals redefined impurity as the state of bondage and ignorance. Here, impurity and purity become illusory categories that bar the individual from the recognition of the divine.[19] Rather than focus on the pure-impure dichotomy, the practitioner is to abolish all distinctions between the two.[20] Flood explains the connection between the monarchy and the *kāpālika*-like practices.

> Although the [*Netra Tantra*] has connections with royalty, it also bears witness to popular possession and exorcism rites which were probably pervasive among lower social levels. Indeed, one of the main tasks of the orthopraxy of Brāhmaṇ was to prevent possession. These "demons" (*bhūta*) and powerful female deities or "mothers" (*mātṛ*) enter through the "hole" (*chidra*) of the shadow of impure men and women whose behavior is bad (*durācāra*) and who have neglected their ritual obligations, so causing the evil eye (*dṛtṣtipāta*) to fall upon them.[21]

Flood argues that possession practices were the dominion of those at the lower end of the social scale. But this statement ignores the scriptural tradition of the Bhūta Tantras, which focuses on exorcism.[22] Sanderson has compiled two lists of the canonical Bhūta Tantras, one taken from the *Śrīkaṇṭhīya* and the other from a text prefixed to the *Jñānapañcāśikā*.[23] Unfortunately, few manuscripts of complete Bhūta texts survive.[24] The *Netra Tantra* is one of the few extant texts to provide examples of the exorcistic and apotropaic rites of the Bhūta Tantras.[25] Despite the loss of the Bhūta Tantras, they were at one time important enough to be classified among the five major categories of Tantric Śaiva literature.[26] Sanderson traces the Gāruḍa and Bhūta Tantras as they became excluded in textual classification systems.[27] The eighth-century[28] *Brahmayāmala Tantra* is an early example of a text that reduces the importance of the Gāruḍa and Bhūta categories.[29] This indicates that the Bhūta Tantras became theologically less important over time. Flood's association of exorcism with lower society is not supported by literary evidence.[30] Though pushed to the margins, the Bhūta Tantras were not dismissed completely. Kṣemarāja turns to the Bhūta *Kriyākālaguṇottara* in his commentary on the *Netra Tantra*.[31] This demonstrates that, though marginalized, the Bhūta Tantras remained an important resource for exegetes.

Apotropaic rites appear early in the textual record. The oldest sections of the *Atharva Veda* contain healing poems, magic, and destructive sorcery.[32] Slouber's study of early Tantric medicine reveals that Gāruḍa Tantras, which focus on snakebite venom and other poisons, share references with the *Atharva Veda*.[33] Further, the *Chāndogya Upaniṣad* mentions *bhūtavidyā* as a possible pre-Tantric tradition of exorcism.[34] These attestations demonstrate that exorcism did not set itself apart from the orthodox praxis of the Brahmanical tradition. Exorcism was not exclusively the domain of the lower classes.

The Vaiṣṇava Pañcarātrin *Viṣṇudharmottarapurāṇa*[35] calls for the king to appoint an Atharvavedin Brahmin as his personal priest.[36] The *Viṣṇudharmottarapurāṇa* aims to convince monarchs of the Pañcarātrins truth rather than that of their Pāśupata Śaiva rivals.[37] However, it also urges the monarch to perform devotional works and build temples in order to displace Vedic sacrificial customs.[38] In other words, the *mantrin* is both an expert in the Vedas and introduces a new sacrificial paradigm to the court. This allows him to perform both Vedic and non-Vedic rites. Sanderson argues that Śaiva officiants legitimized dynastic power through the foundation of temples. They developed specialized rituals that drew on their expertise in the

Atharva Vedic rites to protect the monarch.[39] Further, Geslani demonstrates the brahminical relationship between Arthavedins and monarchs, especially in the lustration (*nīrājanā*) rites.[40]

Vanquishing Death: *mṛtyu vañcana*

Rites that focus on the vanquishment of death appear in many Sanskrit texts. Many rely on mantras for protection from death. The *mṛtyuñjaya* mantra, meaning conquering death, appears in the *Ṛg Veda*. It is unclear when the Vedic mantra was first called *mṛtyuñjaya*.[41] Regardless, the purpose of the mantra is clear. The *mantrin* recites the mantra in ritual so that he or his benefactor overcomes death. The *Atharva Veda* also includes references to rituals that ward off or destroy (*apa-√han*) death.[42] Gonda notes several references to early domestic rites that allow one to overcome death.[43] The *Bṛhadāraṇyaka Upaniṣad* says that the divine is far from death: "the divine is named *dūr* because death is far (*dūra*) from him. Death is far from him who knows this."[44] It then explains how speech becomes fire when it crosses beyond death. Similarly, smell becomes air, sight becomes the sun, hearing becomes the directions, and mental perception becomes the shining moon.[45] In other words, the senses have the ability to pass beyond death without becoming obliterated. The *Bṛhadāraṇyaka Upaniṣad* then instructs the priest to recite the verses: "from the unreal lead me to the real, from darkness lead me to light, from death lead me to immortality."[46] In this verse, death and darkness are the unreal; light and immortality are the real. Death, then, is something that can be bypassed. Einoo[47] charts a variety of verbs used in passages that develop ideas of how to overcome death. His work demonstrates how difficult it is to ascertain what constitutes overcoming death. Some texts simply use conquer (*√ji*); others draw on more complex verbal formulations such as "remove by means of an offering" (*ava-√yaj*), "conceal" or "render invisible" (*antar-√dhā*), or "repulse" (*prati-√nud*).[48] Some Buddhist[49] and Haṭha Yogic[50] texts use conquer (*√ji*) or cheat (*√vañc*) to describe this process.[51]

Tantric Sanskrit texts that describe victory over death through ritual were translated into Tibetan in the tenth and eleventh centuries.[52] These texts became part of Tibet's Buddhist tradition.[53] As a result, these, the *mṛtyu vañcana* rituals found in Buddhist texts and those found in the *Netra* and *Svacchanda Tantra*s have much in common. This includes the goal to control death through mastery of disease and the use of mantras, *maṇḍalas*, and meditative imagery. The mantras, *maṇḍalas*, and meditative imagery in Buddhist and Śaiva traditions are also similar. Sanderson[54] argues that the *Cakrasamvara* is closely related to several early Śaiva Tantras, and that it may itself have originally been a Śaiva work that was transformed to comply with Buddhist conventions.[55] In Tibetan, death ransom rituals are known as *chilu*.[56] *Chilu* rites are prescribed only when the beneficiary of the rite is about to die prematurely. It is a grave sin to perform a *chilu* rite when death is irreversible or occurs at the proper time.[57] Like the practices found in the *Netra Tantra*, *chilu* rituals involve the invocation of the deity, mantras, and *maṇḍalas*,[58] as well as the performance of alchemical medicinal rituals.[59] The Buddhist *Mṛtyuvañcanopadeśa* (tenth or eleventh century)[60] indicates there are always both signs of death and a fixed time for death.[61] The *Mṛtyuvañcanopadeśa* explains how to cheat death if the signs of imminent death are identified early enough. These signs may be external or internal. They include astrological changes, bodily symptoms of illness, and ominous dreams.[62] It claims that "some who have died in a number of ways can be seen to live again."[63] These rituals draw on a variety of impure bodily substances, including blood and urine. Practices listed in the *Mṛtyuvañcanopadeśa* that draw on bodily substances are far more heterodox than anything in the *Netra* or *Svacchanda Tantras*.[64] The *Netra* and *Svacchanda Tantras* allow for impure substances to be mixed (*miśraka*) in ritual.[65] However, neither the *Netra Tantra* nor *Svacchanda Tantra* prescribes antinomian practices. Instead, they hint at such practices and allow for their performance, but do not require them.

> The *Netra Tantra* goes beyond death conquest to include lifespan, strength, victory, loveliness, firmness, wisdom, a beautiful form, and good fortune, the highest kingdom for kings, all of these arise. Tormented by pain, [the ritual beneficiary] will be without pain; someone marked by disease will be without disease; a barren woman [will] obtain a son; a girl [will] attract a husband. [The beneficiary] will surely attain whatever pleasures he wants. (NT 6.46–48ab)[66]

Like immortality, these goals are not easy to attain. Beauty, good fortune, or offspring may appear to be within reach, but in reality they require the same level of ritual intervention as the conquest of death.

Maintaining the Physical Body

The *Netra Tantra* employs the terms *amṛta* or *amṛtatva* to describe its ultimate goal. Both can easily be translated as "immortal" or "immortality." Etymologically, both come from the root √*mṛ*, meaning "to die," with the inclusion of the negative *a-* prefix. Hence, both mean "non-dead," or "immortal." This etymology does little to clarify or add ontological nuance. In Vedic mythology immortality is the preserve of the gods.[67] Their immortality is defined by perpetual life.[68] According to Scharfe, the Vedas also indicate that humans can attain a non-eternal life in heaven.[69] The *Chāndogya Upaniṣad* says, "[He who] stands in Brahman attains immortality."[70] Immortality can also refer to fame or through offspring, though these too run the risk of transiency.[71] The cycle of rebirth (*saṃsāra*) also complicates the idea of immortality. Does immortality mean the cessation of a single death or of *saṃsāra*? As Scharfe demonstrates, there is not one answer to the question "What is immortality?"[72] The *Netra Tantra* does not provide an answer to this question either. Einoo and Scharfe point out that immortality often means a life of 100 years or a life that is lived to its full duration.[73] The *Netra Tantra* often speaks of averting sudden or untimely death (*apamṛtyu*).[74] Therefore, this definition of immortality, as the full duration of one's life, makes sense in the context of the *Netra Tantra* with respect to non-salvific rites. I assume this definition in my focus on the rites to overcome death (*mṛtyu vañcana*) as a supernatural power (*siddhi*) that both avoids sudden death and eliminates illness.[75]

Three chapters of the *Netra Tantra* focus on yoga. The three approaches (*upāya*) are gross (*sthūla*), subtle (*sūkṣma*), and highest (*para*).[76] In this chapter I focus only on the *sthūla* methods because I have set out to explore ritual behavior as it impacts the world. I focus on rites that protect the living king. At the *sūkṣma* and *para* levels, the text emphasizes the metaphysics of yoga and turns its focus away from worldly outcomes.[77] The *sūkṣma* and *para* chapters say little about ritual. Neither chapter refers to the use of *maṇḍala*s. For example, Chapter 7 focuses on the vanquishment of death by the drawing of breath through the channels (*nāḍi*) and centers (*cakra*) of the *sūkṣma* body.[78] Chapter 8 instructs the *mantrin* how to quiet the senses and mind in order to conceive of the universal essence of Amṛteśa.[79]

After brief preliminaries, the *Netra Tantra* introduces the three yogic methods:

> The method is threefold: gross (*sthūla*), subtle (*sukṣma*), and highest (*para*).
>
> The *sthūla* [method consists of] sacrifice, oblation, mantra recitation, [and] meditation, together with *mudrās*, the *mohana yantras*,[80] and so forth. The king of mantras (*mantrarāṭ*) [i.e., *oṃ juṃ saḥ*] brings about [relief].[81]
>
> The *sukṣma* [method contains] yoga of the *cakras*,[82] etc., and by upward momentum [of breath] through the channels (*nāḍī*).[83]
>
> The *para* [method], is Mṛtyujit, which is universal and bestows liberation. (NT 6.6–8)[84]

Rastogi explains that the threefold yoga of the *Netra Tantra* mirrors the tripartite nature of mantra,[85] as discussed in Chapters 1 and 2. *Sthūla* corresponds to the most embodied manifestation of mantra, the limited condition (*aṇu*). It also refers to Netra, as the protector.[86] The etymology of *sthūla* is to become big, to grow, to increase (√*sthūl*).[87] *Sthūla* is synonymous with *pīna*, *pīva*, and *pīvara*, all meaning fat or dense.[88] These gross bodies are "one-time-only aggregations of the gross elements,"[89] and are subject to death and disease. This does not designate the transmigratory body but that which remains at the time of death. *Sthūla* practice focuses on the alleviation of illness and the defeat of death.

> When [the *mantrin*] perceives the power of death, when death touches and sees [a person], then he should worship Amṛteśa with the aim to repulse [death]. He employs the name [of the afflicted],[90] [and] should worship all-pervading *Mṛtyujit* with entirely white ornaments, according to the rule taught before [in previous chapters focused on daily ritual]. He [who is ill] quickly escapes from death. My speech is true and not false. According to the rules for the great protection[91] [rite, the *mantrin*] should make an oblation in the name of [the afflicted] into a fire fueled with holy wood. [This fire burns] in a round pot [adorned] with three girdles. [The *mantrin*] uses sesame seeds soaked in ghee and milk [mixed] together with white sugar. Even for someone gone to Yama's abode [i.e., someone who has died],[92] great peace arises quickly. *Mṛtyujit* is sure to destroy death when pleased with an oblation of fragrant ghee put into a fire fueled by milk-tree wood. (NT 6.9–14)[93]

This passage indicates that the daily rituals described in the *Netra Tantra*'s earlier chapters offer a quick escape from death. Why then another configuration? The rituals the *Netra Tantra* describes here are typical of rites performed to achieve a specific desire (*kāmya karman*) found throughout Indian religious literature.[94] They are optional and practiced to obtain a specific result. Often they relate to the worship of a particular deity.[95] Though escape from death may be quick, it is wholly dependent upon the will of the deity. Thus, the more difficult the objective, the more complex the rite becomes.[96] Larivière points out that the optionality of *kāmya* rites does not mean the ritual specialist is free to perform or omit the rites. Instead, *kāmya* rites can only be performed if the *mantrin* is able to do so completely and to perfection.[97] *Kāmya* rites tend to be long rituals that often last for several days.[98] Public *kāmya* rites are only to be performed by those who have attained the highest level of initiation (*ācārya*). Those who hold a *sādhaka* initiation may perform the rites in private.[99] In the Śrīīvidyā Tantric tradition, those who have not performed the obligatory rites (*nitya karman*) must not perform *kāmya* rites. Therefore, the *mantrin* must fulfill both the Vedic and Tantric obligations first, before he can perform desire-based rites.[100] The royal priest must be an Atharvavedin. This means he too must be able to perform Vedic and Tantric rites. The professional *mantrin* is a person who relies on a visible post-initiatory discipline in order to justify his own professional necessity.[101] Initiation itself confers liberation, but the officiant must continue ritual repetition as proof of his own qualification to perform rituals for clients.[102] It should also be noted that *kāmya* rites are never performed to gain liberation. Kumārila's famous verse confirms this:

> If one desires liberation, one should not engage in motivated (*kāmya*) [rites] or forbidden acts. One should perform [only] one's regular and incidental [duties. But one should do so not in view of any reward but simply] to avoid the negative consequences [of failing to perform them.][103]

Easing the Pain of Death and Disease

The *mṛtyu vañcana* rite begins with a preparatory fire oblation. It consists of standard ritual offerings such as honey, milk, and ghee. The fire is fueled by the wood of milk trees (*kṣīravṛkṣa*).[104] Milk trees come in four types: Indian fig (*uḍumbara*), bodhi (*aśvattha*), banyan (*nyagrodha*), and Ashoka tree (*madhūka*). All have white sap and are commonly used in rites of pacification and prosperity.[105] Additionally, the rites call for guggula resin (bdellium). The seventh-century *Harṣacarita* describes the use of guggula[106] in a rite to avert the death of Harṣa's father, Pabhakaravatdhana.[107] The *Devī Purāṇa*[108] relates how kings should honor Indrāṇī with clothing, ornaments, perfumes, milk-rice, ghee, and guggula resin. In return, the goddess fulfills all desires and gives the king longevity, health, and sovereignty.[109] A donation grant from the seventh century refers to a guggula-pūjā at a temple of the deity Kāpāleśvara,[110] which ties the rites to the charnel ground *kāpālikas*.

Once the offering has been issued, the *mantrin* recites the mantra *oṃ juṃ saḥ* around the name of the rite's beneficiary.

> [Mṛtyujit] instantly destroys fever as a result of an oblation into a fire fueled with milk tree wood. This is the oblation that destroys all bad things. [It] consists of five *amṛtas*: sesame seed, rice, honey, ghee, and milk. Someone with a diminished body quickly becomes nourished through an oblation of chick-pea sized pellets of the resin of the guggula tree [that have been] oiled three times in strict religious observance. When a man is seen to be afflicted with one hundred diseases [and] weak, [he] is released [when the *mantrin*] envelops his name [with the *mṛtyuñjaya* mantra] and recites [it]. (NT 6.15cd–18)[111]

This extract demonstrates that *mṛtyu vañcana* rites aim to alleviate illness as well as untimely death. The text calls for the guru to utilize the *mṛtyuñjaya* mantra to protect the sick. However, it also allows for any mantra to serve as the *mūla* mantra.[112] The act of enveloping (*saṃpuṭa*)[113] protects from the use of an ineffective or mispronounced mantra.[114] To envelop, the *mantrin* simply recites the *mūla* mantra ahead of the name and again at the end, this time in reverse.[115] For example, *oṃ juṃ saḥ* [name] *saḥ juṃ oṃ*. In addition to protection against a performative error, the palindromic enveloping disarms any counter-rituals that one's enemies might undertake.[116] Here the *Netra Tantra* refers to recitation (*japa*) of the mantra. Kṣemarāja adds that enveloping is also used when the *mantrin* writes the mantra and name on the *maṇḍala*.[117]

> Any mantra that a wise man should recite, is enveloped by Amṛteśa. This mantra quickly [brings] him success, even if he is without good fortune. (NT 6.19)[118]

The encapsulation of the name with the mantra or other ritual elements, including script and *maṇḍalas,* marks a transition of the mantra. It shifts from "language to non-linguistic, physical reality from within language itself, therefore virtually and figuratively."[119] In other words, when the *mantrin* envelops the name of the afflicted with the mantra, he surrounds the name (and thus the person himself) with the purified deity. The *Kulārṇava* and *Gandharva Tantra*s explain:

> At the beginning (of the mantra) is the impurity of birth, and at the end, the impurity of death. A mantra which is joined to these impurities does not succeed. Having removed the (impurities of) beginning and end, the wise one should chant the mantra. A mantra which is released from this pair of impurities leads to all success.[120]

The *mantrin* also envelops medicine with the mantra to help to pull this body immediately away from death. For the *mantrin*'s continued spiritual power, the medicine needs to be supplemented by prayer.[121]

> [The *mantrin*] envelops medicine [consisting of herbs][122] with the mantra. [He then] gives [the mantra wrapped medicine] to [the person whose][123] body is weak. At that very moment, his body gains nourishment and [becomes] strong. (NT 6.20)[124]

The *Netra Tantra* does not cite any specific medicinal remedies. Nor does it say that the *mantrin* should diagnose illness or administer medical treatment. The passage does not reveal whether the *mantrin* contributes to some form of medical treatment or diagnosis. Neither does it spell out how closely the *mantrin* worked with an Āyurvedic physician.[125]

8
Maṇḍalas

Maṇḍala: Locating the Divine in the Physical World

The *Netra Tantra* has little to say about the nature of *maṇḍala*. It presumes that the *mantrin*, a highly trained professional religious officiant, is versed in the use of *maṇḍala*. In earlier chapters, I discuss the specific *maṇḍalas* laid out in the *Netra Tantra* for use in its protective rites. Here I introduce *maṇḍala* as a general Tantric concept.

White describes the *maṇḍala* as "the hallmark of Tantric theory and practice, mesocosmic template through which the Tantric practitioner transacts and appropriates the myriad energies that course through every level of the cosmos."[1] In other words, the *maṇḍala* is the cosmos made manifest so that the practitioner can engage with it. Further, he notes that the *maṇḍala* has its origins in royal power, coming from the Vedic notion of the king as *cakravartin*, he who stands at the center of the wheel and turns the kingdom that surrounds him.[2] This means that the king must watch over and expand his kingdom in all directions. In the *maṇḍalas* included in the *Netra Tantra*, the *mantrin* writes the name of the person afflicted with illness in the central space of the *maṇḍala*. He then writes the mantra at each of the eight cardinal and inter-cardinal directions for protection. This allows the *mantrin* to envelop the person with protection. The lotus flowers described in the *Netra Tantra* have either eight, sixteen, or thirty-two petals. This allows the practitioner to place the letters of the alphabet around the afflicted in the same way that he places the deity and his protective elements around him during worship.

Brunner describes the principal elements of *maṇḍalas*. Her work distinguishes *maṇḍala*, *cakra*, and *yantra* and identifies the differences among the three.[3] Bühnemann[4] refines Brunner's distinctions, explaining that the three terms are often used interchangeably within texts.[5] Brunner discusses three types of physical *maṇḍalas*: "seat *maṇḍalas*," "image *maṇḍalas*," and "distributive diagrams," plus a fourth type that consist of

Illness and Immortality. Patricia Sauthoff, Oxford University Press. © Oxford University Press 2022.
DOI: 10.1093/oso/9780197553268.003.0009

mental objects.[6] *Maṇḍalas* of the last type stand apart from the others.[7] Seat *maṇḍalas* lack a clear physical structure and are used to protect the deities or ritual objects that are placed on them.[8] Image *maṇḍalas* are geometric designs made with colored powders that are destroyed after their use. They are also called "powder *maṇḍalas*." Finally, distributive diagrams are surfaces divided into squares into which the *mantrin* invokes a divine or demonic power for placation.[9]

The *Netra Tantra*'s death-conquering rituals use only image *maṇḍalas*. The *Svacchanda Tantra*'s rich visualizations do not draw on *maṇḍalas* at all. The *Netra Tantra* also describes the use of a *cakra* in addition to a *maṇḍala*. The *cakra* here is a diagram that is drawn onto the *maṇḍala* and represents the divinities that are present. Törzsök discusses the use of the terms *maṇḍala* and *cakra* in the *Svacchanda Tantra* and other early Śaiva texts where the distinction between the two is often unclear.[10] In the death-conquering ritual, no such ambiguity exists. *Maṇḍalas* act as surrogates for physical bodies. The *mantrin* invokes the body of an individual by writing his name.

Maṇḍalas of Protection

The *Netra Tantra* does not disclose information like the overall dimensions of *maṇḍalas*, but it does specify the materials the *mantrin* should use to draw it. Once drawn, he places (*nyāsa*) the mantra and the name of the afflicted person on the *maṇḍala*. This empowers the *maṇḍala* and summons the deity.[11]

Törzsök examines the *maṇḍalas* used in the *Svacchanda Tantra*'s initiation process. The moment at which the initiand sees deities on the *maṇḍala* is the point when he transforms into an initiated practitioner.[12] For many, the initiation rite is the only encounter with the *maṇḍala*.[13] Though ritual manuals speak of *maṇḍalas* as optional in daily rites,[14] they are essential in occasional and initiation rites.[15] However, sight of the *maṇḍala* during initiation is not always required. The *Parā-trīśikā-Vivaraṇa* says that one who knows the *bīja mantra* is initiated even if he has not seen the *maṇḍala*.[16]

Maṇḍalas, like mantras, are not symbolic representations of the divine. They are physical structures that function as devices through which a practitioner witnesses deities.[17] During rites, the practitioner views the deities in the *maṇḍala*, not as icons but as literal manifestations of the deities.[18] In the next section, I explain the technicalities of *maṇḍalas* in greater detail.

Let me turn first to the rites described by the *Netra Tantra*. The text first calls for a preliminary visualization in which the living being (*jīva*) is connected to the mantra. In this case, the *jīva* is a diseased or dying person for whom the *mantrin* performs the ritual. The text says that the *jīva* exists in the heart lotus (*hṛtpadma*). This is a common non-dual Śaiva Tantra trope used for internal practice.[19] The *hṛtpadma* is especially important in the *Svacchanda Tantra*'s yogic instruction.[20] It designates the place within the body where the practitioner enshrines the deity. This practice is similar to the initiation (*dīkṣā*) rite described in Chapter 5, where the *mantrin* replaces the body of the initiand with a new, tantricized body. Again, the text calls for a protective enveloping (*saṃputa*) as a preliminary measure:

> The being (*jīva*), is enclosed with [the syllables] *saḥ*, etc. [This rests] in the middle of the lotus of the heart, [which] is in the middle of the orb of the moon. [This done, the *jīva*] escapes from death completely. After [the *mantrin* has] enclosed [the *jīva*] with syllables beginning with *saḥ*, etc.,[21] [the *mantrin*] masters the procedure. [That is, he] should visualize [the encircled *jīva*] in the body. [The afflicted] is sure to become free from all disease, of this there is no doubt. (NT 6.21–22)[22]

After the *mantrin* connects the afflicted's body with the mantra, disease washes away. The *mantrin* then calls to mind the nectar (*amṛta*) that purifies and cleanses the diseased body.

> Delighted, [the *mantrin*] should visualize [the *jīva*] in his own or someone else's [body][23] being flooded by waves of *amṛta*, in the middle of a lotus on the ocean of milk, enclosed between two moons one above and one below, enclosed by the syllables *saḥ*, etc. He [visualizes his] body, beautiful inside and out, filled with nectar. [He is] freed without exertion and without trouble, and liberated from any sickness. (NT 6.23–25ab)[24]

This passage is reminiscent of the *Mālinīvijayottaratantra*:

> And now the supreme secret, the acme of the *amṛta* of Śiva's gnosis is described for the destruction of disease and death in yogins. [The yogin] should visualise Parā in her own form pouring forth *amṛta* in the sixteen-spoked wheel in the void, whose hub is formed by the moon. Armed with the previously[-described] *nyāsa*, for an instant (?) the wise [yogin] should

> then lead his tongue to the uvula and insert it [there]. He should visualise the white heavenly *amṛta*, flowing from the orb of the moon. . . . Drinking it, within six months he effortlessly becomes free of decrepitude and disease; after a year he becomes a conquerer of death. Once it has become sweet-tasting thenceforth his mouth fills up with whatever flowing substance he, with focused mind, visualises in it, such as blood, alcohol or fat or milk to ghee and oil etc."[25]

In both passages the *mantrin* (or yogin) visualizes *amṛta* flooding the body. In the *Netra Tantra* the orbs of the moon envelop the *jīva* in much the same way as the mantric *saṃputa*. They surround and therefore protect him. In the *Mālinīvijayottaratantra* passage, *amṛta* flows directly from the moon. While the *Mālinīvijayottaratantra* is clearly of a more transgressive nature than the *Netra Tantra*, the texts share symbolism. Kṣemarāja often cites the *Mālinīvijayottaratantra* in his exegetical work.[26] The importance of the *Mālinīvijayottaratantra* in the Śaiva system is apparent as Abhinavagupta chose it as the foundational text for his work and for the *Tantrāloka*.[27]

Kṣemarāja says that the *mantrin* should imagine the *jīva* seated on the moon disc at the pericarp of a white lotus, in the center of the ocean of milk. One moon is above and another is below the seated *jīva*. The *amṛta* flows from the upper moon. The *jīva* envisages the waves of the ocean filling his body inside and out, surging up with the brightness of moonlight. The body, enclosed by the mantra, then becomes free of disease.[28] This visualization shares imagery with the *Svacchanda Tantra*'s meditation on *amṛta*.

The *Netra Tantra* next introduces the first *maṇḍala*. Here it instructs the practitioner to draw rather than imagine the image. The text retains its moon imagery through the moon (*candra*) *maṇḍala*. The *candramaṇḍala* occurs in many Śaiva and Buddhist Tantras.[29] In the *Netra Tantra*, the person afflicted with disease is encircled by lotus petals and *vajras*.[30] The *yogin* writes the name of the afflicted person in yellow bile and saffron ink in the middle of a white lotus. This is enclosed by the *candramaṇḍala*, which protects in the same way as the enclosed mantra.

> Enveloped by *saḥ*, etc., [the *mantrin* writes the name of the person] afflicted by all diseases in yellow bile and saffron mixed with milk on the middle of a white lotus with eight petals. [This he] encloses in the *candramaṇḍala*, set in a square, and decorates it with Indra's *vajras*. [The afflicted] is then cured of the torment of all diseases, there is no doubt. (NT 6.25cd–27)[31]

Kṣemarāja explains that the *maṇḍala* should be drawn on birch bark or another appropriate surface using a mixture of cow bile, saffron, and milk. The *mantrin* should write the mantra in full on each petal of a white lotus. He then inscribes the name of the afflicted on the lotus's pericarp and *vajras* in each corner. The *candramaṇḍala* is a moon disc with sixteen faces.[32] The sixteenth phase of the moon is the *amṛtakalā*, which corresponds to the sixteenth *kalā* of the lunar fortnight when the moon is invisible. The *amṛtakalā* is portrayed as an immortal moon and corresponds to the *visarga*.[33] It is the supreme energy of consciousness.[34]

As the *mantrin* draws each *maṇḍala*, lotus petals double in number. The first *maṇḍala* has eight petals, the next sixteen, and the last one thirty-two. In the eight-petaled lotus, each petal points toward the cardinal and intermediate directions. This allows each deity associated with a direction to be placed on the corresponding petal.[35] The structure of these *maṇḍalas* resembles the *siddhi maṇḍalas* in Chapter 9 of the *Svacchanda Tantra*.[36] Here, the *maṇḍalas* and *yantras* protect the practitioner from death[37] by means of Bhairava's various forms. The *maṇḍalas* that ward off death often require the placement of the name of the diseased person at the center. The *mantrin* focuses both on the afflicted and the deity in order to merge them. Though the text leaves room for the mantra to vary, the deity does not. The deity must appear in the most appropriate form of Bhairava for its specific purpose.[38] In other words, the *mantrin* must pray to the correct deity, otherwise death may not be averted. Death rituals of other sects are ruled ineffective.[39]

The *Netra Tantra* then presents another moon *maṇḍala*: the *śaśimaṇḍala*. Its description is less precise than that of the *candramaṇḍala*, though it shares some qualities. The *Netra Tantra* describes the *śaśimaṇḍala* has having sixteen petals and sounds, both common descriptors of the moon. The Tantric moon contains sixteen phases in its waxing and waning cycles.[40] The last of these, again, is the *amṛtakalā*.[41] The sixteen syllables correspond to the Sanskrit vowels[42] and the *ādyanta* pattern consists of the mantra, followed by the name of the afflicted, then the mantra repeated again three times.[43]

> [The *mantrin*] should write the name [of the afflicted] in the middle of a great wheel [that] has sixteen petals. [He] adorns [the petals] with the sixteen vowels, and encloses it with the mantra using the *ādyanta* pattern. The *mantrin* should draw, as before, the *jīva*[44] in the middle of *saḥ*, etc., protected at the end with the covering [i.e., the mantra]. The *amṛteśa*[45]

> mantra envelops [him] on all sides, at each syllable, in the middle of all petals, in the middle of the lunar orb (*śaśimaṇḍala*). The twofold lotus outside follows the sequence [of consonants that] begins with *ka* and ends with *sa*. [This is] enclosed with the syllables *saḥ*, etc. and in that is the name of the person to be healed. Outside [of this, the *mantrin* draws] the disc of the sun (*arkamaṇḍalam*), and below he should completely surround it on all sides beginning in the east. (NT 6.28–32ab)[46]

Once again, the *mantrin* writes the name of the afflicted in the center of the *maṇḍala* and surrounds it with a protective mantra.

This passage reveals that the *Netra Tantra* is very specific about the way to write the mantra. Padoux argues that "in principle mantras cannot be but oral since their nature is that of the word, of the primal *vāc*, identical with the formless absolute."[47] However, there are many instances in which written mantras occur, both in and outside of ritual.[48] In these cases, the written form is linked to the nature of mantras themselves.[49] For example, the *Nayasūtra* of the *Niśvāsatattvasaṃhitā* introduces a series of physical gestures that correspond to the written form of the phonemes.[50] The *Nayasūtra* connects the letters to the *tattva*s and explains:

> Without knowing the *tattva*s [as] situated in the body, and all the letters as they are situated in the body, one cannot be liberated. All these I shall teach you [as they are] written visibly. Some have the shape of parts of the body; some have the shape of the [whole] body [arranged in particular ways].
>
> Putting the hands against [the sides of] the body and the shanks next to one another, [with] the whole body stretched out [straight, one makes one's body] the shape of the "formless" letter *a* (*niṣkalākaravigraham*).[51]

In the *Nayasūtra*, even the formless letter assumes a "written" shape. This formless letter does not correspond to any written script, hence it is called "formless."[52] The *Nayasūtra* then explains how to best position the body so that it corresponds to the written shapes of the characters of the Gupta alphabet.[53]

Similarly, the cosmological basis for *bindu* and *anusvāra* is rooted in their written and verbal articulations. Padoux describes the *bindu* as a "drop" of concentrated phonetic energy. It is the point at which the energy of the word gathers upon itself before it divides itself and spreads outwardly to manifest both its power and the universe.[54] A dot or drop represents the *bindu*.

It constitutes the point that pierces the target at which the mantra aims.[55] The *anusvāra* appears as a dot above a nasalization to indicate its prolongation. It is the graphical and phonetic manifestation of the *bindu*.[56] Likewise, the *visarga*, the sixteenth vowel, is graphically depicted as two dots, the division of *bindu*. It manifests sonically as the escape of breath after a vowel at the end of a word.[57] Graphically then, the written mantra corresponds to the shape of the breath. When the *mantrin* commits the *mṛtyuñjaya* mantra to writing, he places the *śārada* letter, which corresponds to the shape of the mouth made during vocalization, onto the *maṇḍala*.[58] Thus, he connects the sonic with the physical to further empower the mantra and place it within the body of the practitioner.

Maṇḍala and Color

Maṇḍalas rely on the power of mantra to achieve an effect. The mantras that the *mantrin* writes on these diagrams constitute an integral part of *maṇḍalas*.[59] The name of the afflicted, surrounded by petals infused with various phonemes and the mantra *oṃ juṃ saḥ*, appears first. The *mantrin* then encloses this with characters of the alphabet from *ka* to *sa*. The first set of letters consists of the vowel sounds plus *aḥ* and *aṃ*,[60] the second includes the consonants.[61] Finally, the *mantrin* surrounds the whole diagram with the syllables.[62] When the *mantrin* surrounds the name of the afflicted with the mantra, he protects the afflicted person and activates the mantras. Yelle describes the process of enclosure of the central element—in this case, the name used in the ritual—as a transition, "between the 'outside' portions of the mantra and the 'inside' [which] is taken as analogous to the relationship between language and the physical reality: instead of simply stating that 'the word was made flesh,' mantras actually diagram this transition by degrees."[63] In other words, the sounds that surround the mantra lead the *mantrin* into a place where language controls physical reality. The mantra transitions into the body of the afflicted. As it is synonymous with the deity, the divine enters into and transforms the physical body.

A thirty-two-petaled lotus, where each petal represents one of the Sanskrit phonemes, except *ha* and *kṣa*,[64] encircles the *śaśimaṇḍala*. This is the typical *śabdarāśi*, ordering of the alphabet.[65] The *mantrin* merges the name of the afflicted with the mantra and places (*nyāsa*) both on the *maṇḍala*. This fuses the three elements together.

The *Netra Tantra* does not explore the symbolism of its *maṇḍalas*, but other texts do. For example, the Buddhist *Cakrasamvara Tantra* discusses ritual and symbolic elements of *maṇḍalas*. It shares many of these elements with the *Netra Tantra*, such as in its description of a lunar (*śaśin*) *maṇḍala* that brings relief from ailments and disease.[66] The *Cakrasamvara* describes the moon (*śaśin*) as visualized on the left hand of the practitioner.[67] It is a disc that includes a figure with nine parts, eight of which surround a center, which feature the syllable *oṃ*. The parts that surround *oṃ* each contain a syllable.[68] This is similar to the *candramaṇḍala* above, save for the *vajras* and the reference to the four directions. The *Cakrasamvara* says that after visualizing the *śaśimaṇḍala* in the left hand, the "crystalline syllables"[69] appear. The practitioner then places these five syllables "on all areas"[70] presumably on the *maṇḍala*. According to Gray, this creates a diagram of five squares, laid out in the form of a cross, with four more squares at the corners creating a nine-square grid.[71] The points of the cross correspond to the *vajras* of the *candramaṇḍala*. Again, this *maṇḍala* is very similar in composition, though not identical in form to its counterpart in the *Netra Tantra*. These similarities reveal the close relationship between the two texts.

The *Cakrasamvara*, like the *Netra Tantra*,[72] speaks of a "king of mantras" (*mantrarāṭ*). It is this mantra that renders the ritual powerful. Unlike the *Netra Tantra*, in which the *mantrin* inscribes the *mantrarāṭ*, in the *Cakrasamvara* "a king of mantra is born in whatever place to which he directs his thoughts."[73] Rather than an inscription, the *mantrarāṭ* is a mental construct. The *mantrin* does not need to write the mantra but is able to produce it through mediation. In both cases, the deity and the mantra are literally and figuratively identical. Irrespective of the way in which the mantra is generated, its use manifests the divine in the physical world.

The *Cakrasamvara* also explains the symbolic associations of the *maṇḍala*'s colors. The colors white, black, red, and yellow often appear as part of ritual diagrams in Tantric texts, including the *Netra Tantra*. The *Netra Tantra* instructs the *mantrin* to write the name of the afflicted with red lotus and saffron ink mixed with milk. He then mutes yellow pigment with milk. The *Cakrasamvara* describes the symbolism of the colors thus:

> One pacifies with [the color] white, and one kills instantly with black. With red one subjugates and summons in a moment. With yellow, all are subdued—this is the fixed opinion of the teaching. With yellow, one subdues an army with its boats, war machines, and elephants. Just by contemplating the white, the dead are revived. (CS 43.22–25)[74]

This extract contains a selection of the symbols connected with white, black, and yellow. Other texts, both Hindu and Buddhist Tantric associate yellow with the *bhūmaṇḍala* (earth *maṇḍala*) or simply with the Earth itself.[75] Vīravajra's *Padārthaprakāśikā-nāma-śrīsamvaramūlatantraṭīkā*, a commentary on the *Cakrasamvara*, associates yellow with enrichment[76] and the defeat of enemy military forces.[77] Control over armies enriches the monarch and extends his life and legacy. The *Netra Tantra* describes the symbolism of the color of mustard seeds in the *nīrājana* rite. White represents appeasement, red grants a kingdom, yellow causes protection, and black leads to the destruction of an enemy.[78]

The ritual also calls for honey and white, jasmine flowers, camphor dust, sandalwood, and milk.[79] These ingredients add a sensory element to the rite.[80] This rite is associated with the visualization of Rudra found in Chapter 2 of *Svacchanda Tantra*.[81] The *Svacchanda Tantra* also describes a relationship between the ritual described here and the lustration (*nīrājana*), examined in Chapter 6. *Mantrins* perform both rites for the king to protect his life and kingdom.

The *Netra Tantra* then returns to practical matters:

> The *mantrin* should worship the *cakra* with white flowers, after [he] has written the *mantrarāṭ* in grey with camphor dust, together with white sandalwood, and after he has applied milk and yellow pigment, O great goddess. [The *mantrarāt*] provides great protection and bestows good luck and prosperity. [The *mantrin*] should place [the mantra] in the middle of honey, together with completely white offerings. After acting this way for seven days, he becomes Mṛtyujit. [The *mantrin*] explains to kings how best to protect kings. [Protection] removes the enemy's arrogance and grants favors at the time of battle. (NT 6.32cd–36ab)[82]

The *śaśimaṇḍala*, with its center and eight parts, is the locus for the *navātman* mantra.[83] The latter corresponds to nine *tattvas*. Kṣemarāja associates the *tattvas* with the following phonemes: *śiva* (*ha*), *sadāśiva* (*ra*), *īśvara* (*kṣa*), *vidyā* (*ma*), *māyā* (*la*), *kāla* (*va*), *niyati* (*ya*), *puruṣa* (*ū*), and *prakṛti* (*auṃ*).[84] The *Svacchanda Tantra* explains how to place these *tattvas* onto the petals of the lotus.[85] The *mantrin* begins in the northeast (with *prakṛti*) at the upper left, moves clockwise to east, and ends in the center of the flower.[86] Kṣemarāja describes this *maṇḍala*, which he calls *navanābhamaṇḍala*.[87] It is used as part of the purification in the initiation ritual.[88] The *Netra Tantra* reverses the direction of placement. The *mantrin* begins in the center, at *śiva*, and works his way outward. This connects the afflicted with the divine. The *navātman* mantra often appears without its supporting vowels.[89] This renders it inarticulable.

Finally, the *mantrin* prepares a mixture of medicine, water, jewels, and a white lotus in his water pot and anoints the body of the diseased person. The *mantrin* uses additional white elements when he worships on the *maṇḍala*. Here, for the first time, the physical body of the afflicted person is actually present and involved in the ritual.

> The *mantrin* [writes the name of the person] who wishes to become Amṛteśa as well as the nine *tattvas*, starting with *śiva*[90] in the *śaśimaṇḍala*, from the middle going east, etc. When overcome with 100 illnesses or threats of untimely death, then [the *mantrin*] conducts worship with white implements, or with ghee mixed with milk, or with sesame seeds, or [he] uses fuel made of milk[-tree wood]. From [this] oblation [the afflicted] attains peace. Then, after [the *mantrin*] has honored [Mṛtyujit], with a great and auspicious battle-cry, he anoints [the sick person] on the head, [with a substance from] from a pot with a spout that resembles a white lotus, filled with water that contains jewels, [and includes] all kinds of [medicinal] herbs. [Originally] afflicted by various disease, he is [now] liberated, there is no doubt. (NT 6.36cd–45)[91]

The *mantrin* can also perform the ritual on behalf of someone who has already died. The text does not indicate whether a proxy takes the place of the deceased or if the rite takes place prior to or during cremation. Mirnig points out that the Śaiva *mantrin* is deeply involved with Śaiva death rites. As described in early Śaiva sources, initiatory cremation occurs by repeating the initiation rite with the *tattvas* reversed.[92] The use of an effigy in place of the individual is prescribed though the circumstances of that use are not made clear. However, in the brahmanical tradition, an effigy made of *darbha* grass or cow dung may be used in the case of death under inauspicious circumstances or when the corpse is unavailable or badly deformed.[93] Though not made explicit in the text, it is likely that such a proxy may be utilized in the post-death liberatory rites of the *Netra Tantra*.

9
Visualizing Amṛta
SvT 7.207–225

The *Netra Tantra* should not be read as a stand-alone work. It relies on its reader to be familiar with a wide variety of Śaiva works. Further, it was composed after and with much awareness of the *Svacchanda Tantra*. Kṣemarāja comments on the texts together, which further indicates a long-standing connection between the two works.

Unlike the *Netra Tantra*, which assuages the threat of death through ritual, the *Svacchanda Tantra* does so through meditation. The *Netra Tantra*'s seventh and eighth chapters on subtle (*sūkṣma*) and highest (*para*) yoga do teach meditation. However, they focus more on the movement of energy through the subtle body and recognition of Mṛtyujit by suppressing the senses. I focus on the *Svacchanda Tantra* here rather than the *Netra Tantra* as the *Svacchanda Tantra* contains far more details and richer imagery than the *para* chapter of the *Netra Tantra*. In the *Svacchanda Tantra* the practitioner conquers death through contemplation. He visualizes himself moving through the cosmic order (*tattvas*). As he proceeds through the various states, the practitioner defeats both death and time. To do this, he focuses on the deified form of *amṛta*, Amṛteśa.[1]

The *Svacchanda Tantra* teaches *kālamṛtyujaya*. This *tatpuruṣa* compound can be read conquest (*jaya*) of time (*kāla*) and death (*mṛtyu*) or conquest of untimely death (*kālamṛtyu*).[2] Kṣemarāja gives no clarification. He describes *kālamṛtyu* as a supernatural state (*siddhi*) in which the practitioner achieves union with Bhairava.[3] I prefer to leave the term *kāla* untranslated since it can convey both "time" and "death."[4] The *Svacchanda Tantra* speaks of victory over "the three times" (*kālatrayaṃ vijānāti*): the past, present, and future. To conquer them is to vanquish death. Therefore, the ambiguity of the text's use of the word *kāla* reinforces the notion that victory over time and death are synonymous.[5]

Meditation, in the *Svacchanda Tantra*, focuses on breath control, drawing on the *haṃsa* mantra.[6] The *haṃsa* mantra allows the practitioner to move

Illness and Immortality. Patricia Sauthoff, Oxford University Press. © Oxford University Press 2022.
DOI: 10.1093/oso/9780197553268.003.0010

through the *tattvas* in order to conquer past, present, and future.[7] Through this practice, he vanquishes death. In this visualization, the *yogin* manifests *amṛta*, which floods the body.[8] It leads to the attainment of the *siddhis* and knowledge of the *tattvas*. This, in turn, leads to the command over death.[9] This meditation requires a seasoned *yogin* to devote himself to a difficult and esoteric practice that offers him an escape through death by way of liberation.

In order to conquer death, the practitioner must spend six months in meditation.[10] Once achieved, the practice must continue indefinitely so that the practitioner does not risk a return to the world or a return to time. The *Svacchanda Tantra*, like the *Netra Tantra*, sets out the purpose of the practice but conceals the method from the uninitiated. Kṣemarāja writes that it is intended for only the highest, most experienced *yogins*.[11]

Mṛtyu vañcana[12] rituals deploy material objects and physical action to eliminate death. Meditation practice seeks a different kind of bodily transformation.[13] Unlike in the *Netra Tantra* where the *mantrin* enters the body of another to unite them with Śiva, in the *Svacchanda Tantra* the *yogin* cannot perform meditation on behalf of another person. The individual finds release through his own practice.

Much of the meditation imagery of the *Svacchanda Tantra* mirrors what we encountered in the *Netra Tantra*. The *yogin* visualizes either Bhairava or the *haṃsa* mantra in order to gain control over *kāla*. The syllable *haṃsa* manifests as Śiva's creative and destructive breath.[14] *Haṃsa* is combination of *ha* and *sa*, which represent Śiva and Śakti,[15] respectively. It is also a palindrome of *saḥ aham*, or *so 'ham*, meaning "I am that," i.e., the divine.[16] Abhinavagupta proposes *haṃsa* to represent the syllables *ka* to *sa*.[17] The *Svacchanda Tantra*'s *yogin* enunciates the mantric phonemes through his breath. The connection with breathing (*haṃ*/in-breath and *saḥ*/out-breath)[18] enables the *yogin* to emit the mantra constantly as he breathes. With each breath, the *yogin* creates and destroys the entire universe.[19]

> After [the *yogin* has] visualized Bhairava, who is the Lord of Kāla, or [has focused] on *haṃsa*, who is the Lord of All, [the breath], which travels through the pathways of the nostrils, emits and absorbs the universe. (SvT 7.207)[20]

The continual cycle creation and destruction constitutes time. There is no end to the breath as it waxes and wanes. It generates a deity that is both inside and outside the practitioner's body. The life-sustaining nature of breath is the path to *amṛta*. This *amṛta* brings about a state that exists beyond physicality. Once the *yogin* "establishes himself in that state, he can make everything happen,[21] situated among all beings."[22] His presence among the world's beings—including those who have already died and those not yet born—demonstrates the yogin's conquest of time.[23] The *yogin* creates everything through the focus on his breath. This practice spreads the *haṃsa* mantra throughout the world. Time itself has no beginning or end. What is situated in time is located everywhere simultaneously.[24] It is a form of practice that is similar to what is mapped in a later[25] *haṭha* yoga text, the *Khecarīvidyā*. Here, the *yogin* is instructed to worship the *liṅga* "at the place where day and night are suppressed."[26] This allows the *yogin* to conquer death. In the *Khecarīvidyā*, the *yogin* worships and focuses on the *liṅga*, but he cannot create it because it is "free from the process of time."[27] The *liṅga* is, of course, identical with Śiva in the same way as the mantra and *maṇḍala* are synonymous with Śiva.

Returning to the *Svacchanda Tantra*, the text describes the *yogin* situated in his breath so that he can conquer death.

> [The *yogin*] dwells there [in breath]. He should impel all [creation], [and is] situated among all beings. After [he has] meditated upon [*haṃsa*], he conquers death. The powerful Lord does not create that which is not situated in *kāla*. (SvT 7. 208)[28]

The destruction of death is the first step in the meditation process. Once the *yogin* has conquered death, he turns his attention to the higher states of cognition that bring him closer to the divine.

> For one engaged in meditation, after six months, omniscience arises. The knower of yoga is yoked with *kāla*. He recognizes the three times [the past, present, and future]. (SvT 7.209)[29]

The play on *kāla* in this passage is important. When the practitioner transcends time, he simultaneously transcends death. *Kāla* also refers to one of the pure/impure (*śuddhāśuddha*) *tattvas*. When the *yogin* transcends the *tattvas*, and all they represent, he moves up the cosmological map toward the highest *śiva tattva*.

In the next verse, the *yogin* focuses on the *kālahaṃsa*. This mantra, which translates as "time" or "death" *haṃsa*, allows its user to become Śiva. *Kāla* spans time and death: to become Śiva is to be time and death, i.e., to create and to destroy.

In mythology, Śiva appears as Kālāntaka, the Destroyer of Death/Time.

> Śveta was a virtuous king, a devotee of Śiva; everyone in his kingdom was happy. Yama and Kāla came to take him one day when he was worshipping Śiva. Then Śiva, the Destroyer of Kāla, looked at Kāla with his third eye and burnt him to ashes in order to protect the devotee. Śiva said to Śveta, "Kāla eats all creatures, and he came here to eat you in my presence and so I burnt him. You and I will kill evil men who violate dharma, heretics who wish to destroy people." But Śveta said, "This world behaves properly because of Kāla, who protects and creates by destroying creatures. If you are devoted to creation you should revive Kāla, for without him there will be nothing." Śiva did as his devotee suggested, he laughed and revived Kāla with the form he had had. Then Kāla praised Śiva, the Destroyer of Kāla, and Kāla went home and told his wife Māyā and all his messengers never to bring any devotees of Śiva to the world of death, but to bring all other sinners.[30]

This extract, from the *Skanda Purāṇa*, suggests that only a devotee of Śiva is able to escape death fully. It is only possible because Śiva is dedicated to the act of creation. Through the revival of Kāla, he allows time to continue.

Through time (or death, *kāla*) the world continues to flourish. Without the breath nothing is created or destroyed, and nothing at all exists. When the devotee becomes *kāla*, he creates and destroys through the *haṃsa* mantra.

> Either by reciting or meditating on the *kālahaṃsa*, O Goddess, [the practitioner] becomes Śiva [who] has the form of *kāla* and acts freely (or as Svacchanda) like *kāla*. Death has been destroyed, [the *yogin*] has abandoned old age, is free from all danger [caused by] disease, [he] knows, learns, and daydreams. [He] gains the all-supreme *siddhi*s, [which] arise constantly as a result of conquering *kāla*. (SvT 7.210–212ab)[31]

Following the attainment of the *kāla tattva*, the *yogin* moves through the series of hierarchical *tattva*s that confer the powers of the deities. First, he attains those of Brahmā, Viṣṇu, and Rudra before he finally reaches the state of *sadāśiva*. This ranks among the highest of the thirty-six *tattva*s and culminates in the dissolution of the individual into the divine. Once this occurs, a practitioner in "*parāvasthā* (the highest state) of Bhairava is free (*unmukta*) of all notions connected to direction (*dik*) [and] time (*kāla*). He cannot be particularized (*aviśeṣiṇi*) by some definite space (*deśa*) or designation (*uddeśa*)."[32] En route to this unpredicated state, the *yogin* adopts the life span, qualities, and powers of Brahmā, Viṣṇu, and Rudra.[33]

> After [the *yogin*] has meditated [on *haṃsa*] in the right nostril, he obtains the powers of Brahmā. He obtains length of life [and] power equal to [Brahmā].[34] As a result, he [the *yogin*] knows the past. (SvT 7.212cd–213ab)[35]

Brahmā, called Svayambhū, is the self-born or self-created. Now equal in power to Brahmā, the *yogin* is entrusted with the act of creation. He knows the past because he created it. The *yogin* then attains a life span that spans 36,000 Brahmā days.[36] Each Brahmā day consists of two *kalpas*—one for the day and the other for night. Each *kalpa* is made up of 4.32 billion years.[37] The total life span of Brahmā measures 311.04 trillion human years.[38] Although his life will not be infinite, the *yogin* with a life span of Brahmā must continue his meditation in perpetuity.

> Next, the *yogin* acquires the power and life span of Viṣṇu.
>
> When he [visualizes *haṃsa*] in the left [nostril], he knows the future and is equal in strength to Viṣṇu. The king of *yogins* [gains] a life [that] is as long as Viṣṇu's, [and] obtains power [equal to] Viṣṇu's. (SvT 7.213cd–214ab)[39]

Brahmā creates the world; Viṣṇu preserves it. The constituent parts of *haṃsa*—*ha*, *ṃ*, and *sa*—shows Brahmā represented by *ha* and Rudra designated as *sa*. This leaves Viṣṇu as the *anusvāra* between the two phonemes. Viṣṇu is the master over past, present, and future. His life is 1,000 times longer than that of Brahmā.[40]

The *yogin* who attains the life span and power of Viṣṇu then continues his meditation to become equal to Rudra.

> When meditating [on *haṃsa*] in the middle [i.e., the retention of the breath in the central channel][41] or by constant[42] yoga and meditation, the *yogin* knows past, present, and future. He becomes the same as Rudra. (SvT 7.214b–215a)[43]

Again, the phonemes *ha* and *sa* are linked to the states that the *yogin* enters in his meditation. Abhinavagupta connects the phoneme *sa* with the *īśvara tattva*.[44] Here, the practitioner realizes that there is no otherness outside of his own I-ness.[45] However, because his I-ness does not cease, he is not fully released from self, and/or death.

> [He who possesses the] same longevity, strength, beauty, and power as [Rudra] obtains the state of *īśvara*. [He achieves this] because he [has attained] the highest state (*parabhāva*) of Brahmā. (SvT 7.215cd–216ab)[46]

Finally, the *yogin* accomplishes the states of *sadāśiva* and *śiva*. In the *Parātrīśikāvivaraṇa*, Abhinavagupta links *ha* with *sadāśiva*.[47] It closes the mantra.[48] In *sadāśiva*, the *yogin* approaches the end of his practice. Only *tattvas* remain: the inseparable states of *śiva* and *śakti*.[49] At *sadāśiva*, the *yogin* recognizes "I am this." In other words, he cognizes his union with the deity even though he retains a slight notion of I-ness.[50] It is only when he has shed this enduring sense of individuality that he truly conquers death. Only pure knowledge remains; the physical body is irrelevant.

> Because he [attains] the highest state of Viṣṇu, the *yogin* obtains the sovereignty of *sadāśiva*. A person who visualizes the highest state of *rudra* becomes Śiva. Thus, the conquest of death called *amṛta*, is called a "conquering meditation." (SvT 7.216cd–217)[51]

Now that it has laid the groundwork for mantric recitation, the text turns to visualization. In its imagery, the *Svacchanda Tantra* runs parallel to the *Netra Tantra*. However, rather than draw *maṇḍalas*, here, he visualizes the images. In the *Netra Tantra*, the body is represented within the *maṇḍala*, the central image of the rite. In the *Svacchanda Tantra*, the inverse takes place: the body becomes the object of meditation and the imagery springs from within.

> After [this, the *yogin*] visualizes the heart lotus, with sixteen petals, situated in the opening of the channel that pierces the tube [i.e., the lotus stem. He imagines] a white, radiant, completely full moon, endowed with sixteen parts,[52] and with his body in the shape of a lotus pericarp. [Then, he pictures] the self. It is to be imagined [as seated] in the middle of that [moon], and is as spotless as pure crystal. [The self is] pervaded with *amṛta*,

> [which washes over him] in a wave from the ocean of the milky nectar of immortality. (SvT 7.218–220ab)[53]

The heart lotus (*hṛtpadma*) is a common image in Tantric literature. The Śaiva Siddhānta *Parākhya Tantra* describes eight tubes that reach into the eight petals of the *hṛtpadma*. These stems link to various places in the body, all connected with the breath.[54] In the *Netra Tantra* (6.21), the lotus sits in the middle of the moon. The practitioner visualizes the body, enchained by the *mūla* mantra *saḥ*, etc., in the middle of the *maṇḍala*. In *Svacchanda Tantra* 7.220, the practitioner focuses on the seed, itself the body of the moon—one single spot in an ocean of *amṛta*. For true immortality to occur, the seed dissolves into the ocean just as I-ness dissolves into the divine.

The *Netra Tantra* places the *jīva* of the afflicted in the midst of the *amṛta* flooded by two moons: one above and one below (19.89–91). The *Svacchanda Tantra* replaces the *jīva* with an *ātman* and substitutes a lotus for the moon. In the *Netra Tantra*, the *jīva* is encircled with the syllables *saḥ*, etc., while the *Svacchanda Tantra* reverses the mantra and surrounds the *ātman* with *haṃsa*. The *Netra Tantra*'s practitioner visualizes the body, the *Svacchanda Tantra*'s *yogin* imagines *amṛta* as it surrounds and enters him.

> [The *yogin*] should visualize a second lotus above him in the great ocean with the power of *amṛta* as well as a lotus with its full moon mouth[55] pointed downward. In the middle of that, he should visualize *haṃsa* joined with the *bindu* and topknot. He should visualize a divine rain of *amṛta*, falling everywhere and imagine [it to] enter [his body] in the opening above himself [i.e., the path through the center of the body (*suṣumṇā*) through which the *ātman* rises to *śakti tattva*]. (SvT 7.220cd–222)[56]

The *yogin* conquers death through the visualization of his body flooded with *amṛta*. In the *Svacchanda Tantra*, *amṛta* enters the meditative body from above.

> He should visualize a white, very dense, unctuous *amṛta*, which destroys death and himself [when he is] flooded and filled with it. (SvT 7.223)[57]

The *yogin* allows the nectar to overwhelm his body so that the nectar becomes his body. Once *amṛta* has washed over him, he attains his goal of overcoming death.

> He should visualize his entire body flooded with nectar entering through the openings and apertures of his channels, which are set in the stem of the lotus. (SvT 7.224)[58]

When the *yogin* can no longer chant the *haṃsa* mantra, when his breath comes to an end and he has shed his physical body, he conquers death. His body is the mantric body. It secures the conquest of death. A *yogin* "whose self is constantly thus, becomes the same as Amṛteśa."[59]

The text then returns to the physical anxieties concerned with death. Even though the *yogin* continues to breathe, his activity does not exceed the experience of the power he attained through meditation. Since he is yet to shed his body, I-ness continues to exist. The *yogin* is advised to experience as little of that I-ness as possible. He continues his practice, visualizing himself as self, located within the single seed of the moon, reflected in the ocean of milky *amṛta*. "After he has abandoned diseases, death, and becoming old, he plays with minuteness,[60] etc."[61] Through this process, he attains and stays within *sadāśiva*, connected to the world through the slightest sense of an individual self.

> Thus, from his meditation on *amṛta*, the *yogin* conquers time and death or stays in the highest *tattva*. He is no longer bound by any aspect of time (SvT 7.226).[62]

Social Implications

The composers of the *Netra* and *Svacchanda Tantra*s offer two different pathways to immortality. In the former, a professional *mantrin* performs yoga on behalf of a patron afflicted with illness and impending death. In the latter, the *yogin* focuses on his own internal experience through which he visualizes his path to Amṛteśa. Both require a symbolic lexicon that prompts the practitioners to use and understand different ritual elements. They both draw on mantras, *maṇḍala*s, and visualization techniques.

Here, I explore the yoga of immortality in the *Netra* and *Svacchanda Tantra*s to help us understand what the texts mean when they speak of immortality. To this end, I examine a number of theories about purity and the development of *mṛtyu vañcana* practices. I focus on the technical detail of these rites, not on their cosmological underpinnings.

I shall now briefly comment on the social implications that spring from successful *mṛtyu vañcana* rites. For a monarch, the conquest of death means that he can continue to rule his kingdom with the help of the deities. The rites of appeasement that that *yogin* performs on his behalf safeguard his health and allow him to live to the end of his natural life.[63] Even though the *mṛtyu vañcana* rites of the *Netra Tantra* are, in theory, available to all, the chief audience is here the royal chaplain.[64] He benefits from their performance economically and in terms of status. As a side effect, he too gains health and long life. The *yogin* in the *Svacchanda Tantra* does not accrue physical or economic rewards. He achieves liberation. He must already be highly practiced to perform the meditation. He continues with his practice to attain immortality in the highest states of consciousness.

My study of the conquest of death does not go beyond the *Svacchanda* and *Netra Tantras*. Many other texts discuss similar rituals. A thorough study of Buddhist and Hindu *mṛtyu vañcana* rites would provide a more nuanced understanding of immortality in Indian thought. Similarly, an expanded study of the yoga chapters of the *Netra Tantra* is necessary. Bäumer has begun this work through her recently published translation of Chapters 7 and 8 of the *Netra Tantra*.[65]

Finally, I agree, of course, with Sanderson that the literature of Śaiva Tantra reveals little historical information.[66] Ironically, this presents an interesting opportunity for the historian. It is not possible to study the religious practice of women in the *Netra Tantra*, for example. This is so because the text does not speak of female practitioners. However, I can approach the text as a social historian. In this way it is possible to examine the texts in conversation with one another in order to recreate the theological conversations that took place among the members of the different belief systems over time. I have attempted to do just this by comparing sections of texts with one another, such as the *Cakrasamvara* or the works of Abhinavagupta. To recreate the philosophical dialogues in the texts allows us to better understand the world in which our subjects lived.

Conclusion

As I bring this work to a close, I want to first reflect briefly on its development. I began the research on what came to be this work in 2012. Since then five books and articles have been published that deal directly with the *Netra* and *Svacchanda Tantras*. Prior to this work, Sanderson's 2004 article "Religion and the State" and Brunner's 1974 "Un Tantra du Nord" were the only comprehensive studies of the *Netra Tantra*. Arraj's 1988 "The Svacchandatantram" and Törzsök's 2003 "Icons of Inclusivism" provided an entry point to the *Svacchanda Tantra*. This work will join Flood, Wernicke-Olesen, and Khatiwoda's forthcoming translation as the newest scholarship on the *Netra Tantra*. This wave of interest in the text during the research process allowed me to make key decisions, such as to focus only on corporeal yoga rather than the entire system of yoga. As the project has grown, been pared back, and grown again, I have left pages and pages of ideas and translations in boxes under my desk. Some will likely be revised and make it into the world while others will continue to take up precious space. Interesting as they may be, they simply do not fit within the book presented here.

My goal with this work was to examine and contextualize the protective rites laid out in the *Netra Tantra*. As the work developed, I became more and more interested in the practicalities of ritual. Thankfully, I had chosen the right text. The *Netra Tantra* offers rich descriptions of the mantras, *maṇḍala*s, and meditations that lead one away from illness and toward immortality. Though I am not trained as an art historian, my years as an arts journalist drew me time and again to the sculptural record. This is often difficult with Tantra as the physical record rarely matches that of the literary one. Again, I was fortunate to have chosen a text whose descriptions do match a small number of bronze and stone pieces. Not only does this offer practical, historical information but it also allowed me to write a work that is at times heavy on the theoretical and at others filled with colorful stories. My intention is to offer readers various entry points to the text.

In this work I explore several themes: ritual elements and iconography, the development of Tantric identities, and rites related to the conquest of death.

Illness and Immortality. Patricia Sauthoff, Oxford University Press. © Oxford University Press 2022.
DOI: 10.1093/oso/9780197553268.003.0011

On their own, each of these subjects offers new insight into medieval Śaiva Tantra. Together, they provide a comprehensive picture of the position of the *Netra Tantra* relative to other medieval Śaiva Tantric treatises.

In the first three chapters I examine mantra and iconography. This serves to contextualize the text within the corpus of medieval Tantric literature. I argue in Chapter 2 that Kṣemarāja, in his commentary on both the *Netra* and *Svacchanda Tantras*, allows for mantras to be considered actions. This interpretation impacts how mantras are encoded within Tantric literature and their use in ritual. I also explain that the nature of mantra is tripartite: gross (*sthūla*), subtle (*sūkṣma*), and supreme (*para*). This corresponds to the three types of yoga charted by the *Netra Tantra*. The three methods offer the practitioner three levels of mantric practice. I also compare the text's presentation of mantra with other Tantric works, including the *Mālinīvijayottara*, *Svacchanda Tantra*, and *Kulārṇava Tantra*. This allows me to map mantric theory within the wider body of Tantric literature.

In Chapter 3 I examine the visualized representations of deities worshipped as part of calendrical rites.[1] Here, I discuss the factors common to descriptions of these deities in the *Netra Tantra*. Ultimately, the text explains that all deities are to be worshipped as *Netra Tantra*'s main godhead, Amṛteśa or Mṛtyujit. For example, the *mantrin* is to visualize Amṛtalakṣmī, Bhairava, Tumburu, Nārāyaṇa, Māyā, Sūrya, as well as the Buddha with the hand-gestures (*mudrā*) of wish-fulfillment and protection. This allows the *mantrin* to worship Amṛteśa in his various forms while continuing his protective practices. The symbols of the divine in the *Netra Tantra* return time and again to protection and wish fulfillment.

The production of Tantric iconography allows the practitioner to build a Tantric identity that exists in addition to, but separate from, his social self. The deities and *maṇḍala*s that the Tantric practitioner visualizes contain symbolic Tantric elements. Similarly, during the process of initiation (*dīkṣā*), the initiand is exposed to Tantric symbolism. In Chapter 4, I examine how the practitioner attains his Tantric identity and how it shapes his interaction in the non-Tantric world. I argue that the caste erasure that occurs during initiation is limited to the ritual sphere. This is attested in the practice of lustration (*nīrājana*) in which the monarch is honored. Clearly, in this rite the social hierarchy must remain in place. I also argue that caste hierarchies post-initiation are replaced with a hierarchy of initiatory status. Here, disciples hold different responsibilities and reside in different levels of reality (*tattva*) on initiation. Though caste distinction disappears during practice, the *Rājataraṅgiṇī* and other medieval Sanskrit works reveal that engagement across castes remains problematic for members of the upper echelons of court society. As a result, purity and impurity within ritual bleed into the social sphere with real-world consequences.

This leads to a discussion of the practicalities of *nīrājana*, the lustration of arms. In this rite the king, kingdom, and world are both protected and maintained through the constant use of mantras and maṇḍalas. Chapter 6 examines the rite as a microcosm for the worldly realm and discusses the importance of transgression with regard to the monarch. The *Rājataraṅgiṇī* describes the presence of Tantric *mantrins* in medieval Kashmiri courts. Kalhaṇa's descriptions of rites and behaviors demonstrate that he was aware of the influence of Tantric practitioners. The rites then were, at least at court, semi-public. The *mantrin* would have performed rituals for the monarch without suspicion. The *Netra Tantra* describes many of such rites. I focus on those of lustration (*nīrājana*) and death-conquest rituals (*mṛtyu vañcana*). In each, the *mantrin* performs rituals for the monarch to protect him from both worldly and supernatural dangers. The hazards range from military hostility, disease, famine, and poverty to supernatural threats. The *mantrin* also performs protective rites for the king's family. This assures the longevity of the kingdom and the royal line. In both cases, he performs the rituals away from public view. The lustration rite appears in several ancient Indian texts but rarely in a religious treatise. The religionization of the practice legitimizes the *mantrin*'s role in the rite and as a member of elite society.

Stepping away from the monarch, I discuss the *Netra Tantra*'s gross (*sthūla*) yoga practices, which are available to any initiate. Here, the *mantrin* performs rites (*mṛtyu vañcana*) to alleviate illness. I contrast this rite with the visualization found in the *Svacchanda Tantra*. The *Svacchanda Tantra* shares imagery with the *Netra Tantra*, but focuses on the outcome of liberation rather than worldly gain. The *mantrin* performs both *nīrājana* and *mṛtyu vañcana* for the king. To conquer death, the *mantrin* builds protective *maṇḍalas* that appease the deities. These constitute visual representations of the Tantric world. Ritual is a complex system of activity that relies on many layers of symbolism. The symbols imbue the ritual with power. To understand them allows the practitioner to develop his Tantric identity. I then turn to immortality. I compare the ways in which Sanskrit texts approach the conquest of death to produce health, good fortune, and other worldly achievements. This work demonstrates the importance of the *mantrin* to the continued social fabric of the kingdom through his unique circumstances in which he is always engaged in ritual practice.

Notes on Methodology

Scholars embark on the study of Tantra from a range of methodological and theoretical perspectives. Some seek to explore the philosophical questions posted by the texts, others set out to examine the genesis and spread of practice. I have attempted to align these approaches, following the socio-historical approach of Alexis Sanderson. I build upon Sanderson's own study of the *Netra Tantra* by reflecting on the social implications of the practices laid out within the text. Sanderson analyzes the relationship between the *mantrin* and the king; I explore the ritual implications of the practices and how they help tie society together. Tantric texts do not say much about the world outside of their own belief system. Yet, it is important to contextualize them in an attempt to understand their place in the wider society. I agree with Sanderson that academics should attempt to read Tantric texts through a social and historical lens. I do this through textual analysis and by comparing the rites in the work to the available information we have about Tantric practice. Despite the limited availability of historical documents from the period, it is possible to contextualize the rituals and sociopolitical positions of the people who performed the rites cited in the Tantras. Such a technique humanizes both the practitioners and the practice. It reveals the way in which practitioners fit into society. This allows us to trace the development of both ideas and practices over time and to map the emergence of the different religious schools.

Through this approach, I have found the *Netra Tantra* to be a consistent and important work. It clearly lays out an important argument regarding the nature of mantra that adds a nuanced understanding to scholarly arguments and situates the text in a way that demonstrates that the same questions that plague us today—such as health and longevity—were critical to the development of Tantric traditions in the past. While the philological approach has been crucial for the mapping of Tantra as it developed, a purely language-based approach ignores the impact that practices and ideas had on individuals. This reminds us that the text is part of a tradition of real-world practitioners who struggled to make sense of their world in some of the same ways as the modern academic.

Notes

Introduction

1. White 2012: 145.
2. Sanderson 2004: 273.
3. Sanderson 1988: 664.
4. White 2012: 1, 145.
5. Törzsök 2014: 196.
6. Sanderson 2009: 273.
7. Shāstrī 1926: preface.
8. NAK MS 9/32, 5/689, 1/280, 1/1076, 5/1976, 5/689; Microfilm E139/2, E789/47, H 388/18, E 711/17, I 32/22, E 928/25, H 937/20, E 128/41, E 770/2, E 78/9, H 397/8, H 334/19, E 2082/2, A 1298/5.
9. NAK MS 1/285.
10. NAK MS 9/305.
11. NAK MS 5/4866.
12. Bäumer 2018: 4; Flood, Wernicke-Olesen, and Khatiwoda *forthcoming*.
13. Padoux 1990.
14. Sanderson 1988: 688–670; Hatley 2018: 9–10.
15. Staal 1989.
16. Bühnemann 2009: 110.
17. Sanderson 2004: 240.
18. Bäumer 2018: 14, 18, briefly discusses the synonymy of death and time in Chapter 9 of the *Netra Tantra*.
19. Bäumer 2018: 14, 18, briefly discusses the synonymy of death and time in Chapter 9 of the *Netra Tantra*.
20. NT 6. 2b–3: *yathā siddhipradaṃ loke mānavānāṃ hitaṅkaram || 2 ||*

    pūrvoktaduṣṭaśamanam apamṛtyuvināśanam |
    āpyāyanaṃ śarīrasya śāntipuṣṭipradaṃ śubham || 3 ||

Chapter 1

1. Bisschop 2020, 16; Sanderson 1998, 664.
2. Padoux 2011: 1–2.
3. Staal 1996: 223–236.
4. Staal 1996: 225.

5. The Sanskrit term *mantrin* has two overlapping meanings in the context of the NT. First, a *mantrin* is the "knower of mantra." Second, he is a councillor or minister of a monarch. As the *mantrin* of the NT is both, I have retained this term throughout rather than using the more familiar guru or yogin. On the occasion, the text utilizes the term teacher or religious preceptor (*ācārya*) as a synonym for *mantrin*.
6. Padoux 2011: 7. See Chapter 8 for a discussion on the distinction among the three categories of ritual drawing.
7. Including the seventh-century *Kālottara*, written by the Tamil Brahmin writer Yāmunācārya and influential on the development of later Tantric ritual; tenth-century Kaula *āgama Āgamaprāmāṇya*; eleventh- or twelfth-century text on temple worship, *Īśānaśivagurudevapaddhati*; post-twelfth-century Kashmiri *Agnikāryapaddhati*; late medieval period Kashmiri *Devīrahasya*; sixteenth-century *Bṛhat Tantrasāra*. Additionally, a handful of texts that have not yet been studied or dated also include the mantra. These texts include *Siddhilakṣmīkoṭyāhutidinakṛtya*, *Acintyaviśvasādākhyam*, *Ugracaṇḍapūjāpaddhati*, *Kāmikāgama*, *Krīyakramādyotikā*, *Tantracintāmaṇi*, *Dīkṣāprakāśa*, *Vāruṇapaddhati*, *Vimalāvatī Tantra*, *Parākramapūjā*, and *Hāhārāva* Tantra.
8. Brunner 1974: 125.
9. *ṚV* 7.59.12 [*om*] *trayambakaṃ yajāmahe sugandhim puṣṭivardhanam | urvārukam iva bandhanān mṛtyor mukṣīya māmṛtāt* || This mantra is also found at YV 3.60 and AV 14.1.17. The use of both mantras offer the practitioner protection from death. The *mṛtyuñjaya* mantra of the ṚV appeals to Rudra while that in the NT implores Śiva.
10. Biernacki 2016: 71–72.
11. Korberg Greenberg 2018: 183.
12. Michaels 2015: 110–112.
13. LaFleur 1998: 38.
14. Padoux 1990: 63.
15. Here I indicate the physicality of mantric optics because, of course, visualization is an important part of Tantric practice, and practitioners are guided through various practices in which they visualize mantras in various ways.
16. LaFleur 1998: 47.
17. Padoux 2011: 36.
18. Flood 2006: 75.
19. NT 5.20.
20. White 2003: 2.
21. The deity of the NT is also known as Parameśvara, Amṛteśa, Amṛteśvara, Mṛtyujit, Mṛtyuñjaya, Bhairava, and Śiva.
22. NT. 5.20.
23. NT. 1.32–34.
24. NT 2.3.
25. NT 2.9.
26. NT 2.11.
27. The list contains two types of Grahas: seizers and planets.
28. NT 2.13–15a.

29. NT 2.15b–16a.
30. Rastogi 1992: 259.
31. The *mātṛkā* consists of all fifty phonemes of the Sanskrit alphabet though in this case the first letter of each category, save for the aspirate, stands in for the rest.
32. Earth, water, fire, air, and ether.
33. Padoux 1989: 35.
34. The NT uses the terms teacher (*ācarya*) and *mantrin* synonymously.
35. Here called *tritanu*.
36.

bhūpradeśe same śuddhe candanāgurucarcite |
karpūrāmodagandhāḍhye kuṅkumāmodasevite ||*17*||
ācāryas tu prasannātmā candanāgurucarcitaḥ |
uṣṇīṣādyair ābharaṇair bhūṣitaiḥ sumahāmatiḥ ||*18*||
padmam aṣṭadalaṃ kṛtvā mātṛkāṃ tatra cālikhet ||
tritanuṃ madhyato nyasya vargān prāgādito likhet ||*19*||

37. For example, the MT, SvT, *Uttarasūtra*, NS, *Guhyasūtra*, BraYā, SYM, and TĀ.
38. Törzsök 2009: 1.
39. In his translation of Abhinavagupta's YH, Padoux gives several charts associating each phoneme of the *mātṛkā* with the *tattvas*, demonstrating some of the intricacies of the technical meanings associated with the phonemes. See Padoux 2013: 130, 132–133, 145–146.
40. Bühnemann 2003: 21. There are also instances in which one substitutes the lotus with a spoked wheel (*cakra*) on which the deities are assigned to the hub and spokes. Bühnemann 2003: 24. Such a *cakra* appears in Chapter 6 of the NT.
41. Törzsök 2009: 10–11.
42.

pūjayet parayā bhaktyā puṣpadhūpādivistaraiḥ ||
mantrāṇāṃ mātaraṃ devi proddharen mantradevatāṃ ||*20*||
viśvādyaṃ viśvarūpāntaṃ viśvahāmṛtakandalam |
jyotir dhvaniḥ parāśaktiḥ śiva ekatra saṃsthitaḥ ||*21*||
anena grathitaṃ sarvaṃ sūtre maṇigaṇā iva |

43. Wilke and Moebus 2011: 725.
44. Throughout the NT *amṛta* refers to non-death, immortality, the nectar of immortality, and the deity Amṛteśvara. Therefore, I leave the term untranslated throughout the text, indicating a specific meaning of the word only when it clearly refers to one or another meaning.
45. See Bansat-Boudon and Tripathi 2011: 203; Padoux 2003: 75; Silburn and Padoux 2000: 102, 177.
46. This phase, which is added to the moon's fifteen stages of waxing or waning, is the *amṛtakalā*, in which the moon does not die. See Mallinson 2007: 213n277.
47. Kṣemarāja explains, they are called the seventy million (*saptakoṭi*) mantras because they came into being "in the beginning of the world after authority was manifested"

(*saptakoṭyo mantrā iti prathamasarge tāvatāmevādhikāro'bhūt*). Seventy-million here is meant as a stand-in for all.

48. Kṣemarāja adds that this follows the place of fire (*agni*), after the first group of letters, starting with *ka* (*kavarga*). In other words, it is a letter in the second (*tālavya*) group.
49. According to Kṣemarāja, who adds *tathā tiryaggo vāyus tatpatre yo 'ntaḥ pavargāpekṣayā makārastena.*
50.

asmān mantrāḥ samutpannāḥ saptakoṭyo 'dhikāriṇaḥ ||22||
citrabhānupadāntaṃ tu śaśāṅkaśakalodaram |
tadaṅkuśordhvavinyastaṃ tiryaggāntordhvayojitam |||23||
etat tat paramaṃ dhāma etat tat paramāmṛtam |
yat tat paramam uddiṣṭam amṛtaṃ lokaviśtutam ||24||
pīyūṣakalayā yuktaṃ pūrṇacandraprabhopamam |
etat tat paramaṃ dhāma etat tat paramaṃ padam ||25||
etat tat paramaṃ vīryam etat tat paramāmṛtam |
tejasāṃ paramaṃ tejo jyotiṣāṃ jyotir uttamam ||26||
sarvasya jagato devam īśvaraṃ kāraṇaṃ param |
sraṣṭā dhartā ca saṃhartā nāsty asya sadṛśo balī ||27||
mantrāṇāmālayo hy eṣa sarvasiddhiguṇāspadam |

The interpretation of phonemes found in the NT differs greatly from a similar mantric exposition in the *Uttarasūtra* of the *Niśvāsatattvasaṃhitā*. "The syllable JUṂ awakens mantras; with the syllable OṂ he should kindle them; with NAMAḤ he should perform purification [of them] (*amalaṃ kuryāt*); with SVĀHĀ he should make them flame (*dīpayet*); the syllable SAḤ, positioned at the beginning and end, is to be used for 'cutting'. They [*scil*. *Mantras*] bestow all objects of desire when this rite has been performed as prescribed (*yathokte karmmaṇā kṛte*)." Trsl. Goodall 2016: 379.

51. Trsl. Bansat-Boudon and Tripathi 2011: 252–253.
52. Singh 1979b: 20.
53. SvT 7.212b–217.
54. Padoux 2011: 70; Davis 2000: 48.
55. Davis 2000: 49.
56. For a detailed discussion of the *aṅgamantra*s throughout the Śaiva tradition, see Brunner 1986b: 89–132.
57. Davis 2000: 49.
58. The *Kāmikāgama* is a twelfth-century text from South India focused on temple construction.
59. Davis 2000: 49–50.
60. SvT 2.32.
61. Ślączka 2007: 74, 117.
62. Davis 1992: 114.
63. SvT 4b–12a.
64. SvT 2.4b–7a.
65. McCarter 2014: 741.
66. *Ānta* here is used to describe consonants that do not have an adjoining vowel.

67.

adhunāṅgāni vakṣyāmi saṃnaddho yais tu siddhyati ||28||
kṛtāntamadhyamaṃ varṇaṃ svararāṇpañcamānugam |
prabhañjanāntaśirasaṃ hṛdayaṃ sarvasiddhidam ||29||
somāntam analād yena yuktaṃ praṇavayojitam |
etac chiraḥ anilāntena yuktā māyā śikhā smṛtā ||30||
īśāntam īśvarordhvaṃ ca dvādaśārdhordhvayojitam |
śivaśaktyātha nādena yuktaṃ tad varma cottamam ||31||
sabhairavādyaṃ praṇavaṃ sadāgatiśiraḥsthitam |
netramantro mahograś ca sarvakilviṣanāśanaḥ (em. sarvakilbiṣanāśanaḥ)||32||
ajīvakaṭasaṃyuktam astram etat prakīrtitam |
aṅgaṣaṭkaṃ samākhyātaṃ mantrājasya siddhidam ||33||

Chapter 2

1. Burchett 2008: 813.
2. Burchett 2008: 814.
3. Burchett 2008: 814.
4. Padoux 1990: 374.
5. Beck 1993: 31.
6. Timalsina 2005: 214.
7. Timalsina 2005: 214.
8. Burchett 2008: 813; Padoux 1990: 373.
9. Padoux 1990: 373.
10. Burchett 2008: 817.
11. Dundas 2000: 235.
12. Smith 2004: 218 argues that the term "magic" should be abandoned in academic discourse as those things termed "magic" "have better and more precise scholarly taxa." While Smith correctly identifies that there is a problem with the term magic, I believe abandoning it completely denies an important distinction between religion and magic, which exists on a spectrum that is more subjective than many other academic categories. The pejorative nature of the term magic in Western tradition demonstrates how the meaning and usage of the term shifts over time and with perspective. One might apply the term to the actions of another in order to marginalize or condemn such practices and often those who perform them. Consequently, an overlap exists between religion and magic.
13. Dundas 2000: 235.
14. Burchett 2008: 817.
15. Burchett 2008: 817.
16. Cassirer 1925 [1955]: 40.
17. Burchett 2008: 818.
18. Padoux 1990: 381.

19. Burchett 2008: 819.
20. Timalsina 2005: 215. KP 57.88 and LT 39.35 emphasize the importance and prominence of silent *japa*.
21. Austin 1962: 4–14.
22. Staal 1989: 74, 80.
23. Staal 1989: 80.
24. Staal 2008: 250.
25. Staal 2008: 250.
26. Braun 2015: https://plato.stanford.edu/entries/indexicals.
27. Staal 1989: 75–84.
28. Wheelock 1989: 120.
29. Wheelock 1989: 57–58.
30. Staal 1996: 239.
31. KĀ 2.45.93, 2.64.70, 2.65.58, PhT 3.95, 3.99.
32. KĀ 2.75.12.
33. Alper 1989: 260.
34. In a verse not found in the published edition of the *SvT* but, according to Alper 1989: 287n23, may be a variant of *SvT* 2.142[cd–143ab].
35. Trsl. Alper 1989: 259.
36. Alper 1989: 260.
37. Alper 1989: 260.
38. Alper 1989: 260.
39. NTU 16.43, SvT 4–400.
40. *kurvanti mantrakaraṇāni kathaṃ prayuñjīta*. NTU 16.43. Note here that the root √*prayuj* can refer to practice but also to recitation, performance, production, and unification.
41. *mantrakaraṇakriyāyogād yojayāmi pare śive*. SvT 4–400cd.
42. TĀ 19.26–27, 21.34.
43. Staal 1989: 66.
44. Staal 1989: 67.
45. Staal 1989: 67.
46. Staal 1989: 68.
47. Taber 1989: 150.
48. Staal 1996: 224.
49. Staal 1996: 224.
50. Taber 1989: 157.
51. Taber 1989: 158.
52. Taber 1989: 153, 158.
53. Padoux 2011: xi.
54. The phonemes *a*, *ka*, *ca*, *ṭa*, *ta*, *pa*, *ya*, and *śa*.
55. Padoux 2011: 94.
56. Padoux 2011: 93.
57.

mantrāḥ kim ātmakā deva kiṃsvarūpāś ca kīdṛśāḥ |
kiṃprabhāvāḥ kathaṃ śaktāḥ kena vā saṃpracoditāḥ ||1||

58. Padoux 1989: 297.
59. Padoux 1989: 298.
60. TU 2.2.1–5. The five sheaths (*pañcakośa*) that make up the body are food (*anna*), breath (*prāṇa*), mind (*manas*), understanding (*vijñāna*), and bliss (*ānanda*).
61. Larson and Bhattacharya 1987: 49.
62. See Goodall 2016: 77–111 for the development of the *tattva* system within early Śaiva literature.
63. VBh 145.
64. ŚD 7.84–85b.
65. Sanderson 1990: 76; Nemec 2011: 46.
66. Sanderson 1990: 78–80.
67. Sanderson 1990: 78.
68. Sanderson 1990: 78.
69.

śivātmakās tu ced deva vyāpakāḥ śūnyarūpiṇaḥ |
kriyākaraṇahīnatvāt kathaṃ teṣāṃ hi kartṛtā ||2||
amūrtatvāt kathaṃ teṣāṃ kartṛtvaṃ copapadyate |
vigraheṇa vinā kāryaṃ kaḥ karoti vada prabho ||3||
na dṛṣṭo hy aśarīrasya vyāpāraḥ parameśvara |
śarīriṇo yato bandhaḥ kathaṃ baddhasya kartṛtā ||4||
śaktihīnasya kartṛtvaṃ viraddhaṃ sarvavastuṣu |
evaṃ śivātmakā mantrāḥ kathaṃ sidhyanti vastutaḥ ||5||

70. Nemec 2018: 218 demonstrates that Somānanda conceived of Śiva as a disembodied yet active agent and that *amūrtatva* is the immateriality that characterizes both Śiva and all of existence. Nemec 2018: 216n1 also notes that while Somānanda uses the term *amūrtatva* often, those who follow him rarely use it, even by Somānanda's disciple Utpaladeva. This supports the dating given by Sanderson 2004, which places the *Netra Tantra* before Somānanda.
71. Nemec 2018: 217, quoting ŚD 2.76.
72. Nemec 2018: 218.
73. Nemec 2018: 220, Trsl. of ŚD 3.35–36.
74. The *Netra Tantra* describes Śiva and Śakti in their purest forms. As such I have kept the capitalizations of both terms but do not intend for them to refer to their deific forms.
75.

atha cecchaktirūpās te kasya śaktis tu kīdṛśī |
śaktiḥ kiṃ kāraṇaṃ deva kāryaṃ tasyāś ca kīdṛśam ||6||
yāvan na śaktimān kaścit kasya śaktir vidhīyate |
svatantrā na prasidhyet tu vinā siddhena kenacit ||7||
asiddhena tu yat sādhyaṃ
tad asiddhaṃ pracakṣate |
vastuśūnyā na caivātra śaktir vai vidyate kvacit ||8||
śaktirūpās tu te mantrāḥ kevalās tu viparyayaḥ |

76. Singh 1979a: xvii.

77. ŚS 1.19 *śaktisaṃdhāne śarīrotpattiḥ* ||
78. To my knowledge, the only verses we currently have from the *Lakṣmīkaulārṇava* are quoted in Kṣemarāja's commentary on the *Śiva Sūtra*.
79. LK *na saṃdhānaṃ vinā dīkṣā na siddhīnāṃ ca sādhanam* |
na mantro mantrayuktiś ca na yogākarṣaṇaṃ tathā ||
80. NT 7.40 *sā yoniḥ sarvadevānāṃ śaktīnāṃ cāpy anekadhā* |
agnīṣomātmikā yonis tasyāḥ sarvaṃ pravartate ||
81. Gonda 1977: 161.
82. Schomerus 2000 [1912]: 59.
83. NT 21.30 *kāryaṃ tasya parā śaktir yathā sūryasya raśmayaḥ* |
vahner ūṣm eva vijñeyā hy avinābhāvinī sthitā ||
84. NT 21.31–32a *sarvānandakarī bhadrā śivasyecchānuvartinī* |
taddharmadharmiṇī śāntā nityānugrahaśālinī || *21–31* ||
vivarta etat sarvaṃ hi tacchakter nānyato bhavet |
85. The text uses *aṇu* and or *āṇava* synonymously.
86. Singh 1979a: xxii.
87. Trsl. Goodall 1998: 290–291.
88. Rastogi 1992: 252.
89. Rastogi 1992: 252.
90.
atha ced āṇavā mantrā vigrahākārarūpiṇaḥ ||*9*||
ātmasvarūpā vikyāta malinā balino nahi |
malino malinasyeva prakṣālyati kasya kaḥ ||*10*||
na siddhā hy āṇavā mantrā kevalāḥ parameśvara
tattvatrayaṃ vināstitvaṃ viruddhaṃ vastusantateḥ ||*11*||
yuktir evātra vaktavyā prāṇināṃ hitakāmyayā |
dṛśyante balino mantrā apradhṛsyāḥ surāsuraiḥ ||*12*||
sarvānugrāhakatvena sarvadāḥ sarvagāḥ śivāḥ |
saṃkṣepato mahādeva saṃśayaṃ tu vada sva me ||*13*||
tvattaḥ parataro nānyaḥ kaścid asti jagat pate |
brūhi sarvaṃ maheśāna yadi tuṣṭo 'si me prabho ||*14*||
91.
aho praśno mahāgūḍho na pṛṣṭo 'haṃ tu kenacit |
coditaṃ tu mayā sarvaṃ sarvaśāstreṣu sarvadā ||*15*||
na vindanti vimūḍhās tu māyayā cchāditāḥ sadā |
tattvatrayaṃ vinā vas tu mantro vaktuṃ na yujyate ||*16*||
āstāṃ tāvat jagat sarvaṃ tattvahīnaṃ na sidhyati |
tritattvanirmitaṃ sarvaṃ yat kiṃcid iha dṛśyate ||*17*||
tattvatrayaṃ vinā devi na padārtho hi vidyate |
tasmāt tattvatrayaṃ sarvaṃ paraṃ cāparam eva ca ||*18*||
śivātmakāḥ śaktirūpā jñeyā mantrās tathāṇavāḥ |
tattvatrayavibhāgena vartante hy amitaujasaḥ ||*19*||

92. NT 21.35–37.
93. NT 21.46b–47a.
94. NT 21.56.
95. NT 21.80–82.
96.

śrūyatāṃ saṃpravakṣyāmi saṃśayaṃ te hṛdi sthitam |
mantrakoṭyo hy asaṃkhyātā sarvāḥ sarvādhikārikāḥ || 5 ||
śivaśaktiprabhāvāś ca sarvaśaktisamanvitāḥ |
bhogamokṣapradāḥ sarvāḥ svaśaktibalabṛṃhitāḥ || 6 ||
kintu devaḥ paraḥ śānto hy aprameyaguṇānvitaḥ |
śivaḥ sarvātmakaḥ śuddho bhāvagrāhyo hy anuttamaḥ || 7 ||
āśrayaḥ paramas teṣāṃ vyāpakaḥ parameśvaraḥ |
tadicchayā samutpannāstac chaktyā saṃpracoditāḥ || 8 ||
bhavanti saphalāḥ sarve sarvatraivādhikāriṇaḥ |
yadetatparamaṃ dhāma sarveṣām ālayaḥ śivaḥ || 9 ||
asmād eva samutpannā mantrāś cāmoghaśaktayaḥ |

97. NT 22.23b refers to the six causes (*kāraṇa*): Brahman, Viṣṇu, Rudra, Īśvara, Sadāśiva, and Śiva. NT 7.21 introduces the *kāraṇas* as part of its yogic practice. The verse above adds a seventh kāraṇa, that of *laya* or *ālaya*, dissolution or refuge in the divine. Mantras and Śaktis arise from the divine, so at their most powerful and perfect they can lead those who use them back to that unchanging state of Śiva. Śiva here does not refer to the divine Śiva but instead to a state of Śiva that must be surpassed for the attainment of liberation. See NT 7.23–24. Here one might expect to find Śakti among the list of kāraṇas and NT 7.26 does, in fact, list Śakti among them as an implicit part of Śiva. *brahmāṇaṃ ca tathā viṣṇuṃ rudraṃ caiveśvaraṃ tathā |sadāśivaṃ tathā śaktiṃ śivasthānaṃ prabhedayet.*
98. For example, Slouber 2017: 60–63 demonstrates that the *vipati* or Gāruḍa mantra, *kṣi pa oṃ svā hā*, has, in both textual and modern tradition, been associated with the cure of snakebites or immunity to infestation by snakes. As such, the *vipati* mantra is not as versatile as the *mṛtyuñjaya* mantra, though this does not mean it is more or less powerful. Here Slouber also demonstrates how modern practitioners of Tibetan Buddhism have expanded the use of the *vipati* mantra to protect against cancer and other illnesses. Though somewhat more generalized than the original usage, this appears to be a very recent interpretation.
99. NTU 22.11 *ataśca pradhānabhūto nāyako'pi anupaplava ityāṇavādimalebhyo niṣkrāntaste ca niṣkrāntā yataḥ*
100. NUT 22.11.
101. Padoux 2011: 96–99.
102. Padoux 2011: 97.
103. Padoux 2011: 99.
104. Padoux 2001: 96 points out that the pattern for *saṃpuṭa* in the NT differs from that in the eleventh-century *Śāradātilaka* in which the syllables of the two mantric parts make the pattern b1, a1, b2, a2, etc.

105. Kṣemarāja does clarify this further but Padoux 2011: 97 points out that the PhT describes the pattern as b1, a2, b2, a3, b3, etc., whereas the *Agnipurāṇa* describes the pattern as a1, a2, b1, a3, a4, b2, etc. Therefore, from Kṣemarāja's commentary alone we cannot determine the pattern intended here.
106. NTU 18–11 *mantrād anantaraṃ nāma tatas trirnmantra iti ādyantam.*
107. NT 18.10b–11 *saṃpuṭaṃ grathitaṃ grastaṃ samastaṃ ca vidarbhitam || 10 ||*
ākrāntaṃ ca tathādyantaṃ garbhasthaṃ sarvatovṛtam |
tathā yuktividarbhaṃ ca vidarbhagrathitaṃ tathā || 11 ||

See also NTU 18–11 and Padoux 2011: 96–99 for detailed explanations regarding the patterns in the NT and related Tantras. This list is adapted from Padoux 2011: 96–99.
108. Padoux 2011: 100.
109. See Yelle 2003: 21–24.
110. *Nirvacana* help to explain both why a particular word is the right word for the thing that it describes and also why the words used are in harmony with what they say. For Kṣemarāja, this allows him to justify the non-dualistic exegesis and interpretation of the text. He reads the names of both the SvT and NT as demonstrating the lack of true externality that would allow for a dualistic reading. See Kahrs 1999: 61.
111. NTU 22–13 *yathā netraṃ cakṣur bhāvaprakāśakam tathedaṃ cinnetram aśeṣaprakāśakatvān netrabhūtam ity uktam ataḥ sarveṣāṃ jīvanam.*
112.
nityo niyāmako hy eṣāṃ netāraṃ [em. *netāro*] *nirupaplavaḥ || 10 ||*
niṣprapañco nirābhāsas trāyakas tāraṇaḥ śivaḥ |
trāṇaṃ karoti sarveṣāṃ tāraṇaṃ trastacetasām || 11 ||
nayate mokṣabhāvaṃ tu tārayen mahato bhayāt |
nayanāc ca tathā trāṇān netram ity abhidhīyate || 12 ||
jīvanaṃ sarvabhūteṣu netrabhūtaṃ prakīrtitam |
samastamantrajātasya svāmivat parameśvaraḥ || 13 ||
113. Here Kṣemarāja has read *netāraṃ* from verse 22.10b as *netā* + *aram* whereas I suggest *netāraṃ* be emended to *netāraḥ* to agree with *eṣaṃ.*
114. The first of the three *malas*, the other two being karma and *māyā*.
115. *niyataṃ bhavaḥ sarvadikkālākrāntikṛt tadaparāmṛṣṭaś ca, eṣāṃ mantrāṇāṃ niyāmako niyoktā araṃ śīghram icchām ātrādeva netā bahirābhāsakaḥ svātmasātkārakṛc ca ataś ca pradhānabhūto nāyako 'pi anupaplava ity āṇavādi malebhyo niṣkrāntas te ca niṣkrāntā yataḥ | evaṃ niṣprapañco nirābhāsaśceti yojyam prapañco jagadvaicitryam ābhāsāḥ saṃkucitāḥ prakāśāḥ trāyakaḥ sarvarakṣākaras tāraṇo mocakaḥ ataś ca śivaḥ śreyomayaparamaśivasvarūpo mṛtyujinnāthaḥ | etadeva trāṇam ity ardhena sphuṭīkṛtam | trāṇaṃ rakṣā trastacetasāṃ saṃsārabhītānām | etac cākṣaravarṇasārūpyeṇa netranāthasya nirvacanam ||*
116. Kahrs 1999: 57.
117. Kahrs 1999: 62.

118. Though the *Netra Tantra* goes by several other names, most connected to the name of the deity, such as *Netrajñānārṇavatantra*, *Amṛteśatantra*, *Mṛtyujitāmṛtīśamahābhairavatantra*, and *Mṛtyujidamṛteśatantra*.
119. Though the commentary follows the whole of *śloka*s 22.14–28, for ease of reading I have included relevant parts here in tandem with the *śloka*s they explain. The commentary is bracketed and in a slightly smaller font.
120.

praṇavaḥ prāṇināṃ prāṇo jīvanaṃ saṃpratiṣṭhitam |
gṛhṇāti praṇavaḥ sarvaṃ kalābhiḥ kalayec chivam || 14 ||

121. In other words, he internalizes all of the nine levels of sound up to *samanā*, beginning with *bindu*. The nine levels are *unmanā*, *samanā*, *vyāpini*, *śakti*, *nādānta*, *nāda*, *nirodhika*, *ardhacandra*, and *bindu*.
122. Of which there are four levels: *vaikharī* (sounds at the *sthūla* level, i.e., words, sentences, the articulation of air or utterances), *madhyamā* (unarticulated sounds that reside in the mind), paśyanti (sensation without differentiation), and *para* (the supreme or soundless sound). See Joo 1998: 41–43 for detailed descriptions of the four levels.
123. *prāṇināṃ sarvajīvatāṃ sarvajñeyakāryajñānakaraṇaprathamābhyupagamakalpānāhataparāmarśātmasa amānyaspandarūpaḥ praṇava eva prāṇāstaṃ vinā jñānakriyā 'ghaṭanāt | etasmin hi sati teṣāṃ jīvanaṃ prāṇāpānādiprasarātma samyak pratiṣṭhāmeti anyathā bhastrāvāyuvadapratiṣṭhitameva syāt | tadevaṃbhūto 'py ayamantaḥkṛtamaśeṣaṃ vakṣyamāṇākārokārādikalābhiḥ saha svātantryāt pṛthagābhāsya tābhireva gṛhṇāti vimarśayuktyā samanāntamātmasāt karoti śivaṃ ca kalayet parāvāgvṛttyā vimṛśet atha ca kalayed ekaviṃśādhikāranirūpitadṛśā 'varohakrameṇa hṛdante kṣipet tatparāmṛtasiktaṃ viśvaṃ vidadhīta*
124. *tattva*, *bhuvana*, *kalā*, *pada*, *mantra*, *varṇa*. Flood 2006: 129.
125. *brahmā*, *viṣṇu*, *rudra*, *īśvara*, *sadāśiva*, *anāśrita*. Sanderson 2007b: 393n541.
126.

ṣaṭprakāraṃ mahādhvānaṃ ṣaṭkāraṇapadasthitam |
juhoti vidyayā sarvaṃ juṃkāreṇa pracoditam ||15||

127. *madhyamantrākṣarātmanā vidyayā vedanapradhānayā śaktyā pracoditaṃ madhyadhāmordhvārohāvarohayuktyā juhoti paradhāmamahānale kṣipati*
128. See Mallinson and Singleton 2017: 260, for various interpretations of *oṃ* in Vedic and Yogic texts.
129. Here *śuddhavidyā* does not refer to the *tattva* but to pure, divine knowledge.
130. Trsl. Barretta 2012: 208.
131. *pūryate paramaśivatacchaktisāmarasyamāpādyate 'nayā viśvam iti vyutpattyā paripūrṇā pūrṇāhutistayā*
132. This can also be read as a compound, *samyaksaṃtṛpti*, that which has a nature that is true gratification.

133.

svarūpaṃ yatsvasaṃvedyam samyaksaṃtṛptilakṣaṇam |
sarvāmṛtapadādhāraṃ savisargaṃ paraṃ śivam ||16||
pūrṇaṃ nirantaraṃ tena pūrṇāhutyā tu pūrṇayā |

134. Thus, he surpasses *samanā*, which was the highest level reached in the previous mantric constituent part.

135.

tato'pi
pūrvanirṇītasvarūpādiśabdavācyaṃ yat śivaṃ paramaśivākhyaṃ cidghanaṃ dhāma, savisargam iti arasvātantryātmonmanāśaktisamarasaṃ tena tṛtīyabījayuktyavaṣṭam bhāsāditena śivāmṛtarasena

136.

svoccārā yā svabhāvasthā svasvarūpā ca svoditā ||17||
icchājñānakriyārūpā sā caikā śaktir uttamā |
tayā prakurute nityaṃ śaktimān sa śivaḥ smṛtaḥ ||18||

137. *taditthaṃ mantroccārayuktyā prāptaparadhāmā yo mantrī sa sākṣāt śaktimān śiva eva smṛta iti vyavahitasaṃbandhāḥ*
138. See Rastelli and Goodall 2013: 498, for a detailed description of how one is to perform the *pūrṇāhuti*.
139. *sarvarasātmaparaśaktitadvat sāmarasyātma kurute*
140. *pūryate paramaśivatac chaktisāmarasyam āpādyate 'nayā viśvam iti vyutpattyā paripūrṇā pūrṇāhutistayā*
141. Padoux 2000: 43.
142. Dating the *Kulārṇava* is difficult, but Padoux 2000: 43 says it is likely pre-fifteenth century. This means it may be later than Kṣemarāja but the ideas held within the text are likely much earlier than the earliest written text.
143. The *Kulārṇava Tantra*, quoted in Padoux 2000: 48, says, "The glorious mantra that bestows the fruits of all accomplishments is rooted in the grace of the guru. It leads to the supreme Reality."
144. Padoux 2000: 44.
145. Alper 1989: 239.
146. Padoux 2000: 45.

Chapter 3

1. Rabe 2000: 434.
2. White 2003: 136–140.
3. White 2003: 137.
4. At the time of this writing, the British Museum had just opened an exhibition titled *Tantra: Enlightenment to Revolution*. Unfortunately, I was unable to attend due to the coronavirus pandemic. None of the pieces featured on the exhibition website are of Kashmiri provenance and the catalogue (Ramos 2020) lists no Kashmiri pieces.

5. Unknown. Representation of Śiva. Ninth century. Stone. British Museum, London. Museum number 1988,0312.1.
6. Unknown. Mask of Bhairava. Late sixth to seventh century. Copper alloy, possibly brass. Metropolitan Museum of Art, New York City. Accession number 2013.249.
7. Sanderson 2004: 240.
8. Bühnemann, personal email correspondence, November 2017.
9. Bühnemann 2009: 110.
10. Sanderson 2004: 241.
11. Bühnemann 2009, uses the spelling Mṛtyuṃjaya for the deity. I have changed the spelling to conform to that used within this manuscript though have retained the name she uses for the deity despite myself using Mṛtyujit throughout this text. This is, of course, the same deity.
12. Bühnemann 2009: 110.
13. The fountain at Mohancok Hiti is located in a private section of the Hanūmāṇdhokā Palace and is inaccessible. Photographs indicate that many of the seventy-two extant sculptures at Tusā Hiti have counterparts at Mohancok Hiti. Bühnemann 2009; 107.
14. Bühnemann 2009: 110–111.
15. Bühnemann 2017. The Jageshvar Temple in Uttarakhand houses an eighth-century Mṛtyuñjaya temple worshipped in Śiva's liṅga form. Lochtefeld 2002: 309; Jageshwar Temple Organization (accessed February 17, 2018), mahamritunjayjageshwar.com.
16. Bühnemann 2017.
17. Lochtefeld 2002: 633.
18. C. fifth to fourth century BCE, Flood 1996: 153, or sixth to fifth century BCE, Muller-Ortega 1989: 27.
19. Lochtefeld 2002: 633.
20. Michaels 2003: 217.
21. Lochtefeld 2002: 633.
22. Lochtefeld 2002: 633.
23. Michaels 2003: 218.
24. Michaels 2003: 218.
25. Flood 2003: 206.
26. Rastelli and Goodall 2013: 446.
27. C. 2300–1750 BCE. Srinivasan 1975/76: 47.
28. Marshall 1931: 52.
29. Marshall 1931: 52–56.
30. Bryant 2001: 162.
31. Bryant 2001: 163.
32. Bryant 2001: 163.
33. The National Museum of India's website identifies the seal as Śiva and says, the "anthropomorphic form of ithyphallic Shiva is one of the most significant Indus finds attesting the prevalence of Shiva-cult." It further claims, "This seal with [its] buffalo-horned figure [is] almost unanimously identified as Shiva in his form as Pashupati, Lord of animals—Shiva's earliest representation preceding Vedas by far." See Pasupati Seal, National Museum of India, New Delhi, Acc. No. DK 5175/143, http://

www.nationalmuseumindia.gov.in/prodCollections.asp?pid=42&id=1&lk=dp1. Accessed August, 26, 2020.

34. Rocher 1986: 245; Collins 1988: 36.
35. Tagare et al. 1987: 204–205.
36. NT 6.46–48a.
37. Child 2007: 57.
38. Tagare 1987: 205–216; Eck 2012: 194–197; Doniger 1993: 23.
39. Klostermaier 2007: 503. See Rocher 1986: 222–228 for more detail on possible dating of the text.
40. Eck 2012: 195.
41. Kramrisch 1988: 395.
42. Kramrisch 1988: 395.
43. Gray 2005: 53.
44. Olivelle 1999: 18, 80, 163, 282.
45. In the Vedic tradition, a *padapātha* is a rendering of the text without sandhi, dividing the text into separate words.
46. As cited in Einoo 2005: 109.
47. Einoo 2005: 110.
48. Rocher 1991: 188. Here Rocher also notes several other names of the mantra within the text.
49. Rocher 1986: 222–228.
50. Doniger 2010: 473.
51. *Padma Purāṇa*, Chapter 101 as cited in Mani 1975: 220–221. The story continues with another relative killing the fly Karuṇamuni after a hundred years. Again ash and the mantra resuscitate him and he immediately becomes human again.
52. Einoo 2005: 113. Like most early texts, dating the *Arthava Veda* remains a difficult task but the text clearly predates the common era. Olson 2007: 13 says the acceptance of the text as the fourth Veda likely occurred sometime between 200 BCE and 200 CE.
53. Einoo 2005: 118–119.
54. Mann 2012: 187.
55. Dalal 2011: 145.
56. Rocher 1986: 175–178.
57. Einoo 2005: 118.
58. GP 18.18.2.
59. Rocher 1986: 195–196.
60. Mani 1975: 488; Dalal 2011: 245–246.
61. Klostermaier 1985: 144.
62. Von Stietencron, et al. 1992: 405; Dhal 1986: 3.
63. Rocher 1986: 200.
64. NT 7.52a and 8.55a also refer to the deity as Kālajit, Conqueror of Time or Death.
65. Sanderson 2004: 253.
66. NT 19.103.

67. A local text that dates from the beginning of the Kārkoṭa period (c. 626–855), Siudmak 2013: 5, and which Kalhaṇa used as a source in the writing on his *Rājataraṅgiṇī*, Törzsök 2012: 211.
68. Sanderson 2004: 254.
69. See Ratié 2010: 438.
70.

athedānīṃ pravaksyāmi rājarakṣāṃ vidhānataḥ |
mantrasaṃpuṭayogena madhye nāma samālikhet || 39 ||
tadūrdhve bhairavaṃ devam amṛteśaṃ yajet priye |
devyo daleṣu tenaiva tathaivādyantayojitāḥ || 40 ||
dūtyas tathā niyojyante mūlamantreṇa kiṅkarāḥ |
padmabāhye suśulkaṃ tu likhet tac chaśimaṇḍalam || 41 ||
catuṣkoṇaṃ tu tadbāhye vajralāñchanalāñchitam |
rocanākuṅkumenaiva kṣīreṇa sitayā tathā || 42 ||
likhitvā pūjayec chāntau sarvaśvetopacārataḥ |
yathānurūpanaivedyairghasmarairbalināsavaiḥ || 43 ||
sitacandanasaṃmiśrān karpūrakṣodadhūsarān |
sākṣatāṃstaṇḍulatilān sitaśarkarayā saha || 44 ||
ghṛtakṣīrasamāyuktān homayedyas tu yatnadhīḥ |
yatne parāpyāyanādau dhīrdhyānasaṃvidyasya ||
mahāśāntir bhavet kṣipraṃ gṛhīto yadi mṛtyunā || 45 ||

71. NT 21.72–75.
72. NT 3.1–16.
73. Note here that the Sanskrit uses the feminine *amṛtā* as qualified by *mudrā*. This means that here we have the adjectival meaning of *amṛta*, immortal, not dead, or imperishable, and it cannot refer to the deity Amṛta (masculine), nor the nectar (neuter).
74. In *SvTU* 2.32, Kṣemarāja mentions both the *amṛta mudrā* and *padma mudrā* as part of *mūrti*.
75.

mudrāṃ caivāmṛtāṃ baddhvā padmamudrām athāpi vā |
dhyāyed ātmani deveśaṃ candrakoṭisamaprabham ||17||
svacchamuktāphalaprakhyaṃ sphaṭikādrisamaprabham |
kundendugokṣīranibhaṃ himādrisadṛśāṃ vibhum ||18||
śubhrahārendukandādisitabhūṣaṇabhūṣitam |
sitacandanaliptāṅgaṃ karpūrakṣodadhūsaram ||19||
sphuraccandrāmṛtasphārabahulormipāriplutam |
somamaṇḍalamadhyastham ekavaktraṃ trilocanam ||20||
sitapadmopaviṣṭaṃ tu baddhapadmāsanasthitam |
caturbhujaṃ viśālākṣaṃ varadābhayapāṇikam ||21||
pūrṇacandranibhaṃ śubhram amṛtenaiva pūratam |
kalaśaṃ dhārayantaṃ hi jagadāpyāyakārakam ||22||
paripūrṇaṃ tathā candraṃ vāmahaste 'sya cintayet |
sarvaśvetopacāreṇa pūjitaṃ tam anusmaret ||23||

76. A drawing of the Tusā Hiti sculpture shows the gesture of protection in the remaining left hand, which corresponds to the description found here. Bühnemann 2009: 108, 110.
77. I have not translated the descriptions of most of the goddesses described in the *Netra Tantra*. This is because the imagery of the goddesses largely mirrors that of the male deities they accompany.
78. Here the text also makes reference to *saumya*, soma or nectar but it is not clear what the goddess does with this nectar as she only has four hands with which to hold the attributed items.
79.

tadutsaṅgagātāṃ devīṃ śriyaṃ vai viśvamātaram |
viśuddhasphaṭikapradyāṃ himakundendusaprabhām ||63||
candrār budapratīkāśāṃ gokṣīrasadṛśaprabhāṃ |
muktāphalanibhāṃ śvetāṃ śvetavastrānugūhitāṃ ||64||
sitacandraliptāṅgīṃ karpūrakṣodadhūsarāṃ |
śuddhahārendukāntādiratnojjvalavimaṇḍitām ||65||
sitasradgāmamālābhiḥ kamalaiḥ suvibhūṣitām |
harahāsasuśubhrāṅgīṃ sitahāsāṃ manoramām ||66||
suśuklamukuṭopetām ekavaktrāṃ trilocanām |
baddhapadmāsanāsīnāṃ yogapaṭṭavibhūṣitām ||67||
śaṃkhapadmakarāṃ saumyāṃ varadābhayapāṇikām |
canurbhujāṃ mahādevīṃ sarvalakṣaṇalakṣitām ||68||

80. NT 18–74–75 *athavāṣṭabhujā devī cintāratnakarā śubhā |*
kalaśaṃ dhārayennityamamṛtena samanvitam || 74 ||
somasūryakarā devī sitapadmoparisthitā |
nidhīnāṃ copariṣṭāttu gajamaṅgalabhūṣitā || 75 ||
81. NT 18–80b.
82. I have not translated the descriptions of the goddesses and other attendants here because of the redundancy of their attributes. This does not mean that they are unimportant to visualization practices.
83.

tad evaṃ paramaṃ devam amṛteśam anāmayam |
svabhāvas tatsamuddiṣṭaṃ vyāpakaṃ śāśvataṃ dhruvam || 5 ||
na tasya rūpaṃ varṇo vā paramārthena vidyate |
yasmāt sarvagato devaḥ sarvāgamamayaḥ śubhaḥ || 6 ||
vyāpakaḥ sarvamantrāṇāṃ sarvasiddhipradāyakaḥ |
nirmalaṃ sphaṭikaṃ yadvat tantau protaṃ sitādike || 7 ||
pratibimbeta sarvatra yena yena hi rañjitam |
tattad darśayate 'nyeṣāṃ na svabhāvena rañjitam || 8 ||
tathā tathaiva deveśaḥ sarvāgamaniyojitaḥ |
phalaṃ dadāti sarveṣāṃ sādhakānāṃ hi sarvataḥ || 9 ||
tasmāt srotaḥsu sarveṣu cintāmaṇir ivojjvalaḥ |
bhāvabhedena vai dhyātaḥ sarvāgamaphalapradaḥ || 10 ||

śivaḥ sadāśivaś caiva bhairavas tumburus tathā |
somasūryas varūpeṇa vah nirūpadharo vibhuḥ || 11 ||

84. Sanderson 2004: 274, 284.
85.

niyantritānāṃ baddhānāṃ trāṇaṃ tan netram ucyate ||12||
mṛtyor uttārayed yasmān mṛtyujit tena cocyate |
amṛtatvaṃ dadāty evam amṛteśa iti smṛtaḥ ||13||

86. Einoo 2005: 113–114.
87. Rastelli and Goodall 2013: 353.
88. Davis 2000: 49.
89.

candrārbudapratīkāśaṃ himādrinicayopamam || 19 ||
pañcavaktraṃ viśālākṣaṃ daśabāhuṃ trilocanam |
nāgayajñopavītaṃ tu vyāghracarmāmbaracchadam || 20 ||
baddhapadmāsanāsīnaṃ siddhapadmoparisthitam |
triśūlam utpalaṃ bāṇam akṣasūtraṃ samudgaram || 21 ||
dakṣiṇeṣu kareṣv evaṃ vāmeṣu śṛṇvataḥ param|
spheṭakādarśacāpaṃ ca mātuluṅgaṃ kamaṇḍalum || 22 ||
candrārdhamaulinam devam āpītaṃ pūrvavaktrataḥ |
dakṣiṇaṃ kṛṣṇabhīmograṃ daṃṣṭralaṃ vikṛtānanam || 23 ||
kapālamālābharaṇaṃ jagat saṃtrāsakārakam |
paścimaṃ himakundābhaṃ vāmaṃ raktotpalaprabham || 24 ||
ūrdhvavaktraṃ maheśāni sphaṭikābhaṃ vicintayet |
evaṃ dhyātvā tu deveśaṃ pūjayed vidhipūrvakam || 25 ||
svamūrtau sthaṇḍile liṅge jale vā kamalopari |
īśānādyāṃś ca sadyontān svadikṣu pratipūjayet || 26 ||

90. Sanderson 2004: 274.
91. Davis 2000: 117.
92. Törzsök 2015: 133–155.
93. Kinsley 1998: 169.
94. Dev 2001: 55–56.
95.

athedānīṃ pravakṣyāmi bhairavāgamabheditam |
bhinnāñjanacayaprakhyaṃ kalpāntadahanātmakam || 1 ||
pañcavaktraṃ śavārūḍhaṃ daśabāhuṃ bhayānakam |
kṣapāmukhagaṇaprakhyaṃ garjantaṃ bhīṣaṇasvanam || 2 ||
daṃṣṭrakarālavadanaṃ bhrukuṭīkuṭilekṣaṇam |
siṃhāsanapadārūḍhaṃ vyālahārair vibhūṣitam || 3 ||
kapālamālābharaṇaṃ dāritāsyaṃ mahātanum |
gajatvakprāvṛtapaṭaṃ śaśāṅkakṛtaśekharam || 4 ||
kapālakhaṭvāḍgadharaṃ khaḍgakheṭakadhāriṇam |
pāśāṅkuśadharaṃ devaṃ varadābhayapāṇikam || 5 ||

vajrahastaṃ mahāvīraṃ paraśvāyudhapāṇikam |
bhairavaṃ pūjayitvā tu tasyotsaṅgagatāṃ smaret || 6 ||
pralayāgnisamākārāṃ |

96. A pre-tenth-century Kaula text. Törzsök 2015: 5.
97. Törzsök 2015: 5.
98. Goodall 2015: 458. Here Goodall notes that the expression *bahurūpa* may mean that these faces were homologized with the *bramamantras*.
99. See Hatley 2007: 184–1855n176.
100. The name Bhairavī does not appear in the main text of the *Netra Tantra*. I use it here following Kṣemarāja's use in his commentary.
101. The description of a deity with five faces and three eyes is rather unusual. I take this to mean that the goddess has three eyes on each of her five faces, for a total of fifteen eyes. This is still abnormal though the *Siddhayogeśvarīmata* describes Bhairava as having four faces and twelve eyes, three per face. The *Svacchanda Tantra* describes the deity Kālāgnirudra as four-faced with twelve eyes. Törzsök 2015: 10.
102. The *Butea frondosa* or flame-of-the-forest.
103. This may refer to liquor but can also simply be read as nectar or juice.
104.

lākṣāsindūrasaprabhām |
ūrdhvakeśīṃ mahākāyāṃ vikarālāṃ subhīṣaṇām || 7 ||
mahodarīṃ pañcavaktrāṃ netratrayavibhūṣitām |
nakharālāṃ (em. nakhārālāṃ) koṭarākṣīṃ muṇḍamālāvibhūṣitām || 8 ||
bhairavoktabhujāṃ devīṃ bhairavāyudhadhāriṇīm |
icchāśaktir iti khyātāṃ svacchandotsaṅgagāminīm || 9 ||
aghoreśiti vikhyātāmetadrūpadharāṃ smaret |
sarvatantreṣu ca proktaṃ pracchannaṃ na sphuṭīkṛtam || 10 ||
mamāśayo na kenāpi lakṣito bhuvi durlabhaḥ |
vyādhinigrahaṇādyeṣu pāpeṣu kṣayahetave || 11 ||
gobrahmaṇeṣu rakṣārthaṃ śāntau puṣṭau sadā yajet |
athavā himakundendumuktāphalasamadyutim || 12 ||
candrakoṭisamaprakhyaṃ sphaṭikācalasaṃnibham |
kalpāntadahanaprakhyaṃ japākiṃśukasaṃnibham || 13 ||
sūryakoṭisamākāraṃ raktaṃ vā tamanusmaret |
athavā padmarāgābhaṃ haritālasamadyutim || 14 ||
icchārūpadharaṃ devam icchāsiddhiphalapradam |
yādṛśenaiva vapuṣā sādhakastam anusmaret || 15 ||
tādṛśaṃ bhajate rūpaṃ tādṛksiddhipradaṃ śubham |
padmamadhy asthitaṃ dhyāyet pūjayed vidhinā tataḥ|| 16 ||
yathānurūpanaivedyapuṣpadhūpāsavair vibhum |

105. Kinsley 1998: 167.
106. Kinsley 1998: 168.
107. NT 10.17ab–34.
108. NT 37–38.
109. Törzsök 2015: 6.

110. Törzsök 2015: 2, 6.
111. NT 11.13.
112. Samuel 2008: 306.
113. Sanderson 2003–2004: 356.
114. A crocodile, shark, or dolphin.
115.

athedānīṃ pravakṣyāmi Tantram uttaram uttamam |
mantreṇānena yaṣṭavyaṃ sarvasiddhiphalodayam ||1||
sarvopadravaśānty artham aṣṭapatre kuśeśaye |
pūrvāktamaṇḍale devi madhye devaṃ ca tumburum ||2||
daśabāhuṃ sureśānaṃ pañcavaktraṃ trilocanam |
sādāśivena vapuṣā vaktrāṇy asya prakalpayet ||3||
taṃ cārdhacandraśirasaṃ rājīvāsanasaṃsthitam |
himakundendudhavalaṃ tuhinācalasaṃnibham ||4||
nāgayajñopavītaṃ ca sarpabhūṣaṇabhūṣitam |
sarvābharaṇasaṃyuktaṃ vyāghracarmakaṭisthalam ||5||
gajacarmaparīdhānaṃ vṛṣārūḍhaṃ mahābalam |
khaḍgacarmadharaṃ devaṃ ṭaṅkakandalabhūṣitam ||6||
pāśāṅkuśadharaṃ devaṃ cakrahastākṣasūtriṇam |
varadābhayahastaṃ ca sarvakilviṣanāśanam ||7||
sarvadikṣu sthitā devyaḥ pūrvādau dūtya eva ca |
āgneyyādividikṣv evaṃ kiṅkarā dvāradeśataḥ ||8||
jambhanī mohanī caiva subhagā durbhagā tathā |
dūtayas tu samākhyātāḥ kiṅkarān śṛṇvataḥ param ||9||
krodhano vṛntakaś caiva gajakarṇo mahābalaḥ |
savyāpasavye gāyatrīṃ sāvitrīṃ viniveśayet ||10||
adha ūrdhve 'ṅkuśaṃ māyāṃ vinyasyet tad anantaram |
sarvānyetāni yojyāni mūlamantreṇa sarvadā ||11||
sitaraktapītakṛṣṇā devyo vai caturānanāḥ |
caturbhujā trinenetrā ca ṭaṅkakandaladhāriṇī ||12||
daṇḍākṣasūtrahastā ca pretopari virājate |
jayā devī tu vijayā raktavarṇā caturbhujā ||13||
caturvaktrā trinetrā ca śarakārmukadhāriṇī |
khaḍgacarmadhrā devī hyulūkopari saṃsthitā ||14||
ajitā padmagarbhā ca caturvaktrā caturbhujā |
śāktighaṇṭādharā devī carmapaṭṭisadhāraṇī ||15||
aśvārūḍhā mahādevī sarvābharaṇabhūṣitā |
bhinnendranīlasadṛśī caturvaktravibhūṣitā ||16||
caturbhujā trinetrā ca pāśāṅkuśadharā tathā |
ratnapātragadāhastā divyāsanasusaṃsthitā ||17||
sauvarṇāmbarasaṃvītā svarṇabhūṣaṇabhūṣitā |
svadikṣu saṃsthitā iṣṭā dhyātāḥ siddiphalapradāḥ ||18||
dūtyas tadrūpadhāriṇyaḥ kiṃtu vaktraikabhūṣitāḥ |
dvibhujāś ca trinetrāś ca muṇḍakartaribhūṣitāḥ ||19||
matsyaḥ kūrmas tu makaro bhekas tāsāṃ tathāsanam |

kiṃkarāḥ khaḍgahastāś ca dvibhujāś carmadhāriṇaḥ ||20||
ekavaktrās trinetrāś ca bhrukuṭīkuṭilekṣaṇāḥ |
sitādivarṇabhedena dhyātāḥ siddhiphalapradāḥ ||21||
gāyatrī raktavarṇābhā vaktraikena vibhūṣitā |
baddhapadmāsanāsīnā dhyānonmīlitalocanā ||22||
sāvitrī sitavarṇena dhyānāntar gatalocanā |
tathaivāvayavā devī māyā kṛṣṇā caturbhajā ||23||
mahāpaṭāvagūhinyāsampuṭākārayugmataḥ |

116. Sanderson 2013: 32.
117. Sanderson 2013: 50.
118. Seventh century. Hatley 2018: 140.
119. Hatley 2018: 140.
120. Sanderson 2007b: 245n55.
121. Sanderson 2007b: 245n55.
122. Hatley 2007: 144–145; Goudriaan 1985: 4–5.
123. Acri 2016: 346.
124. Törzsök 2013: 180–181.
125. Goudriaan 1985: 21.
126. VŚT 51, 123.
127. VŚT 119–136.
128. VŚT 201.
129. Malla 1996: 43.
130.

evaṃ vai mantrarājasya kaulikaścodito vidhiḥ |
punaranyat pravakṣyāmi vidhānaṃ yatphalapradam || 1 ||
nārāyaṇaṃ caturbāhuṃ padmapatrāyatekṣaṇam (em. padmapattāyatekṣaṇam) |
atasīpuṣpasaṃkāśam ekavaktraṃ dvilocanam || 2 ||
śaṅkhacakragadāpadmasarvābharaṇabhūṣitam |
divyāmbaradharaṃ devaṃ divyapuṣpopaśobhitam || 3 ||
sphuranmukuṭamāṇikyakiṅkiṇījālamaṇḍitam |
divyakuṇḍaladhartāram utthitaṃ tu sadā smaret || 4 ||
athavā pakṣirājasthaṃ suśvetaṃ tu manoramam |
trivaktraṃ saumyavadanaṃ varāhaharibhūṣitam || 5 ||
bhujaiḥ ṣaḍbhiḥ samāyuktaṃ varābhayasamanvitam |
utsaṅge 'sya śriyaṃ dhyāyet tadvarṇāyudhadhāriṇīm || 6 ||
lāvaṇyakāntisadṛśīṃ devadevasya saṃmukhīm |
caturdikṣu sthitā devīr vidikṣv aṅgāni pūjayet || 7 ||
jayā lakṣmīs tathā kīrtir māyā vai dikṣu tā yajet |
pāśāṅkuśadharā devyo varadābhayapāṇikāḥ || 8 ||
devasya saṃmukhe dhyāyec chrīvarṇā rūpadhāriṇīḥ |
devasya sadṛśāṅgāni tadvarṇāstradharāṇi ca || 9 ||

131. The date of this text is unclear. Gonda 1977: 89, notes that it is one of the oldest Pāñcarātra texts, dating perhaps as early as the fifth century.

132. Gonda 1977: 89.
133. Battacharyya 1931: 27.
134. The text here is missing, making it unclear what he holds in the hand. I am also not certain that *ceyāra* is *ceya + ara* and suspect textual corruption. The Muktabodha online transliteration reads *ceyā (kenā) rodyatapāṇikam.*
135. Half Viṣṇu, half Lakṣmī.
136.

athavāṣṭabhujaṃ devaṃ pītavarṇaṃ suśobhanam |
meṣoparisthitaṃ devi digvastraṃ cordhvaliṅginam || 10 ||
śṛṅgaṃ vaṣṭabhya caikena ceyārodyata (?) pāṇikam |
bālarūpaṃ yajen nityaṃ krīḍantaṃ yoṣitāṃ gaṇaiḥ || 11 ||
caturdikṣu sthitā devyo digambaramanoramāḥ |
karpūrī candanī caiva kastūrī kuṅkumī tathā || 12 ||
tadrūpadhārikā devya icchāsiddhiphalapradāḥ |
bahunātra kimuktena viśvarūpaṃ tu taṃ smaret |
anekavaktrasaṃghātair anekāstrabhujais tathā || 13 ||
śayanasthaṃ vivāhastham ardhalakṣmīyutaṃ tathā || 14 ||
kevalaṃ narasiṃhaṃ vā varāhaṃ vāmanaṃ smaret |
kapilo 'py athavā pūjyaś cāvyakto vāpi niṣkalaḥ || 15 ||
yena yena prakāreṇa bhāvabhedena saṃsmaret |
tasya tanmayatāmeti ityājñā pārameśvarī || 16 ||

137. Sanderson 2004: 285.
138. NTU 13.9; Sanderson 2004: 285.
139. Sanderson 2004: 285.
140. Siudmak 2013: 409.
141. Lawrence 1895: 170–172; Fergusson 1899: 285–291.
142. Siudmak 2013: 409–410.
143. Inden 2000: 85–86.
144. Sanderson 2004: 255n60.
145. Inden 2000: 85.
146. RT 4.181–211.
147. Indra, Agni, Yama, Nirṛti, Varuṇa, Vāyu, Kubera, and Īśāna.
148. We often find 27, 28, or 64 Nakṣatras. Von Stietencron 2013: 75, 81, points out that this is problematic because the lunar and solar years do not match. He argues that 64, which corresponds to the number of celestial *yoginī*s, allows for the insertion of a leap month, allowing for solar and lunar calendrical harmonization.
149. Bryant 2001: 253; Von Stietencron 2013: 76–81.
150. Ślączka 2007: 175, 304, 346.
151. Ślączka 2007: 243.
152.

tejomayamato vakṣye yena siddhirbhaven nṛṇām |
raktapadmanibhākāraṃ lākṣārasasamaprabham || 17 ||
sindūrarāśivarṇābhaṃ padmarāgasamaprabham |

kusumbharāgasaṃkāśaṃ dāḍimīkusumaprabham || 18 ||
kalpāntavahnisadṛśam ekavaktraṃ trilocanam |
caturbhujaṃ mahātmānaṃ varadābhayapāṇikam || 19 ||
vajramekena hastena raśmimekena dhārayet |
saptāśvaratham ārūḍhaṃ nāgayajñopavītinam || 20 ||
raktamālyāmbaradharaṃ raktagandhānulepitam |
athavāṣṭabhujaṃ devi lokapālāyudhānvitam || 21 ||
trivaktraṃ ghoravadanaṃ trinetraṃ vikṛtānanam |
aśvoparisamārūḍhaṃ padmamadhye sadā yajet || 22 ||
hṛcchiraś ca śikhā varma locanāstraṃ prapūjayet |
padmamadhye yajed devaṃ grahān aṣṭau dvitīyake || 23 ||
nakṣatrāṇi tṛtīye tu yathā sāṃkhyaṃ tribhis tribhiḥ |
dalāgre tritayaṃ pūjyaṃ lokapālāṃś caturthake || 24 ||
pañcame padmasaṃsthāne astrāṇy aṣṭau prapūjayet |

153. Lee 1967: 48.
154. Lee 1967: 49; Tissot 2006: 355.
155. Lee 1967: 49.
156. Lee 1967: 49; Shimkhada 1984: 226.
157. Shimkhada 1984: 226.
158. Shimkhada 1984: 225.
159.

utthitaṃ kevalaṃ vāpi dvibhujaṃ raśmisaṃyutam || 25 ||
viśvakarmasvarūpaṃ vā viśvākāraṃ jagatpatim |
caturbhujaṃ mahātmānaṃ ṭaṅkapustakadhāriṇam || 26 ||
saṃdaṃśaṃ vāmahastena sūtraṃ vai dakṣiṇena tu |
devaiḥ siddhaiś ca gandharvaiḥ stūyamānaṃ vicintayet || 27 ||
sthale 'nale jale caiva parvatāgre prapūjayet |
yatra vā rocate citte icchāsiddhiphalapradam || 28 |

160. Sanderson 2004: 254, 255n60.
161. Sanderson 2004: 255n60.
162.

śaṅkhakundendudhavalaṃ trinetraṃ rudrarūpiṇam |
sādāśivena rūpeṇa vṛṣārūḍhaṃ vicintayet || 29 ||
caturbhujaṃ mahātmānaṃ śūlābhayasamanvitam |
mātuluṅgadharaṃ devam akṣasūtradharaṃ prabhum || 30 ||
atho bahubhujaṃ devaṃ nāṭyasthaṃ cintayet prabhum |
umārdhadhāriṇaṃ yadvā viṣṇor ardhārdhadhāriṇam || 31 ||
vivāhasthaṃ ca vā dhyāyet samīpasthaṃ prapūjayet |
brahmā caturmukhaḥ saumyo raktavarṇaḥ sulocanaḥ || 32 ||
lambakūrcaḥ sutejāś ca haṃsārūḍhaś caturbhujaḥ |
daṇḍākṣasūtrahastaś ca kamaṇḍalvabhaye dadhat || 33 ||
vedaiś caturbhiḥ saṃyuktaḥ sarvasiddhiphalapradaḥ |
buddhaḥ padmāsanagataḥ pralambaśruticīvaraḥ || 34 ||

padmākṣaḥ padmacihnaś ca maṇibaddho jagaddhitaḥ |
samādhistho mahāyogī varadābhayapāṇikaḥ || 35 ||
akṣasūtradharo devaḥ padmahastaḥ sulocanaḥ |
evaṃ dhyātaḥ pūjitaś ca strīṇāṃ mokṣaphalapradaḥ || 36 ||

163. NT 37–43.

Chapter 4

1. I use the term medieval here to describe the period of Indian history from approximately the eighth century to the early sixteenth. Despite Wedemeyer's 2013: 58–66 many protestations against the use of this term for its lack of absolute construction and pejorative undertones, it allows us to quickly situate a particular place and time.
2. Urban 2010: 52, 57.
3. Urban 2010: 42–44 briefly outlines the history of this debate from the beginning of Western academic study of Tantra.
4. On this point Urban 2010: 43, includes Flood in this camp, though the passage he cites is itself a reference to the viewpoint of Mayer 1990. Flood 2006: 14, concedes that elements of Tantric practice may have their roots in pre-history but argues that "we simply do not have sufficient evidence to speculate in this way." Instead he focuses on the extant evidence as it exists in the textual record.
5. Wedemeyer 2013: 26.
6. Sanderson 2001: 6n3 citing GS 8.11–16.
7. Wedemeyer 2013: 26.
8. Davidson 2002: 234–235.
9. Urban 2010: 45.
10. See Sanderson 2009; Wedemeyer 2013; Ratié 2010; and Gray 2007, 2012. Bühnemann 1996 shows how the *Phetkāriṇī Tantra* not only adopted a Buddhist goddess into the Hindu pantheon but was then cited as an authoritative text by later Hindu Tantras.
11. Wedemeyer 2013: 191–192.
12. The literary record does demonstrate an early connection between the upper castes and the *kāpālika* practitioners. However, this does not prove a complete separation of influence between communities.
13. As Sanderson 2009: 294–295, 294–295n699 notes, religious texts, poems, and chronicles all indicate the participation of people of all castes in Tantric ritual as more than simply a rhetorical device.
14. Sanderson 2009: 298.
15. Minkley and Legassick 2000: 2.
16. This also assumes a binary of openness and secrecy that I believe to be reductive. Often these two concepts appear to be in opposition when in fact they do not exclude one another. Such open secrecy can exist when multiple parties are aware of the existence and often contents of the secret but act as if the secret is still secure. An example of this from modern Hindu practice is found in the recitation of

the Gāyatrī Mantra. Traditionally initiation is required in order for a practitioner to chant this mantra and that initiation has often been limited to Brahmin males. However, an internet search shows that the Gāyatrī is an extremely popular and well-known mantra. In addition to translations of the meaning and articles about its use, the internet holds thousands of recordings of the mantra available for anyone to listen to and the mantra is even featured in the opening theme song of the popular science fiction television series *Battlestar Galactica*.

17. Simmel 1906: 488.
18. Gibson 2014: 286.
19. Simmel 1906: 462.
20. Gibson 2014: 285.
21. Törzsök 2012: 232.
22. Torzsok 2012: 232.
23. See Törzsök 2012; Sanderson 2007b: 280–281.
24. Törzsök 2012: 225.
25. Torzsok 2012: 228.
26. Harṣa Kashmir from 1098–1101 CE. Stein 1900: 6; this Harṣa is not to be confused with the earlier and more well-known Buddhist king by the same name whose empire ruled much of northern India after the fall of the Gupta Empire. That Harṣa reigned from approximately 590 to 647 CE and his kingdom did not include Kashmir. See Kulke and Rothermund 1986: 103–105.
27. Törzsök 2012: 235.
28. RT 8.1331–1339.
29. Warder 1992: 614; Stein 1900: 36. Warder describes Harṣa as "extravagant, easily swayed by ministers and courtiers and unrealistic, even insane." Stein says, "It is Fate to which Kalhaṇa attributes the failing of all resolve and wisdom in Harṣa at the close of his reign. Yet his own account of the latter shows plainly how little such qualities could be expected from a prince manifestly insane. Fate alone is the cause which turns the recipients of royal fortune into enemies of their relatives and trespassers against the moral laws."
30. RT 7.697–699.
31. Törzsök 2012: 222.
32. Törzsök 2012: 232–237. Among these are references to circles of mother deities, mantric powers, the revival of a dead minister by *yoginīs*, forbidden animal oblations, a mock human sacrifice in front of an image of Bhairava, the use of menstrual blood, and rites involving intoxicating liquors.
33. See Sanderson 2003–2004.
34. Sanderson 2004: 232.
35. See Jamwal 2010–2011: 135 for a detailed description in the change of social geography in Kashmir in the *Nila Purāṇa* to the *RT*. Jamwal notes that the *RT* traces the process of tribal communities becoming important landed classes in the valley. For example, a tribal community called the Lavanyas appears in the first three books. Over time, this group settles into peasant communities, becomes established by the

time of Harṣa, and takes on the name Damaras. Another tribe, the Nisadas, also refers to a caste of boatmen in the Kashmir Valley. The *RT* also refers to enslaved Ḍomba women on several occasions. In one story, RT 5.361–386, King Cakravarman becomes enamored with several Ḍomba singers and invites them into his harem, ignoring their low caste.

36. Kalhaṇa expresses surprise at King Yaśakara, whom he describes as performing Vedic purifications but not dismissing attendants who have eaten food abandoned by the low caste Ḍombas. RT 6.69. A few lines later Kalhaṇa explains that Yaśaskara becomes impure through contact with those who have taken the Ḍombas's food. He uses the metaphor of leprosy to explain how the impurity passes through the touch of the impure to the other. RT. 6.84.
37. Törzsök 2013: 196.
38. Marglin 1985: 66.
39. Marglin 1985: 66–67.
40. Marglin 1985: 68.
41. See Torella 2015 for further discussion of the non-duality of the pure-impure categories in Śaiva Tantra.
42. SvTU 4.67.
43. Trsl. Sanderson 2009: 293–294.
44. Sanderson 1985: 203.
45. Törzsök 2014: 200; SvT 2.152cd–153ab.
46. Sanderson 1985: 192.
47. RT 6.108–112.
48. RT 6.108–112; Sanderson 2007b: 281; Kalhaṇa dismisses the effectiveness of the retaliatory ritual in favor of citing a long-standing illness as the king's cause of death.
49. Sanderson 2007b: 282.
50. Törzsök 2012: 232–237.
51. Marglin 1985: 66–68.
52. Young 1999: 50–51.
53. Inden 1985: 31.
54. The *Tantrasāra* describes a slightly different process in which the teacher stays awake all night in an enlightened state. The initiand tells his teacher his dreams but the teacher does not interpret them for the disciple. This assures that the initiand does not become doubtful or afraid of the interpretations. Chakravarty and Marjanovic 2012: 165.
55. SvT 3.
56.

pratyūṣe vimale kṛtvā śaucādyān pūrvavat kramāt |
sakalīkaraṇaṃ kṛtvā pūrvavat praviśed gṛham || 1 ||
śiṣyaś ca śucirācāntaḥ puṣpahastaḥ guruṃ tataḥ
praṇamya śirasā hṛṣṭo guroḥ svapnān nivedayet || 2 ||

57.

svapneṣu madirāpānam āmamāṃsasya bhakṣaṇam || 3 ||
krimiviṣṭhānulepaṃ ca rudhireṇābhiṣecanam |
bhakṣaṇaṃ dadhibhaktasya śvetavastrānulepanam || 4 ||
śvetātapatraṃ mūrdhasthaṃ śvetasragdāmabhūṣaṇam |
siṃhāsanaṃ rathaṃ yānaṃ dhvajaṃ rājyābhiṣecanam || 5 ||
ratnāṅgābharaṇādīni tāmbūlaṃ phalameva ca |
darśanaṃ śrīsarasvatyoḥ śubhanāryavagūhanam || 6 ||

58. SvT 4.7

narendrair ṛṣibhir devaiḥ siddhavidyādharair gaṇaiḥ |
ācāryaiḥ saha samvādaṃ kṛtvā svapne prasiddhyati || 7 ||

59. This is the empowered mantra that becomes effective immediately.

60.

nadīsamudrataraṇam ākāśagamanaṃ tathā |
bhāskarodayanaṃ caiva prajvalantaṃ hutāśanam || 8 ||
grahanakṣatratārāṇāṃ candrabimbasya darśanam |
harmyasyārohaṇaṃ caiva prāsādaśikhare 'pi vā || 9 ||
narāśvavṛṣapotebhataruśailāgrarohaṇam |
vimānagamanaṃ caiva siddhamantrasya darśanam || 10 ||
lābhaḥ siddhacaroścaiva devādīnāṃ ca darśanam |
guṭikāṃ dantakāṣṭhaṃ ca khaḍgapādukarocanāḥ || 11 ||
upavītāñ janaṃ caiva amṛtaṃ pāratauṣadhīḥ |
śaktiṃ kamaṇḍaluṃ padmam akṣasūtraṃ manaḥśilām || 12 ||
prajvalatsiddhadravyāṇi gairikāntāni yāni ca |

61. SvT 15.6a.
62. Sanderson 1985; Wedemeyer 2013.
63. Hatley 2013: 25.
64. White 1996: 282.
65. Sanderson 1995: 84.
66. Also known as Rāmakaṇṭha, the author of the *SpV*, Sanderson 2007b: 411.
67. Trsl. Bansat-Boudon and Tripathi 2011: 257.
68. Bansat-Boudon and Tripathi 2011: 267.
69. Gray 2007; Hatley 2018; Davidson 2002.
70.

dṛṣṭvā siddhyati svapnānte kṣitilābhaṃ vraṇaṃ tathā || 13 ||
kṣatajārṇavasaṅgrāmataraṇaṃ vijayaṃ raṇe |
jvalat pitṛvanaṃ ramyaṃ vīravīreśibhir vṛtam || 14 ||
vīravetālasiddhaiś ca mahāmāṃsasya vikrayam |
mahāpaśoḥ saṃvibhāgaṃ labdhvā devebhya ādarāt || 15 ||
ātmanā pūjayan devam japan dhyāyan stuvannapi |
suhutaṃ cānalaṃ dīptaṃ pūjitaṃ vā prapaśyati || 16 ||

71. According to Lorenzen 1972: 17, the Dravidian was likely a *kāpālika* or other related ascetic practitioner.
72. Lorenzen 1972: 17.
73. Lorenzen 1972: 17.
74. Von Stietencron 2013: 70.
75. Dezsö 2010: 397.
76. SvT 4.18

bhairavaṃ bhairavīṃ dṛṣṭvā siddhyatyatra na saṃśayaḥ |
śubhāḥ svapnā mayākhyātā aśubhāṃśca nibodha me || 18 ||

77. SvT 4.19.
78. SvT 4.19 *tailābhyaṅgas tathā pānaṃ viśanaṃ ca rasātale |*
79. SvT 4.3.
80. SvT 4.19–20

andhakūpe ca patanam atha paṅke nimajjanam || 19 ||
vṛkṣavāhanayānebhyaḥ patanaṃ harmyaparvatāt |

81. Here ear and nose are in dual instrumental or ablative, *karṇanāsābhyām*, but there is nothing to cut off with or from these body parts.
82. SvT 4. 20–21

kartanaṃ karṇanāsābhyām atha vā hastapādayoḥ || 20 ||
patanaṃ dantakeśānām

83. One must be sacrificed but in the dream he cannot sacrifice himself.
84.

ṛkṣavānaradarśanam |
vetālakrūrasattvānāṃ tathaiva kālapūruṣāḥ || 21 ||
kṛṣṇordhvakeśā malināḥ kṛṣṇamālyāmbaracchadāḥ |
raktākṣī strī ca yaṃ svapne puruṣaṃ tv avagūhayet || 22 ||
miryate nātra saṃdeho yadi śāntiṃ na kārayet |
gṛhaprāsādabhedaṃ ca śayyāvastrāsaneṣu ca || 23 ||
ātmano 'bhibhavaṃ saṃkhye ātmadravyāpahāraṇam |
kharoṣṭraśvasṛgāleṣu kaṅkagṛdhrabakeṣu ca || 24 ||
mahiṣolūkakākeṣu rohaṇaṃ ca pravartanam |
bhakṣaṇaṃ pakvamāṃsasya raktamālyānulepanam || 25 ||
kṛṣṇaraktāni vastrāṇi vikṛtātmā prapaśyati |
hasanaṃ valganaṃ svapne mlānasragdāmadhāraṇam || 26 ||
svamāṃsotkartanaṃ bandhaṃ kṛṣṇasarpeṇa bhakṣaṇam |
udvāhaṃ ca tathā svapne dṛṣṭvā naiva prasidhyati || 27 ||

85. Brunner, Oberhammer, and Padoux 2004: 184. Most Śaiva Tantras allow initiation to occur for those who dream of bad omens. To combat the inauspicious, they prescribe extra rituals. However, Brunner, Oberhammer, and Padoux 2004: 184 note that the Pāśupata *SaṃVi*, verse 35, denies initiatory rites to initiands who have bad dreams. The *SaṃVi* does not appear in the *Tāntrikābhidhānakośa*'s list of abbreviations. I believe it refers to the *Saṃvicchodana* but am not completely sure.

Chapter 5

1. Durkheim 1995 [1912]: 37.
2. Durkheim 1995 [1912]: 37.
3. NT 4.1.
4. SvT 5.1–17 mentions only four types of *tattvadīkṣā*, those with three, five, nine, and thirty-six though SvTU 2.150–151 discusses nine, eighteen, and thirty-six, while SvTU 5.17 adds one.
5. I have translated the text and the commentary here in full. The commentary appears in brackets.
6. During *dīkṣā*, the initiand experiences the various levels of the universe and becomes ritually purified upon reaching each *tattva*. Initiation rites that include fewer than the complete set of thirty-six *tattvas* still reaches the same ritual purification, just in a truncated initiation process.
7. The KSTS edition has *śuddhavidyā* and *vidyā* transposed in this list. I have emended this in my translation.
8. This reading is extremely unusual as *tritattvadīkṣā* almost always consists of *ātman*, *vidyā*, and *śiva*. Rastelli and Goodall 2013: 59, 123. SYM 7.7 describes the three as *prakṛti*, *puruṣa*, and *śiva*.
9. SvTU 5.14 says the *ātma*, *vidyā*, and *śiva tattvas* correspond with the more common *śuddhavidyā*, *īśvara*, and *sadāśiva*.
10. This section of commentary includes several oddities that suggest corruption, such as *vyāpīnī* and *vyāptīni*. Here one would expect *vyāptāni* in the second instance. Similarly, in *viśvādi*, we would expect *api* rather than *ādi*. I have not translated the *ādi*.
11.

> *atha dīksāṃ pravakṣyāmi bhuktimuktiphalapradām |*
> *tattvaiḥ ṣaṭtriṃśatārdhena tadardhenātha pañcabhiḥ ||1||*
> *tribhir ekena vā kāryā parāparavibhūtaye |*
> *pṛthvyādi śivāntāni ṣaṭtriṃśat | tadardham aṣṭādaśabhūtāni pañca prakṛtiḥ puruṣo rāgo niyatiḥ śuddhavidyā kālaḥ kalā māyā vidyā īśaḥ sadāśiva śaktiḥ śiva iti | tadardham api prakṛtiḥ puruṣo niyatiḥ kālo māyā vidyā īśaḥ sadāśivaḥ śiva iti nava | pañca pṛthivyādīni nivṛttyādikalāvadviśvavyāpīni | trīṇi bhuvanaśaktiśivākhyāni māyāsadāśivaśivavyāptīni | ekaṃ tv aśeṣaṃ viśvādi śivatattvam |parāparavibhūtir mokṣabhogau saṃpādyau sarvatrāviśiṣṭau ||*

12. Guttural, palatal, retroflex, dental, labial, semivowel, sibilant, and aspirate.
13. See Heilijgers-Seelen 1994: 85n44 for a brief discussion of other texts in which we find ten *padas*.
14. See SvT, KSTS Volume II, page 57 and Padoux 1990: 355 for diagrams showing the distribution of the phonemes.
15. Kahrs 1999: 275.
16. Goodall 2016: 46.
17. Padoux 1990: 353.

18. Padoux 1990: 330.
19. Padoux 1990: 334.
20. Though the text uses *dīkṣā* in the singular, we can see from the following, the text mentions more than one *kalādīkṣā*.
21. cessation, standing still, knowledge, peace, and supreme peace.
22. Here Kṣemarāja spells out the entire vocalic phonemes in reverse. Though Kṣemarāja does not designate how to group the letters, the typical categories of *varga*s can be followed so long as one classifies *kṣa* in its own class. Padoux 1990: 155.
23. SvTU 1–85 describes the mantra as *h-r-kṣ-m-l-v-y-ū-ṃ*. Here, again, Kṣemarāja says to recite the mantra in its inverse. As one cannot begin speech with the sound *ṃ*, he must instead begin with *ū*.
24.

evaṃ ṣaṭprakārāṃ tattvadīkṣām uddiśya kalādi dīkṣām apy uddiśati
kalābhiḥ pañcabhir vātha padair dīkṣāthavā punaḥ ||2||
varṇaiḥ pañcāśatā vāpi mantrair vā bhuvanais tathā |
nivṛttipratiṣṭhāvidyāśāntāśāntyatītāḥ kalāḥ | śrīpūrvādinītyā mātṛkānusāreṇa kṣa ha sa ṣa śa va la ra ya ma bha ba pha pa na dha da tha ta ṇa ḍha ḍa ṭha ṭa ña jha ja cha ca ṅa gha ga kha ka iti nava padāni viśvaviśrāntisthānatvād visargādy akārāntaṃ tu daśamaṃ padam |śrīsvacchandadṛśā tu navātmaprastāroktāny ekāśītir ūkārādīni padāni | śrīsvāyambhuvādiprakriyayā tu vyomavyāpisaṃbandhīni | varṇāḥ kṣādikāntāḥ catustriṃśat pṛthivyādisadāśivāntavācakāḥ visargādyakārāntāstu ṣoḍaśa śaktiśivatattvābhedāmarśinaḥ | śrīpūrvasthityā madhyamavāgvṛttyoktarūpāṇi padāni paśyantīvṛttyā āsū tritabhedābhedāmarśaprādhānyena mantrāḥ | śrīsvacchandaprakriyayā tu hṛt śiraḥśikhe kavacamastraṃ netram ity aṅgānyeva sadya ādivaktramantrāṇi nivṛttyādikalāpañcakavyāptikrameṇāśeṣādhvāma rśīni | mantrā ihatyaprakriyayā vaktramantrāṇāmabhāvādaṅgānyeva | bhuvanāni tu śrīpūrvoktaprakriyayāṣṭādaśottaraśatasaṃkhyāni svacchandadṛśā tu caturviṃśatyadhikadviśatarūpāṇi asya śāstrasya sarvasrotaḥsaṃgraharūpatvāt tattadāgamoktaṣaḍadhvavibhāgakalpana yā dīkṣākramasyāvirodhāt ||

25. White 2012: 1.
26.

etaiḥ sarvaiḥ prakartavyā kāryā hy ekatamā 'thavā || 3 ||
sarvais tu samudāyena śaktivyaktisvarūpataḥ |
ekatamaṃ saṃśodhyādhvānaṃ vyaktirūpeṇa vyāpakatayā prādhānyenāśritya tadantaritamadhvapañcakaṃ śaktirūpeṇa vyāpyaṃ bhāvayedityarthaḥ | yathoktaṃ śrīsvacchande "adhvāvalokanaṃ paścād vyāpyavyāpakabhāvataḥ" (4-95) ityādi ||

27. Brunner, Oberhammer, and Padoux 2004: 138.
28. Rastelli and Goodall 2013: 470.

29.

eṣā ca sarvaiva dīkṣā
yathāvibhavasāreṇa kartavyā daiśikottamaiḥ ||4||
vibhavavatāṃ mahāsaṃbhāraiḥ | itareṣāṃ dūrvām bupallavādibhir api | evaṃ hy analasyanaiḥ spṛhyābhyāṃ daiśikānām uttamatā ||

30.

tatrādau śiṣyadehapāśasūtrāvalambanam adhvasaṃdhānam adhvopasthāpanam adhvapūjāhomāvadhv āntaḥpāśatrayabhāvanām ādhāraśaktinyāsādi ca kṛtvā vāgīśīpūjanaṃ kāryaṃ tadgarbhe yojayet paśum | karmapāśavaśasaṃbhāvyavicitracaturdaśavidhabhogāyatanotpattyartham |

31. SvT 4.539c–545.

32.

garbhādhānaṃ tu jananam adhikāro layas tathā ||5||
bhogaḥ karmārjanaṃ caiva niṣkṛtis tadanantaram |
mūlamantreṇa kartavyaṃ nānāśarīrāṇām antaḥpraroho garbhādhānam bahir niḥsṛtir jananam bhogayogyānāṃ pravṛddhānāṃ saṃpattir adhikāraḥ tadanantaraṃmantramāhātmyaparipakvabhogasādhanatvasyakarmaṇo'rjanaṃ bhogadānaun mukhyarūpam tadanantaraṃ sukhaduḥkhamohaprāptyātmā bhogaḥ tato nivṛtte 'pi bhoge kaṃcitkālaṃ bhogasaṃskāro layaḥ tato 'pi samastajātyāyurbhoganiḥśeṣasaṃpattyātmā niṣkṛtiḥ ity etatsarvaṃ mūlamantrahomais tryādisaṃkhyaiḥ kāryam niṣkṛtistu śatahomā tadante ca dvijatvāpattirudrāṃśāpattī cintayet ||
samāpteṣu bhogeṣu bhoktṛtvābhāvarūpaṃ viśleṣākhyaṃ saṃskāraṃ kṛtvā
pāśacchedas tathā smṛtaḥ || 4-6 ||
astramantreṇa
tato viśleṣānantarabhāvitayā smṛtaṃ pāśasūtrasya chedam astramantreṇa kṛtvā tenaiva pāśasya
dāhas tu

33. A place twelve fingers breadth above the crown of the head where the out breath rests.

34.

tato 'pi
bhasmīkaraṇatatsthite |
bhasmīkaraṇaṃ niḥsaṃskārāṇāṃ pāśānāṃ śamanam astreṇaiva |
tatsthitaṃ tu nivṛttāśeṣaśarīrasya śiṣyacaitanyasya mūlenaikyaṃ
vibhāvya, svahṛtpraveśena dvādaśāntaprāpaṇapūrvaṃ śiṣyahṛtsthatvāpādanarūpaṃ sthānaṃ sthitam tasya sthitam iti vyutpattyā tatsthitam ||

35. Davis 2000: 94.

36. Törzsök 2014: 354–355 notes that the *Svacchanda Tantra* (SvT 4.88) teaches that children, fools, the elderly, women, and the sick do not receive full initiation. Instead they receive a "seedless" initiation, which means they are not obligated to follow post-initiatory rules. The initiation given to these practitioners is less powerful as they are not expected to become full-time practitioners. Further, Kṣemarāja notes at SvT 3.164 that some sources, he does not say which ones, state that male initiands hold the *pāśasūtra* in his right hand while females hold it in their left. Kṣemarāja says this is wrong because the initiand, regardless of gender, holds *darbha* grass as an extension of the *nāḍīs* in both hands. This means the *pāśasūtra* must be tied to the topknot, generally associated with male practitioners.
37. Davis 2000: 94.
38. Davis 2000: 94.
39. Davis 2000: 94.
40. Davis 2000: 94.
41. The *tanmātras*: sound (*śabda*), touch (*sparśa*), form (*rūpa*), essence (*rasa*), and odor (*gandha*)
42. I have left *kevala* untranslated here as the term is somewhat ambiguous and its meaning varies from text to text, sometimes meaning isolation and at others meaning whole. Here it has the sense of a cessation of individual perception.
43.

nordhve dhyānaṃ prayuñjīta nādhastānna ca madhyataḥ |
nāgrataḥ pṛṣṭhataḥ kiñcit pārśvayor ubhayor api || 41 ||
nāntaḥśarīrasaṃsthāne na bāhye bhāvayet kvacit |
nākāśe bandhayellakṣyaṃ nādho dṛṣṭiṃ niveśayet || 42 ||
na cākṣṇor mīlanaṃ kiñcin na kiñcid dṛṣṭibandhanam |
avalambaṃ nirālambaṃ sālambaṃ na ca bhāvayet || 43 ||
nendriyāṇi na bhūtāni śabdasparśarasādi yat |
sarvaṃ tyaktvā samādhisthaḥ kevalaṃ tanmayo bhavet || 44 ||

44. Brunner 1963: 161.
45. Brunner 1963: 161.
46. Bansat-Boudon and Tripathi 2011: 171n738.
47. Bansat-Boudon and Tripathi 2011: 341.
48. SpK 3.19; SpN 3.19.
49. The *Parātrīśikā Vivaraṇa* describes an external ritual in which the guru performs *nyāsa* on the skull, mouth, heart, genitals, and the whole body (of both himself and the *vīra*). The topknot (*śikhā*) is then tied with twenty-seven mantras. PTV 27; See Singh 1988: 247–248 for the list of these mantras. In the PTV, this *japa* is followed by the consecration of flowers with water, further *japa*, and *nyāsa*. This practice also indicates *nyāsa* on the body: the head, mouth, heart, genitals, body, and topknot.

50.

anantaraṃ brahmāder āhvānapūjāhomapuryaṣṭakāṃśārpaṇaśrāvaṇa visarjanādi kṛtvā kalāditattvāntarānusandhipūrvaṃ sarvādhvasaṃśuddhiṃ kṛtvā

śikhācchedaṃ tato homaṃ

kuryāt viśvādhvāśrayaprāṇaśaktirūpaśikhāvyāptyā śikhāṃ chittvā juhuyād ity arthaḥ ||

anantaraṃ brahmāder āhvānapūjāhomapuryaṣṭakāṃśārpaṇaśrāvaṇa visarjanādi kṛtvā kalāditattvāntarānusandhipūrvaṃ sarvādhvasaṃśuddhiṃ kṛtvā

śikhācchedaṃ tato homaṃ

kuryāt viśvādhvāśrayaprāṇaśaktirūpaśikhāvyāptyā śikhāṃ chittvā juhuyād ity arthaḥ ||

atha vidhyan yathā saṃpattivaśasaṃbhāvyaprāyaścittahomānantaram

"jñātvā cārapramāṇaṃ tu prāṇasañcārameva ca" (4–231)

ity ādiśrīsvacchandoktaprameyapañcadaśakasatattvajño jñānayogaśālī

ācāryavaryaḥ praśāntapāśaṃ śisyam

mūlenaiva tu yojayet || 47 ||

"vyāpāraṃ mānasaṃ tyaktvā bodhamātreṇa yojayet |

tadā śivatvam abhyeti paśur mukto bhavārṇavāt ||" (4–437)

iti śrīsvacchandoktadṛśā paratattvasamāveśanayā paramaśivaikarūpaṃ kuryāt || 7 ||

51.

tadāha

saṃyojya parame tattve saṃsthānaṃ tatra kārayet |

tathāsau tanmaya eva syāt ||

atha yojanikānāṃ vibhāgamāha

adhikārārtham ācārye parāparapade sthite || 8 ||

śivatve sādhakānāṃ tu vidyād dīkṣāṃ sadāśive |

putrake parame tattve samayinyaiśvare tathā || 9 ||

parāparapade śivatve iti

"atrārūḍhas tu kurute śivaḥ paramakāraṇam" iti svacchandoktanītyā paramaśivayojanānantaram ācāryāṇām aparaśivayojanā kāryā sādhakānāṃ tu śivayojanānantaraṃ sadāśivayojanā kāryā putrakāṇāṃ paratattva eva samayināmīśvaratattve iti vibhāgāḥ || 9 ||

52. Abhinavagupta, PTV 22 calls this the *brahmadeha* (*brahma* body).
53. Biernacki 2015: 355.
54. Nemec 2011: 178n211.
55.

upasaṃharati

evam uddeśato dīkṣā kathitā vistaro 'nyataḥ || 4-10 ||

uddeśata ity anyata ity anena cātivitato 'pyayaṃ

dīkṣāvidhir ihātisaṃkṣepeṇāsūtritattvāt śrīsvacchandādiśāstrebhyo

vitatya samyagavagamya prayoktavya iti śikṣayati iti śivam ||
jayatyaśeṣapāśaughaploṣakṛd bhaktiśālinām |
paradhāmasamāveśapradaṃ netraṃ maheśituḥ || ||

Chapter 6

1. White 2000: 4–7 discusses the various definitions scholars and practitioners have given Tantra over time. In popular culture, Tantra is often associated with sexual practices. To rehabilitate Tantra's image, scholar-practitioners have emphasized the non-transgressive, philosophical side of Tantra. This makes a definition of Tantra difficult to agree on, as what makes something Tantric depends largely on perspective. As I noted in the introduction and elsewhere in this work, the *Netra Tantra* does not overtly prescribe any transgressive practices. Yet, because it fits into an ontological canon of work that does call for such behaviors, questions of purity and impurity arise in discussion of the text.
2. Taussig 1998: 354–355.
3. Taussig 1998: 355.
4. Douglas 1966: 123.
5. SvT 15.4a.
6. SvT 15.6a.
7. SvTU 15.6.
8. Douglas 1966: 161.
9. Törzsök 2012: 222.
10. Törzsök 2012: 224.
11. Törzsök 2012: 225–227.
12. The authorship and exact dates of the *Arthaśāstra* are unclear, but the text clearly precedes the spread of Tantrism, with allusions to it found as early as the fifth century CE. Scharfe 1993: 1. The text appears to have been influential up to as late as the fourteenth century. Scharfe 1993: 11. The *Arthaśāstra* is only one of many surviving texts that describe the system of law. Among the most influential works of *dharmaśāstra* are *Manusmṛti*, *Bṛhaspatismṛti*, *Nāradasmṛti*, and *Yājñavalkyasmṛti*.
13. Olivelle 2013: 250.
14. Olivelle 2013: 250.
15. Including removal of the penis.
16. Olivelle 2013: 251. Consenting partners are to receive the same punishment.
17. Olivelle 2013: 251–252.
18. Such as the *Brahmayāmala* and *Svacchanda Tantras*. See Törzsök 2013: 148 and Goodall 2004: xxxvii.
19. Flood 2006: 145.
20. Scharfe 1993: 11.
21. Drabu 1986: 185; RT 4.96, 105.
22. McDaniel 2004: 107; Doniger O' Flaherty 1980b: 275.

23. Scharfe 2002: 208.
24. RT 7.1129–1133.
25. RT 7.1147–1148.
26. RT 7.11149.
27. Here likely a reference to them acting as *yoginīs*.
28. Törzsök 2012: 228.
29. Törzsök 2012: 230.
30. Sanderson 2001: 2–14.
31. Sanderson 2009: 252.
32. Sanderson 2009: 250.
33. Sanderson 2009: 252.
34. Geertz 1980: 36–37.
35. Geertz 1980: 37.
36. Geertz 1980: 37.
37. Bisgaard 1994: 56–58. Kṣemendra and Kalhaṇa were literary rivals. Kalhaṇa accused Kṣemendra's father of raiding the royal treasury for his wealth. Bisgaard points out that Kṣemendra gives a contrary account as to the provenance of Kṣemendra's family wealth. If Kṣemarāja's account is correct, such a theft would indicate close proximity to the court via the ability to access such funds. Though in dispute, this demonstrates Kṣemendra's family proximity to governmental affairs.
38. For example, in KV 1.10–95 the adept Mūladeva instructs a merchant's son in religious hypocrisy and deception. See Vasudeva 2005: 95–127; Bisgaard 1994: 59–64. Further, Kṣemendra's *Narmamālā* and *Deśopadeśa* also contain satirical caricatures of Śaiva gurus. See Bisgaard 1994: 64–68.
39. Vasudeva 2005: 17.
40. Muller-Ortega 2000: 574.
41. Also sometimes spelled Maṅkhaka or Maṅkhuka.
42. KC 3.62, 25.61. Jayasimha ruled from 1128 to 1149. Jayaratha, who would later write the commentary on Abhinavagupta's *Tantrāloka*, was the grandson of a minister to a king widely assumed to be Jayasimha. Rastogi 1987: 88.
43. KC 25: 10–20.
44. KC 25: 144–150.
45. KC 25.94b–95a; 102; 106–134; Pollock 2003: 92; Stein 1900 (vol. I): 12; Bhatt 1973: 8–9.
46. Pollock 2003: 92.
47. Pollock 2003: 117–118.
48. Rastogi 1987: 1 points out the *Śrīkaṇṭhacarita*'s clear reference to the Krama school of Tantra. Rastogi argues that this mention demonstrates the popularity of Krama outside of philosophical circles.
49. KC 17.18–28.
50. KC 17.19.
51. Hanneder 1998: 6–7.
52. Wallis 2007: 249.

53. As is common in this text, the object is not named. Here I assume it is *mṛtyujit* from context.

54.

> *rahasyaṃ sampradāyaś ca sarvaśreyaḥ sukhāvahaḥ |*
> *sādhakās tu prasannā ye bhaktā hy ārādhayanti ca || 84 ||*
> *sarvaduḥkhavimuktās te satyaṃ me nānṛtaṃ vacaḥ |*

55. Sanderson 2010: 12.

56. The grammar is unclear. It can be understood either that the *ācārya* [teacher] performs the ritual on behalf of the monarch's devoted wives and children or that he does so on behalf of his own wives and children. Toward the end of this section we see that the *ācārya* receives the benefits of the ritual as a byproduct of performing it on behalf of another, making the first reading of this sentence more likely correct in this context.

57.

> *anenaivātmanaḥ kāryaṃ sarvaduḥkhanivāraṇam || 85 ||*
> *bhaktānāṃ svasutānāṃ ca svadārāṇāṃ ca kārayet |*
> *svaśiṣyāṇāṃ ca bhaktānāṃ nānyathā tu prayojayet || 86 ||*
> *sarvāśramagurutvāc ca bhūpatīnāṃ ca sarvadā |*
> *tatsutānāṃ ca patnīnāṃ kartavyo hitam icchatā || 87 ||*

58. *mātṛdoṣa* here refers to the polluting attacks of female spirits called *mātṛs*. At NT 19.98–99 the mothers appear in a list of dangers that includes the demons *yakṣas*, *rakṣasas*, *piśācas* as well as bad dreams and terror that causes suffering.

> *nitye naimittike kāmye śāntyarthaṃ kārayet sadā |*
> *mukhe prakṣālite nityaṃ tilakaḥ śvetabhasmanā || 88 ||*
> *saptābhimantritaḥ kāryo mātṛdoṣanivṛttaye |*

59. I have translated *hiṃsaka* here as enemies but, as White 2012: 4, points out, in an earlier section of this same chapter of the *NT*, *hiṃsaka* can be read as, "'a Brāhman skilled in the magical texts of the Atharva-veda': in other words, a black magician or sorcerer." I have used the more generic term "enemy" to denote a person or spirit. Sanderson 2004: 247 translates this loosely as spirits.

60. The text uses the term *mantravid*, a knower of mantra. I retain this term in the translation but use *mantrin* as I have in the remainder of this work for the sake of consistency, as it refers to the same guru.

61. In its dual form, *pārśvayoḥ* can be taken to mean heaven and earth. Sanderson 2004: 248 gives the variant reading from the NGMPP NAK MS 1-285, as *candrayor madhye*, in the middle of two moons. Kṣemarāja's commentary also references the two moons, *candradvayamadhyasthitaṃ*.

62.

> *samālambhanapuṣpaṃ vā tāmbūlenābhimantritam || 89 ||*
> *dīyate yasya tasyaiva na hiṃsantīha hiṃsakāḥ |*
> *bhojanaṃ cābhimantreta mantreṇānena mantravit || 90 ||*

ubhayoḥ pārśvayor madhye bhuñjāno 'mṛtam aśnute |
sarvavyādhivinirmuktas tiṣṭhate nṛpatiḥ kṣitau || 91 ||

63. AŚ 5: 3 describes the compensation given to people performing various official duties. These include bureaucrats, soldiers, performers, and *mantrins*. AŚ 5: 3.20 says, "In sacrifices such as the royal consecration, the 'king' should receive double the wage given to those of equal learning." (Trsl. Olivelle) According to Olivelle, this "king" is a guru who plays the role of the king during the ceremony.
64. For example, the *Dharmasūtras* describe this practice at DSĀ 2: 3.22; DSB 6.1–7.10.
65.

atha krīḍanakāleṣu gajāśvasahitasya ca |
astrakrīḍāsu sarvāsu rakṣārthaṃ kalaśaṃ yajet || 92 ||
krīḍārthaṃ vijayārthaṃ ca rakṣārthaṃ hiṃsakādiṣu |
yasmād duṣṭāś ca bahavo jighāṃsanti nṛpādikam || 93 ||
tasmād rakṣā prakartavyā sarvaśreyaskarī śubhā |

66. AŚ 10: 2.17 describes the vulnerabilities of infantrymen, themselves both symbolic and actual protectors of the kingdom.
67. Sumegi 2008: 40–48.
68. AŚ 14: 3 focuses on esoteric practices, many of which cause the target to fall asleep where he is vulnerable.
69.

tataḥ suptasya nṛpate rakṣārthaṃ kalaśaṃ yajet || 94 ||
raupyaṃ cauṣadhisaṃyuktaṃ candanāgurulepitam |
kṣīreṇa cāmbhasā pūrṇaṃ yajenmṛtyujitaṃ param || 95 ||
sarvaśvetopacāreṇa puṣpadhūpārghapāyasaiḥ |
agre sthitā mahānidrā jagatsaṃmohakāriṇī || 96 ||
sukhārthaṃ nṛpate rātrau jīrṇārthaṃ bhojanādike |
ārabdhā devadevena ājñāṃ dattveti bhāvayet || 97 ||
tato rātriṃ samagrāṃ tu tiṣṭhed vai nidrayā saha |
yakṣarakṣaḥpiśācādyair duḥsvapnair mātṛ saṃbhavaiḥ || 98 ||
bhayais santrāsa duḥkhais tu muktas tiṣṭhed yathāsukham |

The KSTS NT for *bhayais santrāsa* reads *bhayais tantrāsa*, likely a typo.

70. In Buddhist imagery, the Lokapālas sometimes trample demons, making them excellent protectors here. Linrothe 1999: 21.
71. The benefits of the ritual.
72.

lokapāleṣu sāstreṣu rakṣārthaṃ nṛpasaṃnidhau || 99 ||
pūjanaṃ cārghapuṣpādyaiḥ kalaśe pūjite sati |
yasyaivaṃ satataṃ kuryāj jñānavān daiśikottamaḥ || 100 ||
pūrvoktaṃ samavāpnoti . . .

73. In this case, Mṛtyujit is a form of Amṛteśa, who acts as a sort of personal deity for the king as worshipped by the *mantrin* on the king's behalf. See Sanderson 2004: 253.

74. Sanderson 2004: 251 gives this festival as occurring on "the twelfth day of the bright fortnight of the month Bhādrapada (July/August)." Most sources list Śrāvaṇa as July–August and Bhādrapada as August–September. See Bühnemann 1988: 124; and Lochtefeld 2002: 93. Sanderson 2004: 251–252, references the Viṣṇudharmottara, Khaṇḍa 2, chapter 155 and its description of a rite during Bhādrapada in which the king worships Indra. In this rite the king ceremonially enters the decorated city. He then fasts and holds a vigil with his chaplain, astrologer, and citizens. The *mantrin* performs a fire sacrifice. A ritual pole, which was erected and consecrated, is disposed of at the end of the rite.
75. I.e., for the harvest.
76. I.e., the palace.
77. The celebration of *Mahānavamī* in medieval India has been most studied as it occurred in the southern capital of Vijayanagara, due to the abundance of epigraphs, travelogues, and descriptions in various literary sources.
78.

prāheti bhagavāñ chivaḥ |
nimitteṣu ca sarveṣu amṛteśaṃ yajeta ca || 101 ||
kāmarūpaṃ (em: kāmarūpe) sadā yasmāt sarvakāmān avāpnuyāt |
prajānāṃ rakṣaṇārthāya śālīnāṃ cāpi sampade || 102 ||
sutapatnīṣu rakṣārthamātmano rāṣṭravṛddhaye |
indrarūpaṃ yajet tatra vijayārthaṃ nṛpasya ca || 103 ||
gobrāhmaṇeṣu rakṣārthamātmanaḥ svajaneṣu ca |
mahānavamyāṃ pūjyeta bhūriyāgena veśmani || 104 ||
pūrvoktaṃ samavāpnoti āyurārogya-saṃpadam |

79. Kulke 2010: 612.
80. See Fritz and Mitchell 1987 and Sinopoli and Morrison 1995.
81. See Fritz and Mitchell 1987; Mitchell 1992, 1993; and Sinopoli and Morrison 1995.
82. Kulke 2010: 614.
83. Geertz 1980: 13.
84. Geertz 1980: 13.
85. Bansat-Boudon and Tripathi,2011: 32.
86. Eaton 2005: 81.
87. Geertz 1980: 76.
88. Eaton 2005: 80.
89. Kulke 2010: 615.
90. Geertz 1980: 13.
91. Geertz 1980: 13.
92. Geertz 1980: 106.
93. Geertz 1980: 106.
94. Geertz 1980: 13.
95. Kulke 2010: 621.
96. NTU 19.105 *divyāny astrāṇi mantraprabhāvāt saṃpādayati.*
97. Balkaran 2015: 99–100.

98.

astrayāgaḥ prakartavyaḥ prayatnāt siddhihetave || 105 ||
astrasiddhim avāpnoti prayoktā phalam aśnute

99. For example, natural disasters.
100.

yadā mṛtyuvaśāghrātaḥ kālena kalito nṛpaḥ || 106 ||
ariṣṭacihnitātmā vai deśo vā tatsutādayaḥ |
brāhmaṇādiṣu sarveṣu nāśe janapadasya ca || 107 ||
śālyādiṣu ca śasyeṣu phalamūlodakeṣu ca |
durbhikṣavyādhikāryeṣu utpāteṣu mahatsu ca || 108 ||
tadā nīrājanaṃ kāryaṃ rājño rāṣṭravivṛddhaye |
pūrvavad yajanaṃ kṛtvā kalaśenābhiṣecayet || 109 ||

101. Such as AŚ 2: 30.51; BS, Chapter 43.
102. AŚ 2: 30.51, trsl. Olivelle.
103. AŚ 4: 3.13–16, trsl. Olivelle.
104. Inden 1985: 32–33.
105. Shastri 1969: 16.
106. For a more complete description of this ritual see Shastri 1969: 181–182.
107.

niḥśaṃko nirjane rātrau śubharakṣe ca tathāṃśake |
jayapuṇyāhaśabdaiś ca vedamaṅgalaniḥsvanaiḥ || 110 ||
abhiṣiñcet tu rājānaṃ siddhārthān juhuyād bahūn |
nīrājanavidhānena nāmāṅke saṃskṛte priye || 111 ||
vahnau saṃruddhamanasā ajāṃś ca prokṣayed bahūn |
tṛptyarthaṃ bhūtasaṅghasya mantrī rakṣārtham udyataḥ || 112 ||
śākunoktyāṃśagatyā vā vijñāya śakunaṃ hitam |
yakṣendraśivavāruṇyā niryātaḥ sarvasiddhidaḥ || 113 ||

108. By public, here I mean a rite more along the lines of the orthodox traditions but still likely small in attendance.
109. Sanderson 2004: 261n79.
110.

atha pūrvoktavidhinā gṛhe yāgaṃ tu kārayet |
yāvat saptāhnikaṃ devi bhūrihomena siddhidam || 114 ||
asyācalā mahālakṣmī rājyaṃ vā yadabhīpsitam |
bhaumāntarikṣa-siddhīś ca prāpnuyān nṛpatiḥ sukhī || 115 ||
tadā nīrājanaṃ khyātaṃ sarvaśreyaskaraṃ param |
pūrvoktān nāśayed doṣān devi nāstyatra saṃśayaḥ || 116 ||

111. Sanderson 2004: 261.
112. NT 19.110 *nirjana iti guptasthāne.*
113. Shastri 1969: 181.

114.

goṣu madhye yajed yasmāt sadā vardheta gokulam |
sindūraṃ gairikaṃ vāpi abhimantryaiva mantravit || 117 ||
yojayed goṣu rakṣārthaṃ śṛṅgordhve sarvadoṣajit |
aśvānām api rakṣārthaṃ pūrvoktavidhinā yajet || 118 ||
abhimantryaiva kalaśaṃ mūrdhni teṣāṃ prapātayet |
siddhārtho mantrajaptas tu kaṇṭhe kāryo 'tha mūrdhani || 119 ||
sarvadoṣavinirmuktān gajāṃś caiva tu rakṣati |
ajādiṣu paśuṣv evaṃ rakṣāṃ sarveṣu kārayet || 120 ||
sarvaprāṇiṣu rakṣārthaṃ yoktavyo nṛpateḥ sadā |

115. This may be best articulated by the Chinese in the idea of the Mandate of Heaven, in which the Gods judge the monarch's right to rule. If the Gods deem the king is just and virtuous, they allow him to continue his rule. If the Gods become displeased they indicate that disapproval through the infliction of environmental and economic calamities.

116. I.e., insanity.

117.

mahāśāntir bhavet teṣāṃ durbhikṣaṃ naśyati kṣaṇāt || 121 ||
mahābhayeṣu sarveṣu bhūkampolkānipātane |
ativṛṣṭāv anāvṛṣṭau mūṣakādibhayeṣu ca || 122 ||
akālotpannapuṣpādau devair naṣṭaiś ca khaṇḍitaiḥ |
jvaralūtādidoṣaiś ca apamṛtyubhir eva ca || 123 ||
duḥkhair nānāvidhaiś caiva āghrātaṃ maṇḍalaṃ yadi |
karmadoṣāś ca ye kecid graha-doṣās tathā gatāḥ || 124 ||
tirobhāvas tathotpanno mantracchidraṃ tathāgatam |
nāgādiviṣadoṣāś ca kīṭavisphoṭakādayaḥ || 125 ||
vātapittavikārāś ca śleṣmadoṣāś ca sarvataḥ |
arśāṃsi cakṣūrogāś ca tathā visarpakādayaḥ || 126 ||
vyādhyantarāṇi doṣāś ca kṣatajādyāḥ sahasraśaḥ |
ābhyantarā vyādhayaś ca śokādyāś cittanāśakāḥ || 127 ||
abhiśaptāś ca devādyair brahmaṇādyā yadā janāḥ |
tadā tu pūrvavadyāgaḥ kartavyaḥ śāntihetave || 128 |

118. RT 8.498.

119. RT 8.668–671.

120. Iyengar, Sharma, and Siddiqui 1999: 187–188.

121. RT 8.116–1168.

122. Known today as the Jhelum River.

123. RT 8.1175, trsl. Stein 1900, vol. 2: 93.

124. RT 8.1181, trsl. Stein 1900, vol. 2: 94.

125. Trsl. Stein 1900, vol. 2: 98.

126. Sanderson 2004: 268.

127.

pratyahaṃ havanaṃ kāryaṃ rājñāṃ rāṣṭravivṛddhaye |
sukhena bhujyate rājyaṃ nātra kāryā vicāraṇā || 129 ||
sakṛtpūjanamātreṇa naśyante hiṃsakādayaḥ |
naṣṭā daśa diśo yānti siṃhasyeva mṛgādayaḥ || 130 ||
satatābhyāsayogena dāridryaṃ naśyati kulāt |
yasmin deśe ca kāle ca nivasen mantravit sadā || 131 ||
ītayo vyādhayaś caiva khārkhodāstasya vā grahāḥ |
śākinyo vividhā yakṣāḥ piśācā rākṣasās tathā || 132 ||
bālagrahāś ca visphoṭā vyantarāś cāparāś ca ye |
sarvāṇi viṣajātāni durbhikṣaṃ grahapīḍanam || 133 ||
sarvaṃ na prabhavet tatra mantravitsaṃnidhānataḥ |

128. Mustard seeds appear in descriptions of Hindu ritual but not with the same frequency as other elements, such as sesame seeds. The *Suśrutasaṃhita* gives various medicinal uses of mustard seed and the *Arthaśāstra* describes it as a very powerful element of esoteric practice. See *Nidānasthāna* 16.5–8, *Cikitsāsthāna* 5.12–14, 14.16, 16.22–23, 22.30, 32.8, 37.38, and 37.44; AŚ 14: 1.33, 14: 1.36, 14: 2.4, 14: 2.8–9.

129.

ataḥ paraṃ pravakṣyāmi sarvarakṣākaro yathā |
mantranātho mahograṃ ca dhūpaṃ rakṣoghnacoditam || 1 ||

If we read *rakṣoghna* in its alternate form the passage can be read, "and how perfume quickly drives back demons." *Rakṣogna* will be elaborated further in NT 15.5.

130. RT 3.338; Beer 2003: 25; Gentry 2010: 136; Shinohara 2014: 52.

131.

saptavārābhijaptas tu rakṣoghno yasya dīyate |
śiraḥsthaṃ dhārayen nityaṃ sarvadoṣaiḥ sa mucyate || 2 ||

132. Yelle 2003: 50.
133. Kahrs 1999: 96.
134. Kahrs 1999, xiv.
135. See Kahrs 1999: 61–63.
136. Yelle 2003: 45.
137.

sarvadaityakṣayārthaṃ tu maduktenaiva brahmaṇā |
serṣyāṇāṃ caiva sarveṣām abhicāro yataḥ kṛtaḥ || 3 ||
tadāsau sarṣapaḥ proktaḥ pāti rakṣati sarvataḥ |

138. In which the name of a thing is substituted with an attribute or adjunct of that thing.
139.

yadā rakṣāṃsi sarvāṇi vidrutāni hatāni ca || 4 ||
tadā devi mayā proktā rakṣoghnāḥ prathitā bhuvi |

āhaveṣu ca sarveṣu daityaiḥ saha surottamaiḥ || *5* ||
niyuktā duṣṭahantāraḥ siddhyarthaṃ ripunāśane |
teṣām artho yadā siddhas tena siddhārthakā bhuvi || *6* ||
khyātā darpaharā devi bhūtānāṃ duṣṭacetasām |

140. It is not clear exactly how the naming is offered.

141.

yadā sarveṣu bhūteṣu bhayatrasteṣu sarvataḥ || *7* ||
nīrājanavidhānena nāmāṅkaṃ juhuyāt priye |
vahnau saṃkruddhamanasā mantrī rakṣārtham udyataḥ || *8* ||
tadā nīrājanaṃ khyātaṃ sarvaśreyaskaraṃ param |

142. I.e., the four colors: white, yellow, red, and black.

143.

sitādir yugabhedena vartate 'nugrahe balī || *9* ||
śuklaḥ sarvapradaḥ khyāto rakto rājyapradāyakaḥ |
pīto rakṣākaraḥ proktaḥ kṛṣṇaḥ śatruvināśakṛt || *10* |
caturyugeṣu sarvatra pītakṛṣṇau dvirūpakau |
rājasarṣapagaurākhyau dvirūpo 'ntarhitaḥ priye || *11* ||

144. *akta* means oil or ointment. Here it likely refers to honey, ghee, and milk as these are the standard divine foods used in ritual alongside mustard seeds or rice, and sesame seeds.

145.

yadā mṛtyuvaśaṃ yātaḥ sarvabhūtair upadrutaḥ |
tadā tu ghṛtasaṃyuktaṃ gokṣīrsitaśarkarā || *12* ||
tilair vimiśritaṃ kṛtvā juhuyāt sarvaśāntidam |
tilaiḥ kṛṣṇaiḥ samāyuktaṃ rājasarṣapam uttamam || *13* ||
tryaktaṃ vai juhuyāt sadyaḥ sarvaśāntiphalapradam |

146.

anenaivābhimantryaitad yasya haste pradīyate || *14* ||
saubhāgyam atulaṃ tasya jāyate nātra saṃśayaḥ |

147.

saptakṛtvo 'bhisaṃmantrya mantreṇānena mantravit || *15* ||
mūrdhni prapātayed yasya sarvadoṣaiḥ sa mucyate |

148.

abhimantrya . . . vāsāṃsi causadham || *16* ||
samālambhena . . . vābhimantritam |
dīyate yasya tasya . . . hiṃsakaḥ || *17* ||

The commentary, too, is incomplete and does not help fill in the gaps.

White 2012, has claimed that these *hiṃsakas* can also be a brahmin practicing black magic. Certainly they should be included among the list of enemies, but there is no evidence in this particular chapter that this specific type of enemy is being discussed rather than a more general one.

149.

digvidikṣu japed yasya rakṣārthaṃ prayatātmanaḥ |
divā vā yadi vā rātrau svapato jāgrato 'pi vā || 18 ||
avadhyaḥ sarvabhūtaiś ca bhuvi tiṣṭhaty asau naraḥ |

150. Törzsök 2012: 217, 221.

Chapter 7

1. Törzsök 2013: 195.
2. Törzsök 2013: 196.
3. Törzsök 2013: 196. Törzsök notes that Siddhānta Tantras do not completely reject the use of impure substances. The *Guhyasūtra* prescribes the use of impure materials when a practitioner performs rites to obtain supernatural powers.
4. Törzsök 2014: 196. The impure substances described in the *Guhyasūtra* of the *Niśvāsatattvasaṃhitā* include offering cow flesh, blood, skulls, and charnel ground ashes.
5. Sanderson 1985: 200–206.
6. Wedemeyer 2013: 155–165.
7. Lorenzen 1972: 13; Mirashi 1947: 300–310.
8. Lorenzen 1972: 13.
9. Buswell 2004: 450.
10. Lorenzen 1972: 14.
11. Lorenzen 1972: 14–24.
12. Goodall 2015: 71.
13. Wedemeyer 2013: 194.
14. Wedemeyer 2013: 187.
15. Sanderson 1985: 203.
16. Sanderson 1985: 203.
17. Sanderson 1985: 203.
18. Sanderson 1985: 203.
19. Sanderson 1985: 198–199, 203.
20. As Törzsök 2014: 221 notes, early Bhairava Tantras struggle with this non-existence of differentiation as non-dual practice ultimately implies the absence of purity and purification. Only anti-ritual texts can logically remove purification altogether without undermining the need for ritual in the first place. The *Kulasāra* takes the position that all differentiation is delusion and initiation a completely mental practice in which one recognizes the non-differentiation of pure and impure.
21. Flood 2003: 215.
22. Slouber 2017: 40.
23. Sanderson 2001: 14.

24. Sanderson 2001: 14.
25. Hatley 2007: 144.
26. The other four are the Siddhānta Tantras, Bhairava Tantras, Vāma Tantras, and Gāruḍa Tantras. Hatley 2007: 144. Each class of literature stems from one of the Sadāśiva's five mouths. The Siddhānta Tantras from the upper Īśāna face; the Vāma Tantras from the northern face, the Bhairava Tantras from the southern face, the Gāruḍa Tantras from the eastern face, and the Bhūta Tantras from the western face. Sanderson 2014: 20.
27. Sanderson 2014: 19–20.
28. Gray 2007: 14.
29. Sanderson 2014: 20.
30. For example, in addition to the Bhūta Tantras, exorcism appears in Vedic, Upaniṣadic, Epic, and Purāṇic literature. Smith 2006: 177–195 examines the root to enter (*ā√viś*) and its derivative forms, which "occurs almost entirely in the sense of entities of different densities or substantialities penetrating and pervading one another." Smith 2006: 177. Smith 2006: 195–232 argues that ṚV 10.30.5, 9.38.5, 9.95.3; AV 6.2.2, 7.79.3; ĀpŚS 5.1.7; TB 1.2.1.5–7, 1.3.6.2; TU 1.4.3, and many other passages refer to an early idea of *brahman*, *soma*, and other entities as able to enter into humans. He also charts early references to deities as able to shape shift and possess heaven and earth. See TB 3.7.4–5; ŚB 2.2.3.1–3; BU 1.4.7; ŚvetU 3.9; ChU 6.3.1–3; ĪU 9, 12; and many others. MBh and Rām also include many instances of possession, especially through references to curses, boons, subtle interventions, the acts of gods, and identity shifts. Smith 2006: 245.
31. NTU 19.182.
32. Witzel 2003: 76.
33. Slouber 2017: 22.
34. Slouber 2017: 40.
35. Siudmak 2013: 497, dates the text to the fifth or sixth century. Inden 2000: 30 dates it to the seventh or eighth century.
36. Sanderson 2007a: 204n28.
37. Inden 2000: 30.
38. Inden 2000: 30.
39. Sanderson 2007a: 233.
40. Geslani 2018: 125–127.
41. Einoo 2005: 109.
42. Einoo 2005: 113.
43. Gonda 1980: 17, 39, 353 identifies ĀgnG 2.5.4–5; YV 49.2.2, BGŚ 3.11, 1.7.1; ĀgnG 2.5.4; ṚVi 1.3.7.6; AVŚ 2.27, Kauś 38.18, 10.16, 58.3, 58.22; PG 2.6.9; JG 2.9, 35.4; VaiG 6.8, 6.10; SVB 3.1.12; BGP 2.7.3 as related to the overcoming of death.
44. BU 1.3.9.
45. BU 1.3.12–16.
46. BU 1.3.28. The BU also indicates that overcoming death comes about from a unification with the divine. "He conquers repeated death, death cannot reach him, death becomes his self [and] he becomes one with the divinities." BU 1.2.7.
47. Einoo 2005: 113.

48. Einoo 2005: 113.
49. Such as the *Cakrasamvara* and *Mṛtyuvañcanopadeśa*.
50. Such as the *Kecharīvidyā*. This text, as well as the Tantric *Mālinīvijayottaratantra* and others, also uses *kālavañcana*, cheating death or time.
51. The latter are synonymous and are not meant in the pejorative sense that exists with the word "cheat" in English. Brunner, Oberhammer, and Padoux 2004: 99.
52. Mengele 2010: 104. Mengele also notes that similar rites were a part of indigenous Tibetan Bön religion prior to the seventh century.
53. Mengele 2010: 112.
54. Sanderson 1994; Sanderson 2001.
55. Sanderson 2001: 42–47 details similarities between the *Cakrasamvara Tantra* and the Śaiva *Picumata*, *Jayadrathayāmala*, *Siddhayogeśvarīmata*, and *Tantrasadbhāva Tantras*.
56. Mengele 2010: 104 explains that *'chi ba bslu ba* is the Tibetan equivalent of the Sanskrit phrase *mṛtyu vañcana*. The Tibetan term can be translated as "ransoming death" as well as "deceiving/cheating death." The exact phrase *mṛtyu vañcana* does not appear in the *Svacchanda Tantra* or *Netra Tantra* but occurs several times in the *Kālottara*, a Śaiva text shown by Sanderson 2009: 144 to be used and mentioned by Buddhist works such as the (probably) eighth-century *Guhyasiddhi*. The connection between Śaiva and Buddhist practice is clear and demonstrates that the practices, while not identical, are related.
57. Mengele 2010: 112.
58. Or yantras.
59. Mengele 2010: 105–107. The *chilu* ritual involves the visualization of Heruka, the chief deity of the CS (among others such as the Mahāmāyā, Hevajra).
60. Samuel 2012: 275.
61. Walter 2000: 611.
62. Walter 2000: 612–616.
63. Walter 2000: 619.
64. The *Mṛtyuvañcanopadeśa* says, "Some who have died in a number of ways can be seen to live again. One example [of a method for achieving this] would be that of a man, or of a woman having her menses: their blood and other bodily elements, which have become mixed when they emerge in the course of their mutual exchange, are not connected strongly together. Extract two drops of such blood immediately upon the death of someone. These two drops will be released via a small, hollow cylinder smeared with butter, so as to be injected into the nostrils. When one drop emerges from a nostril, it should be rolled into the other. This is done, in turn, for each nostril. It has been seen that people become alive again in this way, so this is a recommended procedure for stopping death in this life." Trsl. Walter 2000: 619. This example, though from a Buddhist text rather than a Bhairava Tantra, demonstrates the sort of mixing to which I alluded earlier. Here the *yogin* takes the pure substance, butter, and mixes it with the impure, blood. He then utilizes this new substance in his breath practice.
65. Törzsök 2014: 196.

66.

āyur balaṃ jayaḥ kāntir dhṛtir medhā vapuḥ śriyaḥ |
sarvaṃ pravartate tasya bhūbhṛtāṃ rājyam uttamam || 46||
duḥkhārdito viduḥkhas tu vyādhimān gatarug bhavet |
vandhyā tu labhate putraṃ kanyā tu patim āvahet ||47||
yān yān samīhate kāmās tān sarvān dhruvam āpnuyāt |

Though the ritual is very similar, the aims are very different to those found in the Buddhist *Mṛtyuvañcanopadeśa* in which a practitioner cheats death by prolonging life so that the practitioner can remain in non-attached meditation.

67. Scharfe 2002: 48.
68. Scharfe 2002: 48.
69. Scharfe 2002: 49.
70. CU 2.23.1 *brahmasaṃstho 'mṛtam eti*. The eighth-century writer Śankara interprets *brahman* in this passage to refer to asceticism (*tapas*) while Vṛttkāra (date unclear) interprets the verse to mean "anyone who stands firm in the eternal attains eternal life." Radhakrishnan 1992: 375.
71. Scharfe 2002: 49.
72. Scharfe 2002: 49.
73. Einoo 2005: 117–118; Scharfe 2002: 48, citing KauśS 10.19b, 10.16–18; ŚB 9.5.1.10.
74. NT 2.3, 2.15, 6.3, 6.5, 6.37, 19.123; NTU 1.35, 6.9, 6.38.
75. NT 7.52 describes *mṛtryuvañcana* as a *siddhi* that results from the acquisition of a divine body.
76. NT 6.6–8.
77. For an introduction to the yoga of the *Netra Tantra* and a full translation of the *sūkṣma* and *para* chapters, see Bäumer 2018; Bäumer 2019.
78. Rastogi 1992: 259, Bäumer 2018: 8–12.
79. Rastogi 1992: 259, Bäumer 2018: 12–18.
80. The name of a specific yantra, which is used to perplex an enemy.
81. Throughout Chapter 6, the subject of action must be assumed from previous verses. Here I assume that people who are approached by threats of untimely death, etc., from verse 36 are the ones who are made powerful by sacrifice, etc.
82. NT 7.1cd–2, describes the physical manifestation of these *cakra*s as six circles, sixteen supports (the supporting vowels), three objects, five elements, joined with twelve knots, endowed with three powers, approached by the paths to the three abodes, [and] endowed with three channels.

    NT 7.1cd–2

    ṛtucakraṃ svarādhāraṃ trilakṣyaṃ vyomapañcakam ||1||
    granthidvādaśasaṃyuktaṃ śaktirayasamanvitam |
    dhāmatrayapathākrāntaṃ nāḍitrayasamanvitam ||2||

83. In his discussion of subtle yoga, White 2009: 162 translates the Sanskrit verb *ā√kram* as "attack." In doing so, he interprets the actions of the *mantrin* as hostile. However, the verb can also mean "approach," "visit," "seize," or "enter into." I see no reason to interpret the entry of the guru into another's body as hostile, nor the one being entered into a "victim." Nor does White justify this reading.

84.

trividhaṃ tadupāyaṃ tu sthūlaṃ sūkṣmaṃ paraṃ ca tat || 6 ||
sthūlaṃ tu yajanaṃ homo japo dhyānaṃ samudrakam |
yantrāṇi mohanādīni mantrarāṭ kurute bhṛśam || 7 ||
sūkṣmaṃ cakrādiyogena kalānāḍyudayena ca |
paraṃ sarvātmakaṃ caiva mokṣadaṃ mṛtyujid bhavet || 8 ||

85. Rastogi 1992: 260.
86. Rastogi 1989: 261.
87. Chakravarty 1999: 275.
88. Chakravarty 1999: 276.
89. Larson and Bhattacharya 1987: 53.
90. Though the text does not indicate it, we can safely assume that here the *mantrin* acts on behalf of the dying subject, who, being so close to death, would not be able to perform the oblations himself even if he knew how.
91. It is unclear from this text exactly what this regulation is. There are mentions of *rakṣāvidhāna* at *Netra Tantra* 6.33, 6.35 (preceded by *rājan*), 11.31 (*sarva*), 15.19 (*rājan*), and 17.19 (*rājan*), but they do not go into detail. In TĀ 3.112 and 3.215, Abhinavagupta references a lost text called the *Tattvarakṣāvidhāna*. Various other references exist scattered through the *Tantrarāja Tantra* and *Svacchanda Tantra*.
92. See Mirnig 2019: 23–25 for a discussion of the doctrinal contradictions of post-death liberation rites for those already initiated and therefore already assumed to attain liberation upon death.
93.

yadā mṛtyuvaśāghrātaḥ kālena kalitaḥ priye |
dṛṣṭas tatpratighātārtham amṛteśaṃ yajet tadā || 9 ||
sarvaśvetopacāreṇa pūrvoktavidhinā tataḥ |
yasya nāma samuddiśya pūjayen mṛtyujidvibhum || 10 ||
mṛtyor uttarate śīghraṃ satyaṃ me nānṛtaṃ vacaḥ |
sitaśarkarayā yuktair ghṛtakṣīraplutais tilaiḥ || 11 ||
puṇyadārvindhane vahnau kuṇḍe vṛtte trimekhale |
mahārakṣāvidhānena juhuyād yasya nāmataḥ || 12 ||
mahāśāntir bhavet kṣipraṃ gatasyāpi yamakṣayam
sugandhighṛtahomena kṣīravṛkṣamaye 'nale || 14 ||
tarpito nāśayen mṛtyuṃ mṛtyujin nātra saṃśayaḥ |

94. Gonda 1977: 214; Gonda 1980: 471.
95. Padoux 2011: 21.
96. Yelle 2003: 10.
97. Larivière 1988: 363–364. This differs from the daily rites (*nitya karman*), which are obligatory for initiates and must be performed to the best of one's ability.
98. Brunner, Oberhammer, and Padoux 2004: 158n9. This includes the preparatory rites that precede the public ritual.
99. Brunner, Oberhammer, and Padoux 2004: 158n9.
100. Brooks 1992: 175.

101. Sanderson 2010: 12.
102. Sanderson 2010: 12.
103. Trsl. Sanderson, quoted in Brunner, Oberhammer, and Padoux 2004: 88.
104. Not to be confused with the African milk tree Euphorbia trigona. *Kṣīravṛkṣa* refers to an Indian ecological taxonomy.
105. Wallace 2016: 253.
106. Bentor 1996: 117–118, notes that guggula and white sesame are also used in Tibetan preparatory rituals to empower wrathful deities and eliminate obstructions during consecration.
107. Lorenzen 1972: 27–28; Joshi 2002: 49.
108. The date of the *Devī Purāṇa* is unclear. It has been variously dated to the sixth, ninth-fourteenth, and eleventh centuries. Rocher 1986: 172.
109. Hately 2014: 212.
110. Lorenzen 1972: 27.
111.

kṣīravṛkṣasamiddhomāj jvaraṃ nāśayate kṣaṇāt || 15 ||
tilataṇḍulamākṣīkam ājyakṣīrasamanvitam |
eṣa pañcāmṛto homaḥ sarvaduṣṭanivarhaṇaḥ ||16||
guggulor gulikābhiś ca tryaktābhiś caṇamātrayā |
homāt puṣṭir bhavaty āśu kṣīṇadehasya suvrate ||17||
yadā vyādhiśatākīrṇo hyabalo dṛśyate naraḥ |
tadāsya sampuṭīkṛtya nāma japtvā vimucyate ||18||

112. NT 22.5–10a.
113. As I noted in Chapter 1, the *Netra Tantra* gives eleven different forms one can use to protect the mantra and nullify any counter-magic that may be used against his rite. *Saṃputa* is the most common type used in the *Netra Tantra*. Padoux 2011: 95–96.
114. Padoux 2011: 89–94; Yelle 2003: 20–21.
115. Yelle 2003: 20.
116. Padoux 2011: 95–96.
117. *mantram ādau likhet*. Padoux 2011: 96.
118.

yaṃ yaṃ mantraṃ japed vidvān amṛteśena saṃpuṭam |
tasya siddhyati sa kṣipraṃ bhāgyahīno 'pi yo bhavet ||19||

119. Yelle 2003: 20.
120. KT 15.57–58; GT 29.19–21. Trsl. Yelle 2003: 22.
121. Even today in the West, medicine is seen by many as insufficient for the healing process, and prayers or thoughts are offered to the sick regardless of their own spiritual position. The history of medicine and the history of spirituality are inextricably linked. The ancient version of the Hippocratic Oath began by invoking various healing and other gods while the modern version calls on the medical practitioner to not play God.
122. *bheṣajam auṣadham*
123. Supplied in the commentary by *yasya*.

124. *kṣiṇagātrasya deveśi bheṣajaṃ mantrasaṃpuṭam |*
dīyate tatkṣaṇād devi sa puṣṭiṃ labhate balī ||20||

125. Wujastyk 1998: 16–17 notes that early Vedic literature, especially the *Atharva Veda*, focuses on health and disease. Further, early Āyurvedic texts claim to descend from the Vedas. However, Wujastyk states that the medical ideas in these early texts do not form an obvious precursor to classical Āyurvedic practice. This indicates that the *mantrin* and the physician had very different roles in court and that the *mantrin* had little to no control over the contents of the medicine he administered.

Chapter 8

1. White 2000: 25.
2. White 2000: 25.
3. Brunner 1986a; Brunner 2003.
4. Bühnemann 2003.
5. The terms *maṇḍala*, *cakra*, and *yantra* are each often translated as "mystical diagram." These diagrams serve as spaces for ritual practice and are created so that the deities can appear within them. Each type has its own frequent characteristics, such as *maṇḍalas* usually including lotus petals or being drawn as square grids. These diagrams are regularly, though certainly not always, made for ritual and destroyed afterward. At times they are big enough for practitioners to enter them and the colors used have symbolic ritual meaning. Bühnemann 2003: 15 shows that cities are routinely said to be based on *maṇḍalic* mapping, but the actual connection between architectural or city design and *maṇḍala* is much more tenuous than it is widely assumed. *Yantras* are small, usually portable, diagrams that utilize geometric patterning. Further, *yantras* can be two- or three-dimensional, while *maṇḍalas* are mostly two-dimensional. Finally, *cakras* are diagrams that can be part of *maṇḍalas*, ritual diagrams in their own right, or are used as a synonym for *maṇḍala* or *yantra*. As ritual diagrams, *cakras* can be circles of deities or associated with particular places of energy within the human body.
6. These *maṇḍalas* can be drawn but are not. They are also used for meditation rather than ritual. They can include *maṇḍalas* of the five elements as well as the sun, moon, fire, and *śakti maṇḍalas* that appear on Śiva's throne. Brunner 2003: 161.
7. Brunner 2003: 161.
8. Brunner 2003: 156; Bühnemann 2003: 20.
9. Brunner 2003: 160.
10. Törzsök 2003: 181–182.
11. Padoux 2011: 70; Davis 2000: 48.
12. Törzsök 2009: 185.
13. Törzsök 2003: 184–190.
14. Törzsök 2003: 185.

15. Bühnemann 2003: 14. Brunner 2003: 157 points out that the Trika recommends using *maṇḍala*s in all rites, including the daily, while the Siddhānta advocate their use only in occasional (*naimittika karman*) and optional (*kāmya karman*) rituals.
16. PVT 19.
17. Bühnemann 2012: 560.
18. Rastelli 2003: 142.
19. Muller-Ortega 1989: 157; TSB 6.221–222; KMT 5.134–135; ParT 14.57–60; TĀ 3.112, 3.215, 15.90–92, 16.42, 30.68, PTV 33.
20. SvT 3.24, 4.234–236, 4.370, 7.39, 7.57, 7.63, 7.83, 7.90, 7.111, 7.118, 7.136, 7.218, 15.28.
21. *Saḥ*, etc., refers to the reversed form of the *mūla* mantra *oṃ juṃ saḥ* or here *saḥ juṃ oṃ* according to Kṣemarāja's commentary: *sādyarṇaiḥ savisargasakārahomabījapraṇavair jīvanikaṭāt kramātkramaṃ bahirniḥsṛtaiḥ rodhitam.*
22.

hṛtpadmamadhyagaṃ jīvaṃ candramaṇḍalamadhyagam |
sādyarṇarodhitaṃ kṛtvā mṛtyor uttarate bhṛśam ||21||
sādyarṇarodhitaṃ kṛtvā dhyāyed dehe tu yogavit |
sarvavyādhivinirmuktaḥ sa bhaven nātra saṃśayaḥ ||22||

23. The commentary adds *yasya śarīraṃ.*

Unlike the earlier mantric practice, the *mantrin* can perform this meditation for his own dying body. However, we will see that the *Svacchanda Tantra* has a much more complex death-conquering meditation that offers the practitioner a much less physical release. The *maṇḍala* and meditation offered here are more likely done on behalf of another whose aim is relief from physical ailments and death rather than for liberation, though there is no reason the guru could not perform this meditation first and the more complicated one later.

24.

kṣīrodapadmamadhyastham amṛtormibhir ākulam |
ūrdhvādhaḥśaśiruddhaṃ tu sādyarṇaiḥ saṃpuṭīkṛtam ||23||
dhyāyate suprahṛṣṭātmā ātmano 'pi parasya vā |
sabāhyābhyantaraṃ śubhraṃ sudhāpūritavigraham ||24||
anudvignam anāyāsaṃ sarvarogaiḥ pramucyate |

25. Trsl. Mallinson 2007: 22.
26. Vasudeva 2004: xxvi.
27. Kaul 2018: 243.
28. SvTU 6.25ab *kṣīrābdhimadhyasthasitasaroruhakarṇikāgatendūpaviṣṭam ūrdhvasthendvamṛtaiḥ sicyamānam aindavaprabhābharocchalatkṣīrodataraṅgair antar bahiś cāpūritam suśubhraṃ ca proktayuktyā dhyātamantrarājasaṃpuṭīkṛtaṃ yasya śarīraṃ bhṛśaṃ dhyāyate sa nīrogo bhavati ||*
29. See Pal 1985 208; Huntington and Bangdel 2003: 78–79.
30. The *Svacchanda Tantra* and *Svacchanda Tantra Uddyota*, SvT, SvTU 5.62, 10.807, 10.927, 10.930, 12.87, refer to the *candramaṇḍala* in a section of the text that describes Śaiva cosmology, though there it could simply be a reference to the actual moon. It is also found in the *Netra Tantra Uddyota* at NTU 10.43, 11.28.

31.

rocanākuṅkumenaiva kṣīreṇa ca samanvitaḥ ||25||
sitapadme 'ṣṭapatre tu madhye sādyarṇarodhitaḥ |
sarvavyādhisamākrāntaś candramaṇḍalaveṣṭitaḥ ||26||
catuṣkoṇapurākrānto vajrabhṛdvajralāñchitaḥ|
mucyate nātra saṃdehaḥ sarvavyādhinipīḍanāt ||27||

32. SvTU 6.27 *gorocanākuṅkumakṣīrair bhūrjādau sitakamalamālikhya pratipatram uktayuktyollikhitamantreṇa rodhito 'rthāt karṇikāyāṃ nāmadvārollikhitaḥ sādhyo bahiḥ ṣoḍaśakalendubimbaveṣṭitaḥ savajrakacaturaśrapurastho vyādhyākrānto 'pi sarvavyādhipīḍanānm ucyate*
33. Brunner, Oberhammer, and Padoux 2000: 134.
34. NTU 2.25a *parā vimarśaśaktis.*
35. Bühnemann 2003: 21.

SvT 5.38–39 describes a similar, eight-petaled lotus used during the initiation ritual in which Svacchanda Bhairava sits in the middle, surrounded by eight deities as represented by sounds, beginning with ha, one on each petal.

pūrvoktena vidhānena aṅgaṣaṭkasamanvitam |
patrāṣṭake nyased varṇān pūrvādīśāṃs tataḥ kramāt || 5-38 ||
sadāśivaṃ hakāreṇety evamādi varānane |
prakṛtyantaṃ vijānīyān madhye pīṭheśakalpanā || 5-39 ||

36. See Törzsök 2003: 202–203 for detailed descriptions of these *maṇḍalas*.
37. In both the SvT and the NT rites can also be used to control or kill others though this is more prevalent in the SvT.
38. Törzsök 2003: 203; Barretta 2012: 14.
39. For example, If one were to perform a death ritual described in the CS, which is similar but honored Heruka in the place of Mṛtyujit, the ritual would be ineffective.
40. Brooks 1992: 125; Nemec 2013: 314n58; Flood 1993: 118.
41. See Malinson 2007: 213 n.277 and Padoux 2011: 19.
42. Beginning with *a* and ending with *visarga.*
43. Padoux 2011: 98.
44. The name of the afflicted.
45. *oṃ juṃ saḥ.*
46.

ṣoḍaśāre mahācakre ṣoḍaśasvarabhūṣite |
ādyantamantrayogena madhye nāma samālikhet ||28||
jīvāntaḥ sāntamadhyasthaṃ varṇāntenābhirakṣitam |
pratyarṇam amṛteśena saṃpuṭitvā tu sarvataḥ ||29||
madhye daleṣu sarveṣu śaśimaṇḍalamadhyagam |
bāhye tu dviguṇaṃ padmaṃ kādisāntakrameṇa tu ||30||
pūrvavat tu likhen mantrī prati sādy arṇarodhitam |
varṇaṃ tadantaḥ sādhyasya nāma bāhye 'rkamaṇḍalam ||31||
purandarapureṇādhaḥ samantāt parivārayet|

47. Padoux 2011: 116.

48. Padoux 2011: 116–118.
49. Padoux 2011: 116.
50. NS 1.1–82b.
51. NS 1.29-31. Trsl. Goodall 2015: 406–407.
52. Goodall 2015: 407.
53. See Goodall 2015: 402 for a diagram of this script and 411, 413, 415, 417, and 420 for figures depicting these positions and their corresponding scriptural forms.
54. Padoux 2011: 117.
55. Padoux 2011: 117.
56. Padoux 2011: 117.
57. Padoux 2011: 117–118.
58. Padoux 2011: 101 notes, "the prescription in tantras of such written procedures shows that these texts, though supposedly revealed, were originally written." It is clear that both the *Nayasūtra* and *Netra Tantra* use the scripts of their composition for their written form, thus corroborating Padoux's statement.
59. Padoux 2011: 119.
60. *aḥ, am, ām, im, īm, um, ūm, ṛm, ṝm, ḷm, ḹm, em, aim, om, aum, aṃ*: these syllables are known as *kalās*, a word that is also a synonym for the phases of the moon. In addition to the phases of the moon, the sixteen *kalās* also represent the sixteen phases of Śiva. In the Trika school of non-dual Śaiva Tantra, to which the NT is related (but it is not part of its canon), there is a 17th *kulā*. This additional *kalā* _is transcendent *citkalā*, pure consciousness. TĀ _3.137; PTV 35; Padoux 2011: 91; Mallinson 2007: 213.
61. The consonant *ha* is not included in this set of consonants. We do find it included in the later mantra of *haṃsa* as the beginning of a different ordering of the alphabet. Jayaratha's commentary on the *Tantrāloka* at 5.144 describes *sa* as *amṛtavarṇa*, the letter of *amṛta*.
62. PTV 22 also notes that the phoneme *sa* represents the 31 *tattvas* from *pṛthivī* _[earth] to *māyā*. The remaining *tattvas śuddhavidyā, īśvara*, and *sadāśiva* stand for *au* and *śiva* and *śakti* for *aḥ*, making the mantra *sauḥ*.
63. Yelle 2003: 41.
64. Kṣemarāja adds the missing *ha* and *kṣa* in order to assure the complete set of phonemes.
65. There is another, more secret, Tantric ordering called *mālinī* _or *nādiphāntakrama*, in which the sounds are arranged from *na* to *pha*. The KubjT and MVUT describe this sequence as re-lated to the goddess Mālinī. Alper 1989: 266; Goudriann and Gupta 1981: 53. Vasudeva 2004; Vasudeva, 2007: 1 for variations on the sequence and analysis of the *nādiphāntakrama*. Kṣe-marāja understood this *śabdarāśi* ordering of the alphabet as a Bhairava who is the male coun-terpart to the female alphabet goddess Mātṛkā. Törzsök 2009: 11.
66. Gray 2007: 347.
67. Gray 2007: 347.
68. Gray 2007: 347.
69. *Oṃ, hrīḥ, ha, hūṃ*, and *phaṭ*. Gray 2007: 347n25.
70. Gray 2007: 347.
71. Gray 2007: 347.

72. See NT 6.7.
73. CS 43.21–22; Trlt. Gray 2007: 348.884 *athavā _mantrarājam (xxx) yatra (xxx) cintayet ||21||(xxx) tadā _jāyate [nātra saṃśayaḥ] |*
74. Trsl. Gray 2007: 348. Here I have solely relied upon Gray's translation as there is not enough of the Sanskrit available to attempt any analysis. We have only three words in *ślokas* 22 and 23a and 23b-25 are missing. Gray works with two more complete Tibetan translations. As Gray points out here, there colors are associated with the deities invoked and substances used during various magical rites.
75. Davis 1992: 112; Rambelli 2000: 373; Flood 2006: 142; Dviveda 1992: 123; Silburn 1988: 128.
76. Gray 2007: 312. Here black, a color not used in the drawing of the *maṇḍala* or *yantra*, is as-sociated with the ability to destroy. Further, Vīravajra associates the colors with different castes and elements. Pacifying/white = *kṣatriya*/water, enriching/yellow = *vaiśya/earth*, con-trolling/ red = Brahmin/fire, destroying/black = *śūdra*/wind.
77. Gray 2007: 348.
78. NT 15.9b-11.
79. The materials here differ greatly from tantric charnel ground rites such as those found in the *Hevajra Tantra*, which gives a clear, transgressive origin for the materials used in *maṇḍala* practice. It says, "black colouring is obtained from charcoal of the cemetery, white from ground human bones, yellow from green lac, red from cemetery-bricks, green from caurya leaves and ground human bones, and dark blue from ground human bones and cemetery charcoal." Snell-grove 1959: 51. Further, the text says to measure using a "cemetery thread," which Vajragarbha's commentary *Hevajrapiṇḍārthaṭīkā* _says is made from the intestine of a corpse. Though the *Netra Tantra* only gives a few of the materials used for its *maṇḍalas*, we can see that they are innocuous substances such as saffron and milk. I provide the materials given in the *Hevajra Tantra* to demonstrate that the symbolism of the colors permeated the tradition though the actual organic material could differ greatly. This means the same *maṇḍala* could be drawn using both orthodox and heterodox materials for similar purposes. As the *Netra Tantra* is a largely conservative text I would expect to only find orthodox substances used within its rites.
80. See Wenta 2018 for a discussion of smell in the non-dual Śaiva tradition.
81. Barretta 2012: 58.
82. *sitacandanasaṃyuktaṃ _rocanākṣīrayogataḥ _||32|| likhitvā _mantrarājaṃ _tu karpūrakṣodadhūsaram |mahārakṣāvidhānaṃ _tu puṣṭasaubhāgyadāyakam ||33|| etac cakraṃ _mahādevi sitapuṣpaiḥ _prapūjayet |sarvaśvetopacāreṇa madhumadhye nidhāpayet ||34||anenaiva vidhānena saptāhān mṛtyujid bhavet |rājarakṣāvidhānaṃ _tu bhūbhṛtāṃ _tu prakāśayet ||35|| saṃgrāmakāle varadaṃ _ripudarpāpahaṃ _bhavet |*
83. SvT 5.19 also calls this mantra *vidyārāja*. Brunner, Oberhammer, and Padoux 2004: 255.
84. NTU 4.1; Padoux 1990: 354. Singh 1979a: 7, also gives an alternate of *śiva, śakti, sadāśiva, īśvara, śuddha, vidyā, mahāmāyā, māyā, puruṣa*, and *prakṛti*. He also says the letters for the given *tattvas* are *h, r, kṣ, m, l, y, ṇ*, and *auṃ*. Padoux 1990: 354n62

gives a similar mantra *rhrkṣvlyūṃ* _without the supporting vowels and describes a variant found at TĀ _30.11-16 and YH 3.102. Singh also gives the sixth *tattva* as *kalā*, which is a mistransliteration of the text. According to Heilijgers-Seeleen 1994: 27, it is understood that these nine *tattva*s include the remaining *tattva*s so that the full set of thirty six are represented within the nine. Goudriaan and Gupta 1981: 35 give a different set of *tattva*s from the Uttarasūtra, *prakṛti, puruṣa, niyati, kalā, māyā, vidyā, īśvara, sadāśiva*, and *dehavyāpin*. Padoux's reading of the PTV gives the nine as *sadāśiva (ka), īśvara (kha), śuddhavidyā _(ga), māyā _(gha) kalā _(jña), vidyā _(ca), rāga (cha), niyati (ja)*, and *kāla (jha)*.

85. SvTU 4.103a.
86. Padoux 1990b: 354. Padoux also notes that this is the same layout/order of a nine-by-nine grid that places OṂ _at the eight cardinal and intermediate directions, and in the center. The remainder of the grid is composed of the letters associated with the nine *tattvas*. Padoux also notes that the syllables used (*h, r, kṣ, m, l, v, y, ū*, and *oṃ*) are a variation on the *navātmamantra* (*R H KṢ _L V Y Ū _M*) given in TĀ _30.11-16 or in Padoux, 2013, p. 121 as *H S KṢ _M L V R Y Ū _M*.
87. SvT 4.41 and 5.34.
88. Padoux 1990: 355.
89. See Brunner, Oberhammer, and Padoux 2004: 261–262 for references to the vowelless *navātman*.
90. As noted above, it is unclear exactly to which set of nine *tattva*s the *Netra Tantra* refers.
91. *śivādinavatattvāni pratyekaṃ _śaśimaṇḍalam ||36|| madhyāt pūrvādi aiśyantam amṛteśena mantriṇā _| yadā _vyādhiśatākīrṇam apamṛtyuśatena vā _||37||tadā _śvetopacāreṇa pūjyaṃ _kṣīraghṛtena vā _|tilaiḥ _kṣīrasamidbhir vā _homāc chāntiṃ _samaśnute ||38||evaṃ _saṃpūjya kumbhe tu sarvauṣadhisamanvite |sitapadmamukhodgāre ratnagarbhāmbupūrite ||39||sarvamaṅgalaghoṣeṇa śirasi hy abhiṣecayet |sa mucyate na saṃdehaḥ _sarvavyādhiprapīḍitaḥ _||40||* The section concludes with a description of the end of the ceremony. (NT 6.41–45) This explanation includes various numbers that refer to something not included in the text. I have not found any clues to this numbering system in any other text and do not know to what they refer. I must agree with Brunner 1974: 141, who argues that this is a later addition to the text and does not make any sense within the current context. The numerical references and lan-guage is very different from the rest of the text. Kṣemarāja makes no attempt to explain the section and dismisses it. *dhyātvā _parāmṛtaṃ _nityaṃ _nityoditam anāmayam |prakriyāntastham amṛtam avatārya parāc chivāt ||41||caturnavāmṛtādhāraṃ _navadhā _navapūritam |śatārdhakṣobhitaṃ _nityaṃ _ṣaṭpañcaikasamanvitam ||42||anantādhāragambhīram aṣṭātriṃśadvibhūṣitam |pañcabhir vā _prasiddhyarthaṃ _pūrṇaṃ _tena nirantaram ||43||evaṃ _dhyānaparo yas tu sabāhyābhyantarāmṛtam |vikṣobhya kalaśaṃ _mūrdhni daiśiko mantratatparaḥ _||44||anugrahapadāvastho hy abhiṣiñcet prayatnataḥ _|sa mucyate na sandehaḥ _saṃsārād duratikramāt ||45||*
92. Mirnig 2019: 65.
93. Mirnig 2019: 67.

Chapter 9

1. SvT 7.225a is the only direct reference to the Bhairava in the form of Amṛteśa in the SvT or SvTU.
2. SvT 7.225a.
3. SvTU 7.226a *siddhibhāgamṛteśabhairavatulya.*
4. In its chapter on the highest (*para*) yoga of the *Netra Tantra*, this ambiguity arises at NT 8.21–22a. Bäumer 2018: 27 translates the passage thus: "The one who by this eightfold *yoga* is firmly established in his own supreme nature conquers Time with this realization and becomes the supreme Lord Amṛteśa (Lord of Immortality). O Goddess! He becomes the Conqueror of Death and Time cannot affect him any longer." Kṣemarāja adds at NT 32c–33a that "being established therein, this person knows everything, past and future. With the senses under control, that reality has the quality of Energy." Trsl. Bäumer 2018: 28.
5. Baretta 2012: 197 includes the *mṛtyu vañcana* rites in a list of the six acts (*ṣaṭkarmāni*) found in the SvT. She labels all six "malevolent." However, *mṛtyu vañcana* rites focus on appeasement (*śānti*), which is not generally considered malevolent (*abhicāra*). It is unclear why Barretta describes *mṛtyu vañcana* as malevolent except to link the SVT with heterodoxy. Her assumption that the conquest of death is somehow evil implies that it is unnatural. However, *mṛtyu vañcana* practices occur throughout Indian literature. As far as I know, no text describes *mṛtyu vañcana* as malevolent. Barretta 2012: 197–198 mistakenly says that this practice is found in the SvT's tenth chapter, though she quotes the seventh in her footnotes. The tenth chapter focuses on cosmology, including the thirty-two hells and purification, but it does not focus on ritual or meditation aimed at the vanquishment of death. Thus, I assume the attribution in the text is a simple error.
6. *Haṃsa* literally translates as goose. Yelle 2003: 28–30 describes *haṃsa* as the path of the breath in which *haṃ* is the sound made on inhalation and *sa* on exhalation. These syllables also contain all the sounds of the Sanskrit language as *ha* begins in the back of the throat and *sa* forward in the mouth to the teeth. The image of the goose is then a pun that leads to a visualization of the entirety of the world within the body.
7. SvT 7.209, 213–214.
8. SvT 7.221–222.
9. Svt 7.226.
10. SvT 7.209a *dhyānayuktasya ṣaṇmāsāt sarvajñatvaṃ pravartate.*
11. SvTU 7.227: *cintayet svābhedena vimṛśet, paraṃ tattvaṃ hṛddvādaśāntasphuritaṃ cidānandaghanātmakam, kālacāreṇa bāhyenāntareṇa ca varjitam, kalākalaṅkena kalpanāmalena śūnyam, ata eva catuṣkalavad akārādikalāyogābhāvād niṣkalam paramaṃ padam anuttaraṃ*
    dhāma || 227 ||
12. Sometimes also called *kāla vañcana.*
13. SvT 7.224b: *amṛtāpūritaṃ dehaṃ sarvam eva vicintayet || 224 ||*
14. Padoux 1990: 82, 140; SvT 7.27.

15. Heilijgers-Seelen 1994: 50.
16. Yelle 2003: 26.
17. TĀ 3.148.
18. Yelle 2003: 27.
19. The mantras and their symbolism are encoded within the texts so as to assure correct use by only the *yogins* who can extract them. The practitioner is able to situate the mantra within the meditation through usage and by understanding the underlying meanings of the mantras. Without this knowledge, the meditation cannot be effective.
20.

dhyātvā kāleśasvacchandaṃ haṃsaṃ vā sakaleśvaram |
nāsikārandhramārgasthaḥ sa sṛjet saṃharej jagat || *207* ||

21. I.e., he should impel the entire world into existence.
22. SvT 7.208a: *tatrasthaḥ kalayet sarvaṃ sarvabhūteṣv avasthitaḥ* |
23. While memory is considered a state of consciousness it can be connected with the present in order to transcend time, opening a path to Absolute understanding. Padoux 2013: 178.
24. Mallinson 2007: 132.
25. c. fourteenth century, Mallinson 2007: 3.
26. Mallinson 2007: 132; Mallinson 2007: 232n416 says, "The *yogin* should hold his breath to stop it flowing in Iḍā and Piṅgalā. He thereby forces it into Suṣumṇā." In other words, the *yogin* holds his breath, suppressing the in- and out-breath in order to vanquish death.
27. Mallinson 2007: 132.
28.

tatrasthaḥ kalayet sarvaṃ sarvabhūteṣv avasthitaḥ |
tatsthaṃ dhyātvā jayen mṛtyuṃ nākālasthaṃ kalet prabhuḥ || *208* ||

29.

dhyānayuktasya ṣaṇmāsāt sarvajñatvaṃ pravartate |
kālatrayaṃ vijānāti kālayuktas tu yogavit || *209* ||

30. SP 1.1.32.4–92. Trls. Doniger O'Flaherty,1980a: 234.
31.

kālahaṃsaṃ sa tu japan dhyāyan vāpi maheśvari |
sa bhavet kālarūpī vai svacchandaḥ kālavac caret || *210* ||
hatamṛtyur jarāṃ tyaktvā rogaiḥ sarvabhayojjhitaḥ |
vijñānaṃ śravaṇaṃ dūrān mananaṃ cāvalokanam || *211* ||
sarvaiśvaryaguṇāvāptir bhavet kālajayāt sadā |

32. VBh 4, Trsl. Singh 1979b: 14.
33. MU 5.2.
34. Incidentally, in popular iconography, Brahmā is often shown riding a swan (*haṃsa*), a fitting vehicle for visualization in this particular meditation.

35.

> *dakṣanāsāpuṭe dhyātvā brāhmaiśvaryam avāpnuyāt || 212 ||*
> *tadāyus tatsamaṃ vīryaṃ bhūtakālaṃ ca vetty ataḥ |*

36. Kinsley 1998: 140.
37. Lotchtefeld 2002: 155. A single *kalpa* is also the largest accepted measure of time in Indian cosmology.
38. Kinsley 2000: 140.
39.

> *bhaviṣyajño bhaved vāme viṣṇutulyabalaś ca saḥ || 213 ||*
> *tatsamaṃ caitadaiśvaryaṃ tadāyur yogirāḍ bhavet |*

40. Bonshek 2001: 217.
41. The two previous verses focused on meditation in the right and then left nostril. This type of breath control, called *prāṇāyāma*, is found throughout the textual tradition relating to yogic techniques. The *Niśvāsatattvasaṃhitā*, the earliest extant Tantric Śaiva text, outlines four types of breath control: inhalation through the left, exhalation through the right, and retention of the in-breath. The fourth type is an internal breath control called *supraśāntai* in which one moves the vital energy from the ear to the navel and the mind from sense objects. Mallinson and Singleton 2017: 144. See Mallinson and Singleton 2017: 127–170 for a detailed account of various breath control practices throughout the Indian literary tradition.
42. *Nityam* here can mean "always," "constant," or "immutable" but may also be simply acting as a verse-filler. However, I have retained the word in the translation following SvT 7.59 which states that *haṃsa* cannot be produced or retained, that it is self-uttered, and it lives within the heart of all living creatures. See Padoux 1990: 140–141 for further discussion of *haṃsa* in the SvT and Kṣemarāja's commentary.
43.

> *bhūtaṃ bhavyaṃ bhaviṣyac ca sarvaṃ jāṇāti madhyataḥ || 214 ||*
> *nityaṃ vai dhyānayogena rudrasya samatāṃ vrajet |*

44. Singh 1988: 132, 133, 143, 145, and 146. Certainly, this is not always the case, as these phonemes can be connected to other *tattvas* at various times but for my purpose, it is important to note the relationship between *ha*, *sa*, and the various states of consciousness.
45. Torella 1988: 164.
46.

> *āyuṣā balavīryeṇa rūpaiśvaryeṇa tatsamaḥ || 7–215 ||*
> *brahmāṇaḥ parabhāvena aiśvaraṃ padam āpnuyāt |*

47. Singh 1988: 132, 133, 143, 145, and 146.
48. Bansat-Boudon and Tripathi 2011: 203.
49. These final states are not dealt with at length in the SvT. The Śakti state is not mentioned at all as this state is only discussed in more esoteric Tantric texts. See Chapter 3 for a discussion of the *tattvas* in the SvT.
50. Bansat-Boudon and Tripathi 2011: 120.

51.

viṣṇoḥ sadāśivaiśvaryaṃ parabhāvād avāpnuyāt || 216 ||
rudrasya yaḥ paro bhāvo dhyātvā taṃ tu śivo bhavet |
evaṃ mṛtyujayaḥ khyātaḥ amṛtaṃ dhyāyato jayaḥ || 217 ||

52. I.e., the phases of the moon. See Mallinson 2007: 213; Dupuche 2003: 47.

53.

nāḍibhinnālarandhrasthaṃ hṛtpadmaṃ ṣoḍaśacchadam |
dhyātvā sitaṃ suvikacaṃ kalāṣoḍaśakānvitam || 218 ||
sampūrṇāvayavaṃ candraṃ karṇikākāravigraham |
tanmadhye cintyam ātmānaṃ śuddhasphaṭikanirmalam || 219 ||
kṣīrāmṛtārṇavāvasthakallolāmṛtapūritam |

54. Goodall and Rastelli 2013: 266.

55. I.e., its calyx.

56.

upariṣṭād dvitīyābjaṃ śāktāmṛtamahodadhau || 220 ||
tac cādho mukhapadmaṃ tu paripūrṇendukaṇīkam |
tan madhye cintayed dhaṃsam adho binduśikhānvitam || 221 ||
varṣantam amṛtaṃ divyaṃ samantāt saṃvicintayet |
ātmordhvarandhramārgeṇa praviṣṭaṃ tac ca cintayet || 222 ||

57.

sitaṃ subahulaṃ sāndram amṛtaṃ mṛtyunāśanam |
tenāplāvitam ātmānaṃ pūryamāṇaṃ vicintayet || 223 ||

58.

padmanālanibaddhaiś ca nāḍīrandhramukhaiḥ sadā |
amṛtāpūritaṃ dehaṃ sarvam eva vicintayet || 224 ||

59. SvT 7.225a: *evaṃ vai nityayuktātmā amṛteśasamo bhavet |*

60. I.e., divine powers.

61. SvT 7.225 *vyādhīn mṛtyuṃ jarāṃ tyaktvā krīḍate tv aṇimādibhiḥ*

62. SvT 7: *evaṃ tasyāmṛtadhyānāt kālamṛtyujayo bhavet |*
athavā paratattvasthaḥ sarvakālair na bādhyate || 226 ||

63. Einoo 2005: 114.

64. Sanderson 2004: 241. See Bäumer 2019: 9–11 for the modern-day practitioner's view of self-practiced rites in the NT's sixth, seventh, and eighth chapters.

65. See Bäumer 2018, 2019.

66. Sanderson 2004: 230.

Conclusion

1. Sanderson 2004: 251n48, 253.

Bibliography

Sources (editions and translations)

Arthaśāstra. Trsl. Patrick Olivelle. (2013). *King, Governance, and Law in Ancient India: Kauṭilya's Arthaśāstra*. Oxford: Oxford University Press.

Brahmayāmala Tantra. Partial trsl. Shaman Hatley. (2007). "The Brahmayāmalatantra and Early Śaiva Cult of Yoginīs." Doctoral dissertation, University of Pennsylvania. Retrieved from ProQuest Dissertations and Theses, UMI Number 3292099.

Bṛhat Saṃhitā of Varāhamihira. Trsl. V. Panditabhushana, Subrahmanya Sastri, and Vidwan M. Ramakrishna Bhat. (1946). Bangalore: V. B. Soobbiah and Sons, M.B.D. Electronic Printing Works.

Bṛhat Saṃhitā of Varāhamihira. Trsl. M. Ramakrishna Bhat. (1996). *Bṛhat Saṃhitā of Varahamihira: Text in Sanskrit with English Translation, Exhaustive Notes and Literary Comments*. Delhi: Motilal Banarsidass.

The Cakrasamvara Tantra (The Discourse of Śri Heruka): A Study and Annotated Translation. Trsl. David B. Gray. (2007). New York: American Institute of Buddhist Studies.

The Cakrasamvara Tantra (The Discourse of Śri Heruka): Editions of the Sanskrit and Tibetan Texts. Ed. David B. Gray. (2012). New York: American Institute of Buddhist Studies.

Chāndogya Upaniṣad. Trsl. S. Radhakrishnan. (1992). *The Principal Upaniṣads*. Amherst, MA: Humanity Books.

Dharmasūtras. Trsl. Patrick Olivelle. (1999). *The Dharmasūtras: The Law Codes of Āpastamba, Gautama, Baudhāyana,and Vasiṣṭha*. Oxford: Oxford University Press.

Garuda Purāṇa. Ed. Shri Ramtej Pandey. (n.d.). Varanasi: Chowkhama Vidyabhawan.

Hevajra Tantra. Trsl. David L. Snellgrove. (1959). *The Hevajra Tantra: A Critical Study*. London: Oxford University Press.

Hevajra Tantra. Trsl. G. W. Farrow and I. Menon. (1992). *The Concealed Essence of the Hevajra Tantra with the Commentary Yogaratnamālā*. Delhi: Motilal Banarsidass.

Kalāvilāsa of Kṣemendra. Trsl. Somadeva Vasudeva. (2005). *Three Satires: Nīlakaṇṭha, Kṣemendra, & Bhallaṭa*. New York: Clay Sanskrit Library.

Khecarīvidyā of Ādinātha. Trsl. James Mallinson. (2007). *The* Khecarīvidyā *of Ādinātha: A Critical Edition and Annotated Translation of an Early Text of* Haṭha Yoga. New York: Routledge.

Kiraṇatantra. Ed. and trsl. Dominic Goodall. (1998). *Bhaṭṭa Rāmakaṇṭha's Commentary on the Kiraṇatantra*, vol. 1, chapters 1–6, critical edition and annotated translation. Pondicherry: Institut Français de Pondichéry/École Française d'Extrême-Orient.

Kubjikāmatatantra. Trsl. Dory Heilijgers-Seelen. (1994). *The System of Five Cakras in Kubjikāmatatantra 14–16*. Groningen: Groningen Oriental Studies.

Manusmṛti. Trsl. Wendy Doniger and Brian K. Smith. *Laws of Manu*. (1991). London: Penguin Books.

Maitrī Upaniṣad. Trsl. S. Radhakrishnan. (1992). In *The Principal Upaniṣads*. Amherst, MA: Humanity Books.

Mālinīvijayottaratantra. Trsl. Somadeva Vasudeva. (2004). *The Yoga of the Mālinīvijayottaratantra*, chapters 1–4, 7, 11–17. Pondicherry: Institut Française de Pondichéry École Française D'Éxtrême Orient.

Māṇḍūkya Upaniṣad. Trsl. S. Radhakrishnan. (1992). In *The Principal Upaniṣads*. Amherst, MA: Humanity Books.

Māṇḍūkya Upaniṣad. Trsl. Patrick Olivelle. (1998). *The Early Upaniṣads: Annotated Text and Translation*. Oxford: Oxford University Press.

Mṛtyuvañcanopadeśa. Ed. Johannes Schneider. (2010). *Vāgīśvarakīrtis Mṛtyuvañcanopadeśa, eine buddhistische Lehrschrift zur Abwehr des Todes*. Wein: Verlag der Österreichischen Akademie der Wissenschaften.

Netra Tantra. (1926, 1939). Sanskrit edition by Paṇḍit Madhusudan Kaul Shāstrī, 2 vols. Kashmir Series of Texts and Studies, nos. 46 and 61. Bombay: Tatva Vivechaka Press.

Netra Tantra. (2007). Transliterated e-text. United States: Muktabodha Indological Research Institute.

Niśvāsatattvasaṃhitā. Ed. Dominic Goodall. (2015). *The Niśvāsatattvasaṃhitā: The Earliest Surviving Śaiva Tantra*, vol. 1: *A Critical Edition & Annotated Translation of the Mūlasūtra, Uttarasūtra & Nayasūtra*. Pondicherry: Institut Français de Pondichéry/ École Française d'Extrême-Orient.

Parākhyatantra. Trsl. Dominic Goodall. (2004). *The Parādhyatantra: A Scripture of the Śaiva Siddhānta*. Pondicherry: Institut Française de Pondichéry École Française D'Extrême-Orient.

Paramārthasāra of Abhinavagupta. Trsl. Lynne Bansat-Boudon and Kamaleshadatta Tripathi. (2011). *An Introduction to Tantric Philosophy: The* Paramārthasāra *of Abhinavagupta with the Commentary of Yogarāja*. New York: Routledge.

Parā-trīśikā-Vivaraṇa of Abhinavagupta. Trsl. Jaideva Singh. (1988). *Parā-trīśikā-Vivaraṇa: The Secret of Tantric Mysticism*. New Delhi: Motilal Banarsidass.

Pratyabhijñāhṛdayam of Kṣemarāja. Trsl. Jaideva Singh. (1990). *The Doctrine of Recognition: A Translation of* Pratyabhijñāhṛdayam *with an Introduction and Notes*. Albany: State University of New York Press.

Ṛg Veda. Trsl. Wendy Doniger. (2005). *The Rig Veda*. New York: Penguin.

Ṛg Veda. Eds. R. L. Kashyap and S. Sadagopan. (1988). *Rig Veda Samhita*. Bangalore: Sri Aurobindo Kapali Sastry Institute of Vedic Culture; uploaded by Ulrich Stiehl. sanskritweb.net/rigveda. Accessed July 11, 2017.

Rājataraṅgiṇī of Kalhaṇa. *The Rājataraṅgiṇī of Kalhaṇa*, vols. 1–3. Eds. Durgaprasada Dvivedi and Peter Peterson. (1892, 1894, 1896). Bombay: Bombay Sanskrit Series Nos. 44, 51, and 54.

Rājataraṅgiṇī of Kalhaṇa. *Kalhaṇa's Rājataraṅgiṇī: A Chronicle of the Kings of Kaśmīr*. Trsl. M. A. Stein. (1900). 3 vols. London: Archibald Constable.

Śiva Sūtra of Vasugupta. Ed. J. C. Chatterji. (1911). *The Shiva Sūtra Vimarshinī*. Kashmir Series of Texts and Studies, no. 1.

Śiva Sūtra of Vasugupta. Trsl. Jaideva Singh. (1979a). *Śiva Sūtras: The Yoga of Supreme Identity*. Delhi: Motilal Banarsidass.

Śiva Sūtra of Vasugupta. Trsl. Mark S. G. Dyczkowski. (1992). *The Aphorisms of Śiva: The* Śiva Sūtra *with Bhāskara's Commentary, the* Vārttika. Albany: State University of New York Press.

Śiva Sūtra of Vasugupta. Trsl. Swami Lakshmanjoo. (2007). *Śiva Sūtras, The Supreme Awakening: With commentary of Kshemaraja*. New Delhi: Universal Shaiva Fellowship.

Somaśambhupaddhati. Trsl. Hélène Brunner-Lachaux. (1963). *Somaśambhupaddhati*, vol. 1. Pondicherry: Institut Français d'Indologie.

Spanda Kārikās and *Spanda Nirṇaya*. Trsl. Jaideva Singh. (1980). Spanda-Kārikās: *The Divine Creative Pulsation*. New Delhi: Motilal Banarsidass.

Śrīkaṇṭhacarita of Maṅkha. Ed. Bankim Chandra Mandal. (1983). *Śrīkaṇṭhacaritam* of Maṅkhaka with the Sanskrit Commentary of Jonarāja. Calcutta: Sanskrit Pustak Bhandar.

Svacchandatantram. Ed. Madhusūdan Kaul Shāstrī. (1921–1935). 7 vols. Kashmir Series of Texts and Studies, nos. 31, 38, 44, 48, 51, 53, and 56. Bombay: Tatva Vivechaka Press.

Svacchandatantram. Ed. V. V. Dwivedi. (1985). *Svacchandatantram with commentary "Uddyota" by Kṣemarāja*. Parimal Sanskrit Series No. 16. 2 vols. New Delhi: Parimal Press.

Svacchandatantram. Transliterated e-text. (2006). United States: Muktabodha Indological Research Institute.

Taittrīya Upaniṣad. Trsl. S. Radhakrishnan. (1992). In *The Principal Upaniṣads*. Amherst, MA: Humanity Books.

The Tantrāloka of Abhinavagupta with commentary by Rājānaka Jayaratha. Ed. Madhusūdan Kaul Shāstrī. (1918–1935). 12 vols. Kashmir Series of Texts and Studies, nos. 23, 28, 30, 35, 36, 35, 29, 41, 47, 59, 57, and 58.

The Tantrāloka of Abhinavagupta. (2000). Trsl. Lilian Silburn and André Padoux. *Abhinavagupta: La Lumière sur les Tantras: Chapitres 1 à 5 du Tantrāloka*. Paris: Collège de France: Publications de L'Institut de Civilisation Indienne.

Tantrasadbhāva. (2006). Devanāgarī etex. United States: Muktabodha Indological Research Institute.

Tantrasāra. Trsl. H. N. Cakravarty. Ed. Boris Marjanovic. (2012). *Tantrasāra of Abhinavagupta*. Portland: Rudra Press.

Vāyu Purāṇa. Trsl. G. V. Tagare. (1987). Delhi: Motilal Banarsidass.

Vāyu Purāṇa. Ed. Rājendralāla Mitra. (1880). Calcutta: Bibliotheca Indica.

Vijñānabhairava. Trsl. Jaideva Singh. (1979b). *Vijñānabhairava, or Divine Consciousness*. Delhi: Motilal Banarsidass.

Vīṇāśikha Tantra. Trsl. Teun Goudriaan. (1985). *Vīṇāśikhatantra: A Śaiva Tantra of the Left Current*. Delhi: Motilal Banarsidass.

Yoginīhṛdaya. Trsl. André Padoux with Roger-Orphé Jeanty. (2013). *The Heart of the Yogini: The Yoginīhṛdaya, a Sanskrit Tantric Treatise*. Oxford: Oxford University Press.

Visual Images

Mandala of Chandra, God of the Moon. Late 14th–early 15th century. Distemper on cloth. Accession Number 1981.465. New York: Metropolitan Museum of Art.

Pashupati Seal (c. 2500–2400 BC). National Museum of India, New Delhi. Accession number DK 5175/143. http://www.nationalmuseumindia.gov.in/prodCollections.asp?pid=42&id=1&lk=dp1. Accessed February 17, 2018.

Unknown. Mask of Bhairava (Late 6th–7th century). Copper alloy, possibly brass. Metropolitan Museum of Art, New York City. Accession number 2013.249.

Unknown. Representation of Śiva. (9th century). Stone. British Museum, London. Museum number 1988,0312.1.

Secondary Sources

Acri, Andrea. (2016). "Once More on the 'Ratu Boko Mantra': Magic, Realpolitik, and Bauddha-Śaiva Dynamics in Ancient Nusantara." In *Esoteric Buddhism in Mediaeval Maritime Asia: Networks of Masters, Texts, Icons*. Ed. Andrea Acri. Singapore: ISEAS-Yusof Ishak Institute.

Alper, Harvey P. (1989). "The Cosmos as Śiva's Language-Game: 'Mantra' According to Kṣemarāja's *Śivasūtravimarśinī*." In *Understanding Mantras*. Ed. Harvey Alper. Albany: State University of New York Press.

Arraj, William James. (1988). "The Svacchandatantram: History and Structure of a Saiva Scripture." Doctoral dissertation, University of Chicago. Retrieved from ProQuest Dissertations and Theses (UMI Number T-30619).

Austin, J. L. (1962). *How to Do Things with Words*. Oxford: Oxford University Press.

Balkaran, Raj. (2015). "Mother of Power, Mother of Kings: Reading Royal Ideology in the *Devī Māhātmya*." Doctoral Dissertation, University of Calgary.

Barretta, Simone. (2012). "Tantric Selves: Body, Mind, and Society in the Religious Cultures of Medieval Kashmir." Doctoral dissertation, University of Pennsylvania. Retrieved from ProQuest Dissertations and Theses. (UMI Number 3542777).

Battacharyya, B. (1931). "Conclusion." In *Jayākhyasaṃhitā*. Ed. Embar Krishnamacharya. Baroda: Oriental Institute.

Bäumer, Bettina Sharada. (2018). "The Yoga of the Netra Tantra: A Translation of Chapters VII and VIII with Introduction." In *Tantrapuspāñjali: Tantric Traditions and Philosophy of Kashmir*. Ed. Bettina Sharada Bäumer and Hamsa Stainton. New Delhi: Aryan Books.

Bäumer, Bettina Sharada. (2019). *The Yoga of the Netra Tantra: Third Eye and Overcoming Death*. Ed. Shivam Srivastava. Shimla: Indian Institute of Advanced Study; New Delhi: DK Printworld.

Beck, Guy L. (1993). *Sonic Theology: Hinduism and Sacred Sound*. Columbia: University of South Carolina Press.

Beer, Robert. (2003). *Handbook of Tibetan Buddhist Symbols*. Chicago: Serindia.

Bentor, Yael. (1996). *Consecration of Images and Stūpas in Indo-Tibetan Tantric Buddhism*. Leiden: Brill.

Bhatt, B. N. (1973). *Śrīkaṇṭhacaritam: A Study*. Baroda: M. S. University of Baroda Research Series. 14.

Biernacki, Loriliai. (2015). "Conscious Body: Mind and Body in Abhinavagupta's Tantra." In *Beyond Physicalism: Toward Reconciliation of Science and Spirituality*. Ed. Edward F. Kelly, Adam Crabtree, and Paul Marshall. Lanham, MD: Rowman & Littlefield.

Biernacki, Loriliai. (2016). "Words and Word-Bodies: Writing the Religious Body." In *Words: Religious Language Matters*. Ed. Ernst van den Hemel and Asja Szafraniec. New York: Fordham University Press.

Bisgaard, Daniel James. (1994). *Social Conscience in Sanskrit Literature*. New Delhi: Motilal Banarsidass.

Bisschop, Peter. (2020). "From Mantramārga Back to Atimārga: Atimārga as a Self-Referential Term." In *Śaivism and the Tantric Traditions: Essays in Honour of Alexis G.J.S. Sanderson*. Ed. Dominic Goodall, Shaman Hatley, Harunaga Isaacson, and Srilata Raman. Gonda Indological Studies No. 22. Leiden: Brill.

Bonshek, Anna J. (2001). *Mirror of Consciousness: Art, Creativity, and Veda*. New Delhi: Motilal Banarsidass.

Braun, David. (2015). "Indexicals." Stanford Encyclopedia of Philosophy. https://plato.stanford.edu/entries/indexicals/.

Brooks, Douglas Renfrow. (1992). *Auspicious Wisdom: The Texts and Traditions of Śrīvidyā Śākta Tantrism in South India*. Albany: State University of New York Press.

Brunner, Hélène. (1974). "Un Tantra du Nord: le Netra Tantra." *Bulletin de l'Ecole française d'Extrême-Orient* 61: 125–197.

Brunner, Hélène. (1986a). "Maṇḍala et Yantra Dans le Śivaïsme Āgamique: Définition, Description, Usage Rituel." In *Mantras et Diagrammes Rituels Dans L'Hindouisme*. Paris: Centre National de la Recherche Scientifique.

Brunner, Hélène. (1986b). "Les membres de Śiva." *Asiatische Studien/Études Asiatiques* 40(2): 89–132.

Brunner, Hélène. (2003). "Maṇḍala and Yantra in the Siddhānta School of Śaivism: Definitions, Descriptions and Ritual Use." In *Maṇḍalas and Yantras in the Hindu Traditions*, Trsl. Raynald Prévèreau, Ed. Gudrun Bühnemann. Brill: Leiden.

Brunner, Hélène, Gerard Oberhammer, and Andre Padoux, eds. (2000). *Tāntrikābhidhā nakośa*, vol. 1: *A Dictionary of Technical Terms from Hindu Tantric Literature*. Vienna: Verlag Der Österreichischen Akademie der Wissenschaften.

Brunner, Hélène, Gerard Oberhammer, and Andre Padoux, eds. (2004). *Tāntrikābhidhā nakośa*, vol. 2: *A Dictionary of Technical Terms from Hindu Tantric Literature*. Beitrage zur Kultur- und Geistesgeschichte Asiens, no. 44. Vienna: Verlag Der Österreichischen Akademie der Wissenschaften.

Bryant, Edwin. (2001). *The Quest for the Origins of Vedic Culture: The Indo-Aryan Migration Debate*. Oxford: Oxford University Press.

Bühnemann, Gudrun. (1988). *Pūjā: A Study in Smārta Ritual*. Vienna: Nobili Research Library, Institute for Indology, University of Vienna.

Bühnemann, Gudrun. (1996). "The Goddess Mahācīnakrama-Tārā (Ugra-Tārā) in Buddhist and Hindu Tantrism." *Bulletin of the School of Oriental and African Studies* 59(3): 472–493.

Bühnemann, Gudrun. (2000). "The Six Rites of Magic." In *Tantra in Practice*. Ed. David Gordon White. Princeton, NJ: Princeton University Press.

Bühnemann, Gudrun. (2003). "Maṇḍala, Yantra and Cakra: Some Observations." In *Maṇḍalas and Yantras in the Hindu Traditions*. Ed. Gudrun Bühnemann. Leiden: Koninklijke Brill NV.

Bühnemann, Gudrun. (2009). "The Identification of a Sculpture of Mṛtuṃjaya/Amṛteśa and Amṛtalakṣmī in the 'Royal Bath' in Patan (Nepal)." In *Prajñādhara: Essays of Asian Art, History, Epigraphy and Culture in Honour of Gouriswar Bhattacharya*, vol. 1. Ed. Gerd J. R. Mevissen and Arundhati Banerji. New Delhi: Kaveri Books.

Bühnemann, Gudrun. (2012). "Maṇḍalas and Yantras." In *Brill's Encyclopedia of Hinduism*. Ed. Knut A. Jacobson, Helene Basu, Angelika Malinar, and Vasudha Narayan. Leiden: Brill.

Bühnemann, Gudrun. (2017). "The Iconography of Śiva Mṛtyuṃjaya." Presentation, Boston, American Academy of Religion Annual Meeting.

Burchett, Patton E. (2008, December). "The 'Magical' Language of Mantra." *Journal of the American Academy of Religion* 76(4): 807–843.

Buswell, Robert E. (2004). *Encyclopedia of Buddhism*, vol. 1: *A–L*. New York: Macmillan Reference.

Cassirer, Bruno. Trsl. Ralph Manheim. (1925 [1955]). *The Philosophy of Symbolic Forms: Volume Two: Mythical Thought*. New Haven: Yale University Press.

Chakravarty, H. N. (1999). "Sthūla-Sūkṣma-Para." In *Kalātattvakośa: A Lexicon of Fundamental Concepts of the Indian Arts*, vol. 4: *Manifestation of Nature Sṛṣṭi Vistāra*. Ed. Advaitavadini Kaul and Sukumar Chattopadhyay. New Delhi: Motilal Banarsidass.

Chakravarty, H. N., trsl. and Boris Marjanovic, ed. (2012). *Tantrasāra of Abhinavagupta*. Portland: Rudra Press.

Child, Louise. (2007). *Tantric Buddhism and Altered States of Consciousness: Durkheim, Emotional Energy and Visions of the Consort*. Hampshire, UK: Ashgate.

Collins, Charles Dillard. (1988). *The Iconography and Ritual of Siva at Elephanta: On Life, Illumination, and Being*. SUNY Press.

Dalal, Roshen. (2011). *Hinduism: An Alphabetical Guide*. New York: Penguin.

Davidson, Ronald M. (2002). *Indian Esoteric Buddhism: A Social History of the Tantric Movement*. New York: Columbia University Press.

Davis, Richard H. (1992). "Becoming a Śiva, and Acting as One, in Śaiva Worship." In *Ritual and Speculation in Early Tantrism*. Ed. Teun Goudriaan. Delhi: Sri Satguru.

Davis, Richard H. (2000). *Ritual in an Oscillating Universe: Worshipping Siva in Medieval India*. Princeton, NJ: Princeton University Press.

DeLeo, Jennifer L., and Yun Tsai. (2008). "Battlestar Galactica's Cylon Dream Kit." *P.C. Magazine*, May 2. http://www.pcmag.com/article2/0,2817,2290393,00.asp.

De Simini, Florinda. (2016). *Of Gods and Books: Ritual and Knowledge Transmission in the Manuscript Cultures of Premodern India*. Berlin: De Gruyter.

Dev, Sukh. (2001). "Ancient-Modern Concordance in Ayurvedic Plants: Some Examples." In *Development of Plant-Based Medicines: Conservation, Efficacy and Safety*. Ed. Praveen K. Saxena. Dordrecht: Springer Science+Business Media.

Dezsö, Csaba. (2010). "Encounters with *Vetālas*: Studies of Fabulous Creatures I." *Acta Orientalia Academiae Scientiarum Hung* 63(4): 391–426.

Dhal, Upendra Nath. (1986). *The Ekāmra Purāṇam*. New Delhi: Nag.

Doniger O'Flaherty, Wendy. (1980a). *The Origins of Evil in Hindu Mythology*. Berkeley: University of California Press.

Doniger O'Flaherty, Wendy. (1980b). *Women, Androgynes, and Other Mythical Beasts*. Chicago: University of Chicago Press.

Doniger O'Flaherty, Wendy. (1988). *Textual Sources for the Study of Hinduism*. Manchester, UK: Manchester University Press.

Doniger, Wendy. (1993). *Purāṇa Perennis: Reciprocity and Transformation in Hindu and Jaina Texts*. Albany: State University of New York Press.

Doniger, Wendy. (2010). *The Hindus: An Alternative History*. London: Penguin Books.

Douglas, Mary. (1966). *Purity and Danger: An Analysis of the Concepts of Pollution and Taboo*. New York: Routledge.

Drabu, V. N. (1986). *Kashmir Polity (c. 600–1200 A.D.)*. New Delhi: Bahri.

Dundas, Paul. (2000). "Jain Monk, Nath Yogi." In *Tantra in Practice*. Ed. David Gordon White. Princeton, NJ: Princeton University Press.

Dupuche, John R. (2003). *Abhinavagupta: The Kula Ritual: As Elaborated in Chapter 29 of the Tantrāloka*. New Delhi: Motilal Banarsidass.

Durkheim, Emile. (1995 [1912]). *The Elementary Forms of Religious Life*. Trsl. Karen E. Fields. New York: Free Press.

Dviveda, Vrajavallabha. (1992). "Having Become a God, He Should Sacrifice to the Gods." In *Ritual and Speculation in Early Tantrism*. Ed. Teun Goudriaan. Delhi: Sri Satguru.

Eaton, Richard M. (2005). *A New Cambridge History of India: A Social History of the Deccan, 1300–1761: Eight Indian Lives*. Cambridge: Cambridge University Press.

Eck, Diana L. (2012). *India: A Sacred Geography*. New York: Harmony Books.

Einoo, Shingo. (2005). "Mṛtyuṃjaya or Ritual Device to Conquer Death." In *Indische Kultur im Kontext. Festschrift für Klaus Mylius*. Ed. L Göhler. Weisbaden: Harrassowitz Verlag.

Fergusson, James. (1899). *History of Indian and Eastern Architecture*, vol. 1. New York: Dodd, Mead.

Flood, Gavin D. (1989). "Shared Realities and Symbolic Forms in Kashmir Śaivism." *Numen* 36(2): 225–247.

Flood, Gavin D. (1993). *Body and Cosmology in Kashmir Śaivism*. San Francisco: Mellen Research University Press.

Flood, Gavin D. (1996). *An Introduction to Hinduism*. Cambridge: Cambridge University Press.

Flood, Gavin D. (2003). "The Śaiva Traditions." In *The Blackwell Companion to Hinduism*. Ed. Gavin Flood. Oxford: Blackwell.

Flood, Gavin D. (2004). *The Ascetic Self: Subjectivity, Memory and Tradition*. Cambridge: Cambridge University Press.

Flood, Gavin D. (2006). *The Tantric Body: The Secret Tradition of Hindu Religion*. New York: I. B. Tauris.

Flood, Gavin D. (2012). "Body, Breath and Representation in Śaiva Tantrism." In *Images of the Body in India: South Asian and European Perspectives on Rituals and Performativity*. Ed. Axel Michaels and Christoph Wulf. New York: Routledge.

Flood, Gavin, Bjarne Wernicke-Olesen, and Rajan Khatiwoda. (Forthcoming). *The Lord of Immortality: An Introduction, Critical Edition, and Translation of the Netra Tantra*, vol. 1, chapters 1–8. London: Routledge.

Fritz, John M., and George Michell. (1987). "Interpreting the Plan of a Medieval Hindu Capital, Vijayanagara." *World Archaeology* 19(1) (June): 105–129.

Geertz, Clifford. (1980). *Negara: The Theatre State in Nineteenth-Century Bali*. Princeton, NJ: Princeton University Press.

Gentry, James. (2010). "Representations of Efficacy: The Ritual Expulsion of Mongol Armies in the Consolidation and Expansionof the Tsang (Gtsang) Dynasty." In *Tibetan Ritual*. Ed. José Ignacio Cabezón. Oxford: Oxford University Press.

Geslani, Marko. (2018). *Rites of the God-King: Śānti & Ritual Change in Early Hinduism*. Oxford: University of Oxford Press.

Gibson, David R. (2014). "Enduring Illusions: The Social Organization of Secrecy and Deception." *Sociological Theory* 32(4): 283–306.

Gonda, Jan. (1977). *A History of Indian Literature*, vol. 2: *Medieval Religious Literature in Sanskrit*. Wiesbaden: Otto Harrassowitz.

Gonda, Jan. (1980). *Vedic Ritual: The Non-Solemn Rites*. Leiden: Brill.

Gray, David B., trsl. (2007). *The Cakrasamvara Tantra (The Discourse of Śri Heruka)*: A Study and Annotated Translation. New York: American Institute of Buddhist Studies.

Gray, David B., ed. (2012). *The Cakrasamvara Tantra (The Discourse of Śri Heruka): Editions of the Sanskrit and Tibetan Texts*. New York: American Institute of Buddhist Studies.

Dominic Goodall. (1998). *Bhaṭṭa Rāmakaṇṭha's Commentary on the Kiraṇatantra*, vol. 1, chapters 1–6, critical edition and annotated translation. Pondicherry: Institut Français de Pondichéry/École Française d'Extrême-Orient.

Goodall, Dominic. (2004). *The Parākhyatantra: A Scripture of the Śaiva* Siddhānta. Pondicherry: Instutut Français de Pondichéry/École Français D'Extrême-Orient.

Goodall, Dominic. (2007). "A First Edition of the Śatika-Kālajñāna, the Shortest of the Non-Eclectic Recensions of the Kālottara." In *Mélanges tantriques a la mémoire d'Heléne Brunner / Tantric Studies in Memory of Heléne Brunner*. Ed. Dominic Goodall and André Padoux. Pondicherry : Institut français d'Indologie/École française d'Extrême-Orient. Collection Indologie.

Goodall, Dominic, trsl. (2015). *The Niśvāsatattvasaṃhitā: The Earliest Surviving Śaiva Tantra*, vol. 1: *A Critical Edition & Annotated Translation of the Mūlasūtra, Uttarasūtra & Nayasūtra*. Pondicherry: Institut Français de Pondichéry/École Française d'Extrême-Orient.

Goodall, Dominic. (2016). "How the Tattvas of Tantric Śaivism Came to Be 36: The Evidence of the *Niśvāsatattvasaṃhitā*." In *Tantric Studies: Fruits of a Franco-German Project on Early Tantra*. Ed. Dominic Goodall and Harunaga Isaacson. Pondicherry: Institut Français de Pondichéry/École Française d'Extrême-Orient.

Goodall, Dominic, and Harunaga Isaacson. (2011). "Tantric Traditions." In *The Continuum Companion to Hindu Studies*. Ed. Jessica Frazier. London: Continuum.

Goudriaan, Teun, and Sanjukta Gupta. (1981). *Hindu Tantric and Sākta Literature*. Wiesbaden: Harrassowitz.

Goudriaan, Teun, trsl. (1985). *Vīṇāśikhatantra: A Śaiva Tantra of the Left Current*. Delhi: Motilal Banarsidass.

Gray, David B. (2005). "Eating the Heart of the Brahmin: Representations of Alterity and the Formation of Identity in Tantric Buddhist Discourse." *History of Religions* 45: 45–69.

Greenberg, Yudit Korberg, ed. (2008). *Encyclopedia of Love in World Religions*. Santa Barbara, CA: ABC-CLIO.

Greenberg, Yudit Korberg. (2018). *The Body in Religion: Cross-Cultural Perspectives*. London: Bloomsbury.

Hatley, Shaman. (2007). "The *Brahmayāmalatantra* and Early Śaiva Cult of Yoginīs." Doctoral dissertation, University of Pennsylvania. Retrieved from ProQuest Dissertations and Theses. (UMI Number 3292099).

Hatley, Shaman. (2013). "What Is a *Yoginī*? Towards a Polythetic Definition." In '*Yoginī*' *in South Asia: Interdisciplinary Approaches*. Ed. István Keul. London: Routledge.

Hatley, Shaman. (2014). "Goddesses in Text and Stone." In *Material Culture and Asian Religions: Text, Image, Object*. Ed. Benjamin J. Fleming and Richard D. Mann. New York: Routledge.

Hatley, Shaman. (2018). *The* Brahmayāmalatantra *or* Picumata, vol. 1, chapters 1–2, 39–40, and 83. Pondicherry: Insitut Français de Pondichéry, École française d'Extrême-Orient. Hamburg: Universität Hamburg.

Hanneder, Jürgen. (1998). *Abhinavagupta's Philosophy of Revelation: Mālinīślokavārttika I*, 1–399. Groningen: Egbert Forsten.

Heilijgers-Seelen, Dory, trsl. (1994). *The System of Five Cakras in Kubjikāmatatantra 14–16*. Groningen: Groningen Oriental Studies.

Huntington, John C., and Dina Bangdel. (2003). *The Circle of Bliss: Buddhist Meditational Art*. Chicago: Serindia.

Inden, Ronald. (1985). "Kings and Omens." In *Purity and Auspiciousness in Indian Society*. Ed. John B. Carman and Frédérique A. Marglin. Leiden: Brill.

Inden, Ronald. (2000). "Imperial Purāṇas: Kashmir as Vaiṣṇava Center of the World." In *Querying the Medieval: Texts and the History of Practices in South Asia*. Ed. Ronald Inden, Jonathan Walters, and Daud Ali. Oxford: Oxford University Press.

Iyengar, R. N., Devendra Sharma, and J. M. Siddiqui. (1999). "Earthquake History of India in Medieval Times." *Indian Journal of History of Science* 34(3): 181–237.

Jageshwar Temple Organization. mahamritunjayjageshwar.com. Accessed February 17, 2018.

Jamwal, Suman. (2010–2011). "Change and Continuity in the Historical and Cultural Geography of Kashmir from Nilamatapurana to Rajatarangini." *Proceedings of the Indian History Congress* 71: 129–139.

Johns Hopkins University, Sheridan Libraries. (September 2015). "Hippocratic Oath, Modern Version—Bioethics—Guides at Johns Hopkins University." *Guides.library.jhu.edu*.

Joo, Swami Laksman. (1998). *Kashmir Shaivaism: The Supreme Secret*. Albany: State University of New York Press.

Joshi, M. C. (2002). "Historical and Iconographic Aspects of Śākta Tantrism." In *The Roots of Tantra*. Ed. Katherine Anne Harper and Robert L. Brown. Albany: State University of New York Press.

Kahrs, Eivind. (1999). *Indian Semantic Analysis: The* Nirvacana *Tradition*. Cambridge: University of Cambridge Press.

Kaul, Manohar. (1971). *Kashmir: Hindu, Buddhist & Muslim Architecture*. New Delhi: Sagar.

Kaul, Mrinal. (2018). "Ontological Hierarchy in the *Tantrāloka* of Abhinavagupta." In *Tantrapuṣpāñjali*. Ed. Bettina Sharada Bäumer and Hamsa Stainton. New Delhi: Aryan Books.

Kinsley, David R. (1998). *Tantric Visions of the Divine Feminine: The Ten Mahavidyas*. New Delhi: Motilal Banarsidass.

Klostermaier, Klaus K. (1985). *Mythologies and Philosophies of Salvation in the Theistic Traditions of India*. Ontario: Wilfrid Laurier University Press.

Klostermaier, Klaus K. (2007). *A Survey of Hinduism*, 3rd ed. Albany: State University of New York Press.

Kramrisch, Stella. (1988). *The Presence of Śiva*. New Delhi: Motilal Banarsidass.

Kulke, Hermann. (2010). "Ritual Sovereignty and Ritual Policy: Some Historiographic Reflections." In *Ritual Dynamics and the Science of Ritual: State, Power, and Violence*. Ed. Axel Michaels. Weisbaden: Harrassowitz Verlag.

Kulke, Hermann, and Dietmar Rothermund. (1986). *A History of India*. London: Routledge.

LaFleur, William R. (1998). "Body." In *Critical Terms for Religious Studies*. Ed. Mark C. Taylor. Chicago: University of Chicago Press.

Larivière, Richard W. (1988). "Adhikāra—Right and Responsibility." In *Languages and Cultures: Studies in Honor of Edgar C. Polomé*. Ed. Mohammad Ali Jazayery and Werner Winter. Berlin: Walter de Gruyter.

Larson, Gerald James. (1969). *Classical Sāṃkya: An Interpretation of its History and Meaning*. New Delhi: Motilal Banarsidass.

Larson, Gerald James, and Ram Shankar Bhattacharya, eds. (1987). *Encyclopedia of Indian Philosophies*, vol. 4: *Sāṃkhya: A Dualist Tradition in Indian Philosophy*. Princeton, NJ: Princeton University Press.

Lawrence, Walter R. (1895). *The Valley of Kashmír*. London: Henry Frowde.

Lee, Sherman E. (1967). "Clothed in the Sun: A Buddha and a Surya from Kashmir." *Bulletin of the Cleveland Museum of Art* 54(2) (February): 42–63.

Linrothe, Robert. (1999). *Ruthless Compassion: Wrathful Deities in Early Indo-Tibetan Esoteric Buddhist Art*. Boston: Shambhala Press.

Lochtefeld, James. (2002). *The Illustrated Encyclopedia of Hinduism*. New York: Rosen.

Lorenzen, David N. (1972). *The Kāpālikas and Kālāmukhas: Two Lost Śaivite Sects*. Delhi: Motilal Banarsidass.

Malla, Bansi Lal. (1996). *Vaiṣṇava Art and Iconography of Kashmir*. New Delhi: Abhinav.

Mallinson, James, and Mark Singleton. (2017). *Roots of Yoga*. London: Penguin Books.

Mandal, Bankim Chandra. (1991). *Srīkaṇṭhacarita: A Mahākāvya of Maṇkhaka: Literary Study with an Analysis of Social, Political and Historical Data of Kashmir of the 12th Century A.D.* Calcutta: Sanskrit Pustak Bhandar.

Mani, Vetta. (1975). *Purāṇic Encyclopedia: A Comprehensive Dictionary with Special Reference to the Epic and Purāṇic Literature*. New Delhi: Motilal Banarsidass.

Mann, Richard D. (2012). *The Rise of Mahāsena: The Transformation of Skanda-Kārttikeya in North India from the Kuṣāṇa to Gupta Empires*. Leiden: Brill.

Marglin, Frédérique Apffel. (1985). "Types of Oppositions in Hindu Culture." In *Purity and Auspiciousness in Indian Society*. Ed. John B. Carman and Frédérique A. Marglin. Lieden: Brill.

Marshall, Sir John. (1931). *Mohenjo-Daro and the Indus Civilization*, vol. 1. London: Arthur Probsthain.

Mayer Robert. (1990). "The Origins of the Esoteric Vajrayāna." *Buddhist Forum*, October, 1–57.

McCarter, Simone. (2014). "The Body Divine: Tantric Śaivite Ritual Practices in the *Svacchandatantra* and Its Commentary." *Religions* 5: 738–750.

McDaniel, June. (2004). *Offering Flowers, Feeding Skulls: Popular Goddess Worship in West Bengal*. Oxford: Oxford University Press.

McDermott, Rachel Fell. (2011). *Revelry, Rivalry, and Longing for the Goddesses of Bengal: The Fortunes of Hindu Festivals*. New York: Columbia University Press.

Mengele, Irmgard. (2010). "Chilu ('Chi bslu): Rituals for 'Deceiving Death.'" In José Ignacio Cabezón. *Tibetan Ritual*. Oxford: Oxford University Press.

Michaels, Axel. (2003). *Hinduism Past and Present*. Princeton, NJ: Princeton University Press.

Michaels, Axel. (2015). *Homo Ritualis: Hindu Ritual and Its Significance for Ritual Theory*. Oxford: Oxford University Press.

Michell, George. (1992). "The Mahanavami Festival at Vijayanagara." In *India International Centre Quarterly* 19(3): 150–161.

Michell, George. (1993). "Reflections of Vijayanagara." *Journal of South Asian Studies* 16, sup. 1: 15–32.

Minkley, Gary, and Martin Legassick. (2000). "'Not Telling': Secrecy, Lies, and History." *History and Theory* 36(4). Theme Issue 39 (December): 1–10.

Mirnig, Nina. (2019). *Liberating the Liberated: Early Śaiva Tantric Death Rites*. Vienna: Austrian Academy of Sciences Press.

Mirashi, Vasudev Vishnu. (1947). "Date of the *Gāthāsaptaśatī*." *Indian Historical Quarterly* 23: 300–310.

Muller-Ortega, Paul E. (1989). *The Triadic Heart of Śiva: Kaula Tantricism of Abhinavagupta in the Non-dual Shivaism of Kashmir*. Albany: State University of New York Press.

Muller-Ortega, Paul E. (1992). "Tantric Meditation: Vocalic Beginnings." In *Ritual and Speculation in Early Tantrism: Studies in Honor of André Padoux*. Ed. Teun Goudriaan. Albany: State University of New York Press.

Muller-Ortega, Paul E. (2000). "On the Seal of Sambhu: A Poem by Abhinavagupta." In *Tantra in Practice*. Ed. David Gordon White. Princeton, NJ: Princeton University Press.

Muller-Ortega, Paul E. (2003). "Ciphering the Supreme: Mantric Encoding in Abhinavagupta's Tantrāloka." *International Journal of Hindu Studies* 7(1–3): 1–30.

Nemec, John. (2011). *The Ubiquitous Śiva: Somānanda's Śivadṛṣṭi and His Tantric Interlocutors*. Oxford: Oxford University Press.

Nemec, John. (2013). "On the Structure and Contents of the *Tridaśaḍāmaratantra*, a Kaula Scriptural Source of the Northern Transmission." *Journal of Hindu Studies* 6: 297–316.

Nemec, John. (2018). "The Body and Consciousness in Early Pratyabhijñā Philosophy: Amūrtatva in Somānanda's Śivadṛṣṭi." In *Tantrapuspāñjali: Tantric Traditions and Philosophy of Kashmir*. Ed. Bettina Sharada Bäumer and Hamsa Stainton. New Delhi: Aryan Books.

Olivelle, Patrick, trsl. (1999). *The Dharmasūtras: The Law Codes of Āpastamba, Gautama, Baudhāyana,and Vasiṣṭha*. Oxford: Oxford University Press.

Olivelle, Patrick, trsl. (2013). *King, Governance, and Law in Ancient India: Kauṭilya's Arthaśāstra*. Oxford: Oxford University Press.

Olson, Carl. (2007). *The Many Colors of Hinduism: A Thematic-Historical Introduction*. New Brunswick, NJ: Rutgers University Press.

Padoux, André. (1989). "Mantras—What Are They?" In *Understanding Mantras*. Ed. Harvey P. Alper. Albany: State University of New York Press.

Padoux, André. (1990). *Vāc: The Concept of the Word in Selected Hindu Tantras*. Trsl. Jacques Gontier. Albany: State University of New York Press.

Padoux, André. (2000). "The Tantric Guru." In *Tantra in Practice*. Ed. David Gordon White. Princeton, NJ: Princeton University Press.

Padoux, André. (2003). "Maṇḍalas in Abhinavagupta's Tantrāloka." In *Maṇḍalas and Yantras in the Hindu Traditions*. Ed. Gudrun Bühnemann. Leiden: Koninklijke Brill NV.

Padoux, André. (2011). *Tantric Mantras*. London: Routledge.

Padoux, André. Trsl. Roger-Orphé Jeanty. (2013). *The Heart of the Yoginī: The Yoginīhṛdaya, a Sanskrit Tantric Treatise*. Oxford: Oxford University Press.

Pal, Pratapaditya. (1985). *Art of Nepal: A Catalogue of the Los Angeles County Museum of Art Collection*. Berkeley: University of California Press.

Pollock, Sheldon. (2003). "Sanskrit Literary Culture from the Inside Out." In *Literary Cultures in History: Reconstructions from South Asia*. Ed. Sheldon Pollock. Berkeley: University of California Press.

Rabe, Michael D. (2000). "Secret Yantras and Erotic Display for Hindu Temples." In *Tantra in Practice*. Ed. David Gordon White. Princeton, NJ: Princeton University Press.

Rambelli, Fabio. (2000). "Tantric Buddhism and Chinese Thought in East Asia." In *Tantra in Practice*. Ed. David Gordon White. Princeton, NJ: Princeton University Press.

Ramos, Imma. (2020). *Tantra: Enlightenment to Revolution*. London: Thames and Hudson.

Rangachari, Devika. (2011). "Women and Power in Early Medieval Kashmir." In *Rethinking Early Medieval India*. Ed. Upinder Singh. Oxford: Oxford University Press.

Rastelli, Marion. (2003). "Maṇḍalas and Yantras in the Pāñcarātra." In *Maṇḍalas and Yantras in the Hindu Traditions*. Ed. Gudrun Bühnemann. Leiden: Koninklijke Brill NV.

Rastelli, Marion, and Dominic Goodall, eds. (2013). *Tāntrikābhidhānakośa*, vol. 3: *A Dictionary of Technical Terms from Hindu Tantric Literature.* Beitrage zur Kultur- und Geistesgeschichte Asiens, no. 44. Vienna: Verlag Der Österreichischen Akademie der Wissenschaften.

Rastogi, Navjivan. (1987). *Introduction to the Tantrāloka: A Study in Structure.* New Delhi: Motilal Banarsidass.

Rastogi, Navjivan. (1992). "The Yogic Disciplines in the Monistic Śaiva Tantric Traditions of Kashmir: Threefold, Fourfold, and Six-Limbed." In *Ritual and Speculation in Early Tantrism*. Ed. Teun Goudriaan. Delhi: Sri Satguru.

Rastogi, Navjivan. (1996). *The Krama Tantricism of Kashmir: Historical and General Sources*, vol. 1. New Delhi: Motilal Banarsidass.

Ratié, Isabelle. (2010). "The Dreamer and the Yogin: On the Relationship Between Buddhist and Śaiva Idealisms." *Bulletin of the School of Oriental and African Studies* 73: 437–478.

Rocher, Ludo. (1986). *The Purāṇas.* Weisbaden: Otto Harrassowitz.

Rocher, Ludo. (1991). "Mantras in the *Śivapurāṇa*." In *Understanding Mantras*. Ed. Harvey Alper Delhi: Motilal Banarsidass.

Samuel, Geoffrey. (2008). *The Origins of Yoga and Tantra: Indic Religions to the Thirteenth Century*. Cambridge: Cambridge University Press.

Samuel, Geoffrey. (2012). "Amitayus and the Development of Tantric Practices for Longevity and Health in Tibet." In *Transformations and Transfer of Tantra in Asia and Beyond*. Ed. István Keul. Berlin: de Gruyter.

Sanderson, Alexis. (1985). "Purity and Power Among the Brahmans of Kashmir." In *The Category of the Person: Anthropology, Philosophy, History*. Ed. Michael Carrithers, Steven Collins, and Steven Lukes. Cambridge: Cambridge University Press.

Sanderson, Alexis. (1986). "Maṇḍala and Āgamic Identity in the Trika of Kashmir." In *Mantras et Diagrammes Rituelles dans l'Hindouisme*. Ed. Andre Padoux. *Équipe no. 249, L'hindouisme: textes, doctrines, pratiques*. Paris: Éditions du Centre National de la Recherche Scientifique.

Sanderson, Alexis. (1988). "Śaivism and the Tantric Traditions." In *The World's Religions*. Ed. S. Sutherland, L. Houlden, P. Clarke, and F. Hardy. London: Routledge and Kegan Paul.

Sanderson, Alexis. (1990). "The Visualization of the Deities of the Trika." In *L'image divine: Culte et meditation dans l'hinduisme*. Ed. André Padoux. Paris: Éditions du CNRS.

Sanderson, Alexis. (1994). "Vajrayāna: Origin and Function." In *Buddhism into the Year 2000. International Conference Proceedings*, 87–102. Bangkok: Dhammakaya Foundation.

Sanderson, Alexis. (1995). "Meaning in Tantric Ritual." In *Essais sur le Rituel III: Colloque du Centenaire de la Section des Sciences religieuses de l'École Pratique des Hautes Études*. Ed. A.-M. Blondeau and K. Schipper. Bibliothèque de l'École des Hautes Études, Sciences Religieuses, vol. 102, pp. 15–95. Louvain-Paris: Peeters.

Sanderson, Alexis. (2001). "History through Textual Criticism in the Study of Śaivism, the Pañcarātra and the Buddhist Yoginītantras." In *Les Sources et le temps* (*Sources and Time: A Colloquium*). Ed. François Grimal, 1–47. Pondicherry, January 11–13, 1997. Pondicherry: Institut Français de Pondichéry/École Française d'Extrême-Orient.

Sanderson, Alexis. (2003–2004). "The Śaiva Religion Among the Khmers (Part 1)." *Bulletin de l'École française d'Extrême-Orient* 90–91: 349–462.

Sanderson, Alexis. (2004). "Religion and the State: Saiva Officiants in the Territory of the King's Brahmanical Chaplain." *Indo-Iranian Journal* 47: 29–300.

Sanderson, Alexis. (2005). "A Commentary on the Opening Verses of the Tantrasāra of Abhinavagupta." In *Sāmarasya: Studies in Indian Arts, Philosophy, and Interreligious Dialogue in Honour of Bettina Bäumer*. Ed. Sadananda Das and Ernst Fürlinger. New Delhi: D. K. Printworld.

Sanderson, Alexis. (2007a). "Atharvavedins in Tantric Territory: The Āngirasakalpa Texts of the Oriya Paippalādins and Their Connection with the Trika and the Kālīkula, with Critical Editions of the Parājapavidhi, the Parāmantravidhi, and the Bhadrakālī-mantravidhiprakarana." In *The Atharvaveda and Its Paippalāda Śākhā: Historical and Philological Papers on a Vedic Tradition*. Ed. Arlo Griffiths and Annette Schmiedchen. Aachen: Shaker Verlag.

Sanderson, Alexis. (2007b). "The Śaiva Exegesis of Kashmir." In *Mélanges tantriques a la mémoire d'Hélène Brunner / Tantric Studies in Memory of Hélène Brunner*. Ed. Dominic Goodall and André Padoux. Pondicherry: Institut français d'Indologie/École française d'Extrême-Orient. Collection Indologie.

Sanderson, Alexis. (2009). "The Śaiva Age: The Rise and Dominance of Śaivism During the Medieval Period." In *Genesis and Development of Tantrism*. Ed. Shingo Einoo. Tokyo: Institute of Oriental Culture, University of Tokyo, Institute of Oriental Culture Special Series, 23.

Sanderson, Alexis. (2010). "Ritual for Oneself and Ritual for Others." In *Ritual Dynamics and the Science of Ritual*, vol. 2: *Body, Performance, Agency, and Experience*. Ed. Angeles Chaniotis et al. Wiesbaden: Harrassowitz Verlag.

Sanderson, Alexis. (2013). "The Śaiva Literature." *Journal of Indological Studies* 25: 1–113.

Sanderson, Alexis. (2014). "Śaiva Texts." In *Brill's Encyclopedia of Hinduism*. Ed. J. Bronkhorst and A. Malinar. Leiden: Brill.

Scharfe, Hartmut. (1993). *Investigations in Kauṭilya's Manual of Political Science*. Wiesbaden: Harrassowitz Verlag.

Scharfe, Hartmut. (2002). *Education in Ancient India*. Leiden: Brill.

Schomerus, H. W. ([1912] 2000). *Śaiva Siddhānta: An Indian School of Mystical Thought*. Trsl. Mary Law. Delhi: Motilal Banarsidass.

Shastri, Ajay Mitra. (1969). *India as Seen in the Bṛhatsaṃhitā of Varāhamihira*. New Delhi: Motilal Banarsidass.

Shinohara, Koichi. (2014). *Spells, Images, and Mandalas: Tracing the Evolution of Esoteric Buddhist Rituals*. New York: Columbia University Press.

Shimkhada, Deepak. (1984). "The Masquerading Sun: A Unique Syncretic Image in Nepal." *Artibus Asiae* 45(2/3): 223–229.

Shulman, David, Whitney Cox, Yigal Bronner, Lawrence McCrea, Chitralekha Zutshi, Luther Obrock, and Daud Ali. (2013). *Indian Economic and Social History Review* 50(2).

Silburn, Lilian. (1988). *Kundalini: The Energy of the Depths*. Trsl. Jacques Gontier. Albany: State University of New York Press.

Silburn, Lilian, and Andre Padoux. (2000). *Abhinavagupta La Lumière Sur Les Tantras chapitres 1 à 5 du Tantrāloka*. Paris: Collège de France.

Simmel, Georg. (1906). Trsl. Albion W. Small. "The Sociology of Secrecy and of Secret Societies." *American Journal of Sociology* 11(1): 441–498.

Singh, Jaideva, trsl. (1979a). *Śiva Sūtras: The Yoga of Supreme Identity*. Delhi: Motilal Banarsidass.

Singh, Jaideva, trsl. (1979b) *Vijñānabhairava, or Divine Consciousness*. Delhi: Motilal Banarsidass.

Singh, Jaideva, trsl. (1988) *Parā-triśikā-Vivaraṇa: The Secret of Tantric Mysticism*. New Delhi: Motilal Banarsidass.

Sinopoli, Carla M., and Kathleen D. Morrison. (1995). "Dimensions of Imperial Control in the Vijayanagara Capital." *American Anthropological Association* 97(1) (March): 83–96.

Siudmak, John. (2013). *The Hindu-Buddhist Sculpture of Ancient Kashmir and Its Influences*. Leiden: Brill.

Ślączka, Anna Aleksandra. (2007). *Temple Consecration Rituals in Ancient India: Text and Archaeology*. Leiden: Brill.

Slouber, Michael. (2017). *Early Tantric Medicine: Snakebite, Mantras, and Healing*. Oxford: Oxford University Press.

Smith, Frederick M. (2006). *The Self-Possessed Deity*. New York: Columbia University Press.

Smith, Johnathan Z. (2004). *Relating Religon: Essays in the Study of Religion*. Chicago: University of Chicago Press.

Srinivasan, Doris. (1975/76). "The So-Called Proto-śiva Seal from Mohenjo-Daro: An Iconological Assessment." *Archives of Asian Art* 29: 47–59.

Staal, Frits. (1989). "Vedic Mantras." In *Understanding Mantras*. Ed. Harvey P. Alper. Albany: State University of New York Press.

Staal, Frits. (1996). *Ritual and Mantras: Rules Without Meaning*. Delhi: Motilal Banarsidass.

Staal, Frits. (2008). *Discovering the Vedas: Origins, Mantras, Rituals, Insights*. New York: Penguin Books.

Stein, M. A., trsl. (1900). *Kalhaṇa's Rājataraṅgiṇī: A Chronicle of the Kings of Kaśmīr*. 3 vols. London: Archibald Constable.

Sumegi, Angela. (2008). *Dreamworlds of Shamanism and Tibetan Buddhism: The Third Place*. Albany: State University of New York Press.

Taber, John. (1989). "Are Mantras Speech Acts? The Mīmāṃsā Point of View." In *Understanding Mantras*. Ed. Harvey P. Alper. Albany: State University of New York Press.

Tagare, G. V. , J. L. Shastri, and G. P. Bhatt. (1987). *Ancient Indian Tradition & Mythology, Vol. 37: The Vāyu Purāṇa, Part 1*. Delhi: Motilal Banarsidass.

Tagare, G. V. (2002). *The Pratyabhijñā Philosophy*. Delhi: Motilal Banarsidass.

Tarabout, Gilles. (2012). "Sin and Flaws in Kerala Astrology." In *Sins and Sinners: Perspectives from Asian Religions*. Ed. Phyllis Granoff and Koichi Shinohara. Leiden: Brill.

Taussig, Michael. (1998). "Transgression." In *Critical Terms for Religious Studies*. Ed. Mark C. Taylor. Chicago: University of Chicago Press.

Timalsina, Sthaneshwar. (2005). "Meditating Mantras: Meaning and Visualization in Tantric Literature." In *Theory and Practice of Yoga: Essays in Honour of Gerald James Larson*. Eds. Gerald James Larson and Knut A. Jacobsen. Leiden: Brill.

Tissot, Francine. (2006). *Catalogue of the National Museum of Afghanistan: 1931–1985*. Paris: UNESCO Publishing.

Torella, Raffaele. (1988). "A Fragment of Utpaladeva's '*Īśvarapratyabhijña-vivṛti*.'" *East and West* 38(1/4) (December): 137–174.

Torella, Raffaele. (2015). "Purity and Impurity in Nondualistic Śaiva Tantrism." In *Proceedings of the International Conference: "Religions: Fields of Research, Method and Perspectives." Studia Religiologica*, vol. 48, No. 2, pp. 101–115.

Törzsök, Judit. (2003). "Icons of Inclusivism: Maṇḍalas in Some Early Śaiva Tantras." In *Maṇḍalas and Yantras in the Hindu Traditions*. Ed. Gudrun Bühnemann. Leiden: Koninklijke Brill NV.

Törzsök, Judit. (2009). "The Alphabet Goddess Mātṛkā in Some Early Śaiva Tantras." Second International Workshop on Early Tantras, Pondicherry, India. <hal-00710939>.

Törzsök, Judit. (2012). "Tolerance and Its Limits in Twelfth Century Kashmir: Tantric Elements in Kalhaṇa's *Rājataraṅgiṇī*." *Indologica Taurinensia*: 1–27.

Törzsök, Judit. (2013). "Yoginī and Goddess Possession in Early Śaiva Tantras." In *South Asia: Interdisciplinary Approaches*. Yoginī. New York: Routledge.

Törzsök, Judit. (2014). "Nondualism in Early Śākta Tantras: Transgressive Rites and Their Ontological Justification in a Historical Perspective." *Journal of Indian Philosophy* 42: 195–223.

Törzsök, Judit. (2015). "The Heads of the Godhead: The Number of Heads/Faces of *Yoginīs* and Bhairavas in Early Śaiva Tantras." *Indo-Iranian Journal* 56: 133–155.

Tsuda, Shiníchi. (1970). "The Saṃvarodaya-tantra: Selected Chapters." Doctoral thesis, Australian National University. Retrieved from ANU Open Research Repository (http://hdl.handle.net/1885/11247).

Urban, Hugh B. (2010). *The Power of Tantra: Religion Sexuality, and the Politics of South Asian Studies*. London: I. B. Tauris.

Vasudeva, Somadeva, trsl. (2004). *The Yoga of the Mālinīvijayottaratantra*, chapters 1–4, 7, 11–17. Pondicherry: Institut Française de Pondichéry École Française D'Extrême Orient.

Vasudeva, Somadeva, trsl. (2005) *Three Satires: Nīlakaṇṭha, Kṣemendra, & Bhallaṭa*. New York: Clay Sanskrit Library.

Vasudeva, Somadeva. (2007). "Synaesthetic Iconography: 1. Nādiphāntakrama." In *Mélanges tantriques à la mémoire d'Hélène Brunner*. Ed. Dominic Goodall and André Padoux. Pondicherry: Institut français d'Indologie/École française d'Extrême-Orient, Collection Indologie.

Von Stietencron, Heinrich. (2013). "Cosmographic Buildings of India: The Circles of the Yoginīs." In *Yoginī' in South Asia: Interdisciplinary Approaches*. New York: Routledge.

Von Stietencron, Heinrich, P. Flamm, J. L. Brockington, A. Malinar, P. Schreiner, K. P. Gietz, A. Kollman, S. Dietrich, R. Söhnen-Thieme, A. S. Pfeiffer, et al. (1992). *Epic and Purāṇic Bibliography (up to 1985) annotated and with indexes: Part I A–R*. Weisbaden: Otto Harrassowitz.

Wallace, Vesna A. (2016). "*Homa* Rituals in the Indian *Kālacakra-tantra* Tradition." In *Homa Variations: The Study of Ritual Change Across the* Longue Durée. Ed. Richard K. Payne and Michael Witzel. Oxford: Oxford University Press.

Wallis, Christopher. (2007). "The Descent of Power: Possession, Mysticism, and Initiation in the Śaiva Theology of Abhinavagupta." *Journal of Indian Philosophy* 36(2): 248–249.

Walter, Michael. (2000). "Cheating Death." In *Tantra in Practice*. Ed. David Gordon White. Princeton, NJ: Princeton University Press.

Warder, A. K. (1992). *Indian Kāvya Literature*, vol. 6. New Delhi: Motilal Banarsidass.

Wayman, Alex. (1967). "Significance of Dreams in India and Tibet." *History of Religions* 7(1) (August): 1–12.

Wedemeyer, Christian. (2013). *Making Sense of Tantric Buddhism*. New York: Columbia University Press.

Welbon, Guy R. (1987). "Secrecy in Indian Tradition." In Kees Bolle. *Secrecy in Religions*. Leiden: Brill.

Wenta, Aleksandra. (2018). "Smell: The Sense Perception of Recognition." In *Tantrapuṣpāñjali: Tantric Traditions and Philosophy of Kashmir*. Ed. Bettina Sharada Bäumer and Hamsa Stainton. New Delhi: Aryan Books.

Wheelock, Wade T. (1982). "The Problem of Ritual Language: From Information to Situation." In *Journal of the American Academy of Religion* 50(1) (March): 49–71.

Wheelock, Wade T. (1989). "Mantra in Vedic and Tantric Ritual." In *Understanding Mantras*. Ed. Harvey Alper. Albany: State University of New York Press.

White, David Gordon. (1996). *The Alchemical Body*. Chicago: University of Chicago Press.

White, David Gordon. (1998). "Transformations in the Art of Love: Kāmakalā Practices in Hindu Tantric and Kaula Traditions." *History of Religions* 38(2) (November): 172–198.

White, David Gordon, ed. (2000). *Tantra in Practice*. Princeton, NJ: Princeton University Press.

White, David Gordon. (2003). *Kiss of the Yogini: "Tantric Sex" in Its South Asian Contexts*. Chicago: University of Chicago Press.

White, David Gordon. (2009). *Sinister Yogis*. Chicago: University of Chicago Press.

White, David Gordon. (2012). "*Netra Tantra* at the Crossroads of the Demonological Cosmopolis." *Journal of Hindu Studies* 5(2): 145–171.

Wilke, Annette, and Oliver Moebus. (2011). *Sound and Communication: An Aesthetic Cultural History of Sanskrit Hinduism*. Berlin: De Gruyter.

Winternitz, Moritz, and V. Srinivasa Sarma. (1983). *Buddhist Literature and Jaina Literature*. Delhi: Motilal Banarsidass.

Witzel, Michael. (2003). "The Vedas and Upaniṣads." In *The Blackwell Companion to Hinduism*. Ed. Gavin Flood. Oxford: Blackwell.

Wujastyk, Dominik. (1998). *The Roots of Āyurveda*. New Delhi: Penguin Books India.

Yelle, Robert A. (2003). *Explaining Mantras: Ritual, Rhetoric, and the Dream of a Natural Language in Hindu Tantra*. New York: Routledge.

Young, Serinity. (1999). *Dreaming in the Lotus: Buddhist Dream Narrative, Imagery, and Practice*. Boston: Wisdom Publications.

Young, Serinity. (2004). *Courtesans and Tantric Consorts: Sexualities in Buddhist Narrative, Iconography, and Ritual*. New York: Routledge.

Index

For the benefit of digital users, indexed terms that span two pages (e.g., 52–53) may, on occasion, appear on only one of those pages.